AF812805

Amit Agrawal • Rakesh Mishra
Ajay Halder
Editors

Special Considerations in Trauma Care

Springer

Editors
Amit Agrawal
Department of Neurosurgery
All India Institute of Medical Sciences
Bhopal, Madhya Pradesh, India

Rakesh Mishra
IMS, Department of Neurosurgery
Banaras Hindu University
Varanasi, Uttar Pradesh, India

Ajay Halder
Department of Obstetrics and Gynecology
All India Institute of Medical Sciences
Bhopal, Madhya Pradesh, India

ISBN 978-981-99-9661-2 ISBN 978-981-99-9662-9 (eBook)
https://doi.org/10.1007/978-981-99-9662-9

© The Editor(s) (if applicable) and The Author(s), under exclusive license to Springer Nature Singapore Pte Ltd. 2024

This work is subject to copyright. All rights are solely and exclusively licensed by the Publisher, whether the whole or part of the material is concerned, specifically the rights of translation, reprinting, reuse of illustrations, recitation, broadcasting, reproduction on microfilms or in any other physical way, and transmission or information storage and retrieval, electronic adaptation, computer software, or by similar or dissimilar methodology now known or hereafter developed.
The use of general descriptive names, registered names, trademarks, service marks, etc. in this publication does not imply, even in the absence of a specific statement, that such names are exempt from the relevant protective laws and regulations and therefore free for general use.
The publisher, the authors and the editors are safe to assume that the advice and information in this book are believed to be true and accurate at the date of publication. Neither the publisher nor the authors or the editors give a warranty, expressed or implied, with respect to the material contained herein or for any errors or omissions that may have been made. The publisher remains neutral with regard to jurisdictional claims in published maps and institutional affiliations.

This Springer imprint is published by the registered company Springer Nature Singapore Pte Ltd.
The registered company address is: 152 Beach Road, #21-01/04 Gateway East, Singapore 189721, Singapore

If disposing of this product, please recycle the paper.

Preface

This manual covers special considerations in trauma care. The chapters will deliberate on the clinical management of trauma in a particular population group or situation, which is often not covered in other books on trauma care. Accordingly, there will be chapters on trauma as per different body regions, geriatric, paediatric, foetal, and trauma with pregnancy. Separate chapters will focus on basic sciences related to craniocerebral and spinal trauma. Each chapter will provide key learning points, highlights, a detailed discussion on the pathophysiology, special considerations, the evidence base available, management protocols, recommendations, a summary, and opportunities for further research studies. Numerous helpful photographs and anatomical drawings will accompany the text in the chapters. In addition, clear flow charts and tables are included to aid in diagnostic and surgical decision-making and identify surgical indications. Essential information is provided on anatomy, physiology, and pathology, and an individual chapter is devoted to lab investigations and radiology and imaging in trauma. This book will assist practitioners in neurology, neurosurgery, anaesthesia, orthopaedics, obstetrics, paediatrics, scientists, postgraduate students, and researchers in trauma management in negotiating the difficult-to-find information regarding different aspects of trauma. This book will be a key reference point for the latest available scientific evidence, controversies, recommendations, and updated knowledge on trauma care in a single volume. This book is suitable for practitioners managing trauma patients and encompasses specialities of neurology, neurosurgery, orthopaedics, paediatrics, obstetrics, geriatrics, and others. In addition, it will also be suitable for postgraduate students, physiotherapy and rehabilitation experts, and researchers in trauma care.

Bhopal, India — Amit Agrawal
Varanasi, India — Rakesh Mishra
Bhopal, India — Ajay Halder

Contents

1 **Epidemiology of Trauma and Injuries** 1
Ankit Mittal and Neeti Rustagi

2 **Laboratory Investigation in Trauma Patients** 11
Nidhi Prasad and Binay Kumar

3 **Radiology and Imaging in Neurotrauma** 23
Deep Yadav, Krishan K. Yadav, and M. S. Sridhar

4 **Neuroimaging and Its Application in the Diagnosis and Early Prognostication of Traumatic Brain Injury (TBI)** 41
Hardik Siroya and Anil Kumar Sharma

5 **Airway Management in Acute Trauma** 65
B. D. Vaishnavi, Palak Gupta, Shilpa Goyal, and Amit Goyal

6 **Anesthetic Considerations** 77
Anuj Jain and Ashutosh Kaushal

7 **Craniocerebral Trauma** 93
Chirag Solanki

8 **Trauma to the Skull Base** 105
Abhinav Srivastava

9 **Temporal Bone Fractures** 115
Vishudh Mohan, Vidhu Sharma, and Amit Goyal

10 **Facial Trauma** 129
Kuldeep Vishwakarma, Ravi Sankar Manogaran, Govind Bhuskute, Saurabh Kumar Rawat, and Abhishek Dubey

11 **Trauma to Neck** 151
Abhinav Srivastava

12 **Battered Baby Syndrome: Diagnosis and Management** 159
Rakesh Mishra, Nityanand Pandey, and Amit Agrawal

13 Military Injuries: Special Considerations 167
M. S. Sridhar and Krishan K. Yadav

14 Algorithm for the Management of Craniocerebral Injuries 177
Rewati Raman Sharma, Apollina Sharma,
and Kalpana Devi Kariyappa

15 The Paradigm Shift in the Incidence of Post-trauma Complications 209
K. L. Sampath Kumar

16 Intracranial Pressure Monitoring in Traumatic Brain Injury 215
Raghu Samala and Ramesh Doddamani

17 Decompressive Craniectomy for Severe Traumatic Brain Injury: CSF Dynamics, Cerebral Perfusion, and Cognitive Outcome 225
Manish Agrawal, Gaurav Purohit, and Rohit Babal

18 Decompressive Craniotomy in Children 239
Nazmin Ahmed and Md. Moshiur Rahman

19 Posttraumatic Stress Disorder 255
Chirag Solanki and Iti Shukla

20 Rehabilitation Aspects in Trauma Patients 267
Rishabh Kumar Rana

21 Community Integration and Holistic Rehabilitation for Traumatic Brain Injuries 279
Vinoth Rajendran, Ankit Mittal, and Neeti Rustagi

Epidemiology of Trauma and Injuries

1

Ankit Mittal and Neeti Rustagi

1.1 Introduction

The word trauma is a wide entity that can be defined as "any type of distressing event or experience that can have an impact on a person's ability to cope and function." Trauma may cause injury in the form of physical harm as well as emotional or psychological harm. In this chapter, we are concerned with trauma resulting in physical harm or injury. The word injury is loosely defined as the adverse effect of physical force upon a person. However, this definition is focused only on certain types of events involving energy transfer. Many public health-focused injury texts believe that the "energy definition," in which "injury" is defined as "harm to the body caused by energy exchanges that have relatively sudden, observable effects", best reflects the causes and pathologies of interest [1]. This definition does describe the events leading to tissue damage (or damage to the body) because of physical force but finds difficulty in including the common events classified as injury like ingestion of foreign body (coin, battery, etc.), or a case of poisoning, where there is no evident tissue damage or transfer of energy. Now, coming to "sudden discernible effects," this excludes the events due to a slow chronic transfer of energy, such as stress fractures, carpal tunnel syndromes, etc. [2]. The best way to define any injury would be by defining both the etiology and the outcome of the event. This eliminates major concerns faced with most definitions. For example, if we classify the bruise as an injury, this will exclude the bruises resulting from sepsis. At the same time, if we describe bruise with its etiology, such as the result of blunt external force, this will exclude the case of sepsis. Similarly, a surgical incision will not be defined as intentional trauma or injury. These theoretical definitions are of lesser use to a surgeon, and a much more fitting operational definition is provided in the

A. Mittal · N. Rustagi (✉)
Department of Community Medicine and Family Medicine, All India Institute of Medical Sciences, Jodhpur, Jodhpur, India

© The Author(s), under exclusive license to Springer Nature Singapore Pte Ltd. 2024

A. Agrawal et al. (eds.), *Special Considerations in Trauma Care*,
https://doi.org/10.1007/978-981-99-9662-9_1

International Classification of Diseases (ICD) versions. The ICD-10 classifies the injuries in Chap. 19 "Injury, Poisoning and Certain Other Consequences of External Causes," and Chap. 20 "External Causes of Morbidity and Mortality." The trauma or injury of our interest in this chapter is the ones resulting from accidents, defined as "an unexpected, unplanned occurrence which may involve injury" [3]. The aim of studying epidemiology of trauma and injury is to understand the agent, host, and environment interactions involved in the process.

1.2 The Problem Statements

Injuries generally can be categorized as intentional and unintentional. This categorization of injuries came to practice only after 1990, post collaboration of the US Centre for Disease Control and Prevention, and the American Public Health Association. This collaboration resulted in changes in the ICD 9 classification, further carried to the ICD 10 as well. Apart from the presence or absence of direct intent for injury, they are also classified by causes of injury, e.g., road traffic accidents, drowning, suicide or attempt at suicide, homicide or assault, or fire injuries, etc. Among these injuries, road traffic accidents contribute most to the burden in form of morbidities, mortalities, and DALYs.

Road traffic accidents endanger the lives of millions globally and in India. The impact of it on society was so huge that the United Nations General Assembly proclaimed the decade of 2011–2022 as decade of action for road safety. Sustainable Development Goals also included two targets for road safety—Target 3.6: which calls for a 50% reduction in the number of road traffic deaths globally by 2020, and Target 11.2: to provide access to safe, affordable, accessible, and sustainable transport systems for all by 2030. Now, before directly going to the burden of the problem, it is very important to understand the way data was generated and the degree to which it represents the actual problem.

1.3 Source of Data

The true estimation of the disease magnitude and burden is completely dependent on the availability of reliable and representative data. Globally, every country has its own system of recording morbidity and mortality by means of hospital-based data on cause of death, utilization of health services for specific causes, and record of reported crimes. All these data sources are independent and incomplete picture of the true problem. There have been efforts to combine global data on mortality in the form of incidence, disability-adjusted life years (DALYs), and years of potential life lost, that has helped us better understand the burden of this problem. One such effort is the Global Burden of Disease (GBD) study that attempts to collect quality data that is consistent as well as comparable and has become the most reliable and consistent source of data on mortality due to injuries. However, these data lack the details of risks and circumstances for injury. The presence of such complete data will help to understand and prioritize the risks and provide a base for planning safer environmental conditions. Compared to mortality data, morbidity data is much more difficult to collect because the data on nonfatal injuries is seldom reported, especially in developing countries. Data with this kind of quality and consistency is only possible from a trauma registry with both facility and community-based listing of events. Few of the developed countries have made such registries like US National Trauma Data Bank and Canadian National Trauma Registry. Apart from these databases, it also requires linking multiple data sources to take a complete picture of the event, its risk, and resultant injuries. For example, data from traffic enforcement will describe the cause and nature of accidents and motor crashes, while the data from the health system will provide the nature of injury resulting from those accidents.

In India, the data related to injuries is majorly recorded and reported by the National Crime Records Bureau (NCRB). Apart from the NCRB, such data is also recorded in the India State-Level Disease Burden Initiative by Public Health Foundation of India, and multiple studies by researchers across the nation. Majority of published literature on morbidity and mortality due to injuries in India is from GBD study. All these estimates undermine the actual burden of accidents and injuries. To attain the true burden, and to identify risk factors of the trauma and injuries, it is required to develop population and hospital-based registries of injuries and link them with data on their mechanism and outcomes.

1.4 Global Burden

Globally, by number of deaths, road traffic injuries (RTI) alone ranked as eighth leading cause of death in 2018. The RTI was pushed out of the top 10 leading cause of death in 2019, majorly due to the increasing burden of noncommunicable diseases in high-income countries, but it still ranked the seventh leading cause of death in low-income countries, and tenth leading cause in lower-middle and upper-middle income countries in 2019 [4]. The true impact of injuries cannot be assessed by the number of deaths alone, instead, the measure of burden in terms of DALYs will provide a better picture of the same. As per the reports of Global Burden of Disease, RTIs ranked up from eighth to seventh place for all ages from 1990 to 2019 contributing to 2.9% of DALY loss. Among other causes of injuries, falls (rank 21), self-harm (rank 22), interpersonal violence (rank 26), and drowning (rank 46) are among the top 50 causes of DALY loss in 2019. The age distribution of injury patterns shows an increased risk of specific injuries for specific age groups. In the age group of 0–9 years road injuries, drowning, foreign body, and falls were among most common causes of DALY loss. The age group of 10–24 years was most prone to road injuries, followed by self-harm, interpersonal violence, falls, drowning, and conflict and terrorism leading to DALY loss. The most productive age group of 25–49 years had road injuries, self-harm, interpersonal violence, and falls among leading causes (Fig. 1.1). With advancing age beyond 75 years, the falls was a more prominent cause of DALY loss [5].

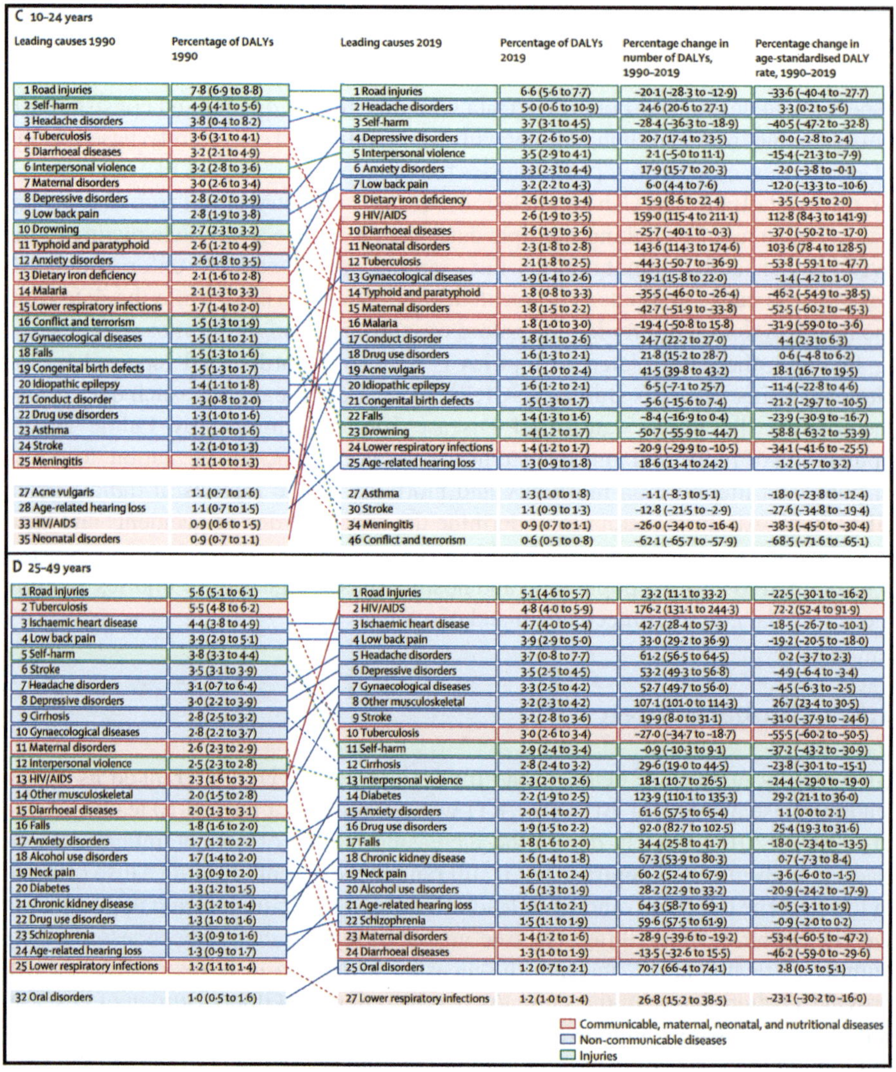

Fig. 1.1 Leading cause of death based on DALY in 1990 and 2019. (Figure C and D from study "Global burden of 369 diseases and injuries in 204 countries and territories, 1990–2019: a systematic analysis for the Global Burden of Disease Study 2019")

1.5 Burden in India

When compared to high-income countries, the probability of a traffic accident is three times higher in low-income nations. India has 1% share of world's vehicles, but accounts for 11% RTIs [6]. However, the RTIs are not the only kind of injuries contributing to the burden of injuries. In India, the majority of data on all injuries is available from NCRB, reported in Accidental Deaths & Suicides in India (ADSI).

The data is well classified for statistical purpose into "Accidental Deaths due to Forces of Nature" which are due to forces/factors of the nature, and "Other causes of Accidental Deaths" which are due to deliberate or negligent conduct of human beings. As per the ADSI-2020 Report, the trend of accidental injuries-related mortalities in India has been declining from 2016 to 2020. In year of 2020, the total number of accidental deaths in India was 374,397. Out of which, 7405 (2.0%) deaths were due to forces/factors of nature and 366,992 (98.0%) deaths were due to causes other than forces/factors of nature. Gender-wise analysis of these mortalities revealed that males (80.5%) were predominant victims. Majority of victims of accidental deaths were between ages of 30 and 45 years accounting for 30.1% of all accidental deaths in country during the year 2020. A total of 41,015 (11.0%) geriatric age group people (60 years and above) died in various accidents during same year. Compared to previous year, 2020 had witnessed a decrease of 9.1% deaths (from 8145 in 2019 to 7405 in 2020) due to forces of nature, and a decrease of 11.1% deaths (from 412,959 in 2019 to 366,992 in 2020) due to causes other than forces of nature.

1.5.1 Accidental Death Due to Forces of Nature

Among 7405 accidental deaths due to forces of nature in 2020, the leading cause was deaths due to Lightning (38.6%), followed by floods (13.0%), exposure to cold (10.5%), and heat/sun stroke (7.2%). Landslides and cyclones were two causes with least mortality at 4.0% and 0.5%, respectively. The age-wise classification of deaths due to forces of nature revealed that the age group of 30–45 years had the highest mortality followed by 60 years and above. The key findings from ADSI-2020 report are shown in Fig. 1.2.

1.5.2 Other Causes of Accidental Deaths

Unlike force of nature, accidents caused as result of "Other Causes" are preventable and can be lowered by taking effective measures toward safety and generating

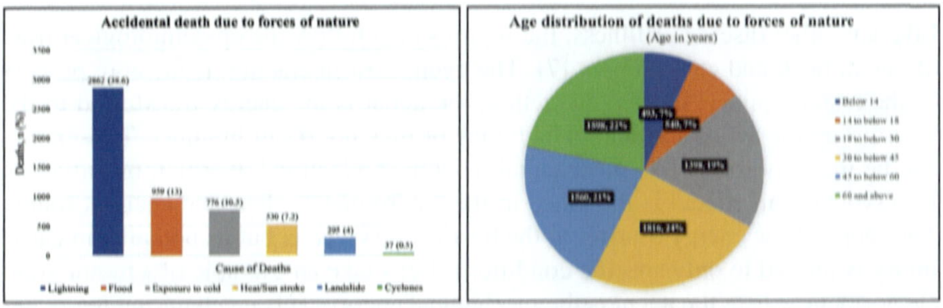

Fig. 1.2 Distribution of accidental death due to forces of nature by cause of death and age groups

general safety consciousness in masses. In year of 2020, a total of 588,738 cases of Accidents were reported due to "Other Causes" which resulted in 366,992 deaths and 338,903 injured persons. The analysis on cause of these deaths revealed that a large proportion of these deaths were due to road traffic accidents accounting for 39.9% (146,354) during 2020. Among other noticeable causes, "Sudden Deaths," "Drowning," "Poisoning," and "Falls" attributed to 13.6% (49,925), 10.1% (37,238), 6.1% (22,221), and 5.6% (20,579) of deaths, respectively. Similar to all accidental deaths, majority of victims for deaths due to other causes were in age groups 30–45 years accounting for 30.3% (111,058 deaths), followed by ages 18–30 years contribution 26.0% (95,340 deaths) of total such deaths.

1.5.3 Economic and Societal Burden of Injuries [6]

The data on the effect of all injury-related morbidity and mortality on the economic state of India is not generated. The data related to economic impact of RTI is available, and since RTI being the leading cause of injuries in India, this can be used to represent economic burden of injuries. According to a 2018 data from the Ministry of Road Transport and Highways, 76.2% of those killed in car accidents were between the ages of 18 and 45, also known as the prime working age group for any country. The World Bank has also conducted a study with the objective of analyzing the socio-economic impacts of road crashes in India, providing us with more measurable outcomes in terms of economic burden. The study revealed that a low-income household (LIH) witnesses 75% loss of income due to road crash, and 54% drop for high-income households (HIH) leading to three times more debt rates in LIH. Poor households also suffer from a decline in quality of life, psychological anguish, and emotional misery in addition to financial difficulties. Women typically take on the majority of caregiving responsibilities in households, which results in a twofold workload and mental strain and exacerbates opportunity gaps for going back to work and generating income. All these findings help us to better understand the direct and indirect cost associated with RTIs.

1.6 Epidemiological Triad of Injuries and the Causal Model

Like any other disease or illness, the injuries also follow the epidemiological triad of agent, host, and environment [7]. The agent-host interaction is the core process of the result—injury. In this interaction, the agent is the energy transferred to the host during the act of accident, which may or may not result in injury. This energy can be in many forms like mechanical, chemical, electrical, thermal, or radiation. Reservoir in this model is the place in the environment where the agent is found. The scope of the energy transfer to the host is everywhere, but its potential to cause injury is limited to only specific conditions. Let's take an example of a motor vehicle accident, where the agent is the mechanical energy. This mechanical energy has a scope of energy transfer when the car is moving, but this only has potential of injury if the car is crashed.

In the given causal model of injuries, the vehicle and the vector are the mechanism of energy transfer. Vehicle is an inanimate object, and the vector is the animate object. For example, the car in a road traffic accident is a vehicle, and an animal in animal bite is a vector. In certain cases, both vehicle and vector can be present such as in a case of gunshot injury—the person discharging the firearm is vector and the firearm itself is a vehicle. These vehicles and the vectors are representations of the environment in this interaction.

As we discussed earlier, the potential of energy transfer to cause injury is less compared to the scope of energy transfer. This is due to certain factors playing a role in the interaction of agent, host, and environment. These factors might be related to the agent or host or environment, and constitute the risk factors for presence or absence of outcome injury. For example, age, medical condition, consumption of psychoactive substances, etc. make the risk factors and may decide the outcome of energy transfer as injury or no injury. These risk factors are different for each agent-host-environment interaction, and this makes it impractical to enumerate all of these risk factors, but a basic model can give in-depth understanding to be able to identify these risk factors.

1.7 Socio-Ecological Model of Risk Factors

For understanding risk factors and prevention of injuries, socio-ecological models are very helpful. The most commonly used model is the one proposed by Dahlberg and Krug in 2002 and has four levels—individual, interpersonal, community, and society [8]. The model has four levels, namely, individual, relationship, community, and societal level.

According to this model, the individual-level decisions and behaviors are determined by all other three levels. Age, gender, socioeconomic status, health status, and personality traits including risk tolerance and the use of safety practices are individual-level factors that affect the risk of injury. For example, male gender has more risk of road traffic injuries, whereas the female gender is at higher risk of burns. Use of psychotropic substances, rash driving, not using a helmet or seatbelt are all individual-level risk factors. Individual-level interventions frequently emphasize raising awareness and promoting behavior change.

Influences from families and other relationships, including the setting in which these relationships take place, are relationship-level factors that predict damage. Role of these factors is bidirectional—it may either increase or decrease the risk of injuries. Teens' risk-taking driving attitudes have been linked to parental communication style, and parental driving may have an impact on their kids' driving habits [9]. High and disparate rates of home injury are correlated with low socioeconomic position, unkempt housing conditions, and failure to address home dangers [10]. Interventions at this level focus on influential communication or changes in the home environment.

Schools, workplaces, and neighborhoods are all examples of community elements that impact local social norms and circumstances. Community elements show high variation and need to be studied in local contexts. Intervention in community-level preventive measures typically aims to alter the culture, procedures, and laws of a certain locality.

Societal level comprises cultural practices and socio-political characteristics of the population. For example, the differences in road traffic accident rates in high, upper-middle, lower-middle, and lower-income countries are due to societal-level risks. Interventions at this level focus on policy making and implementations.

1.8 The Basis of Injury Prevention

The causal model of injuries also divides the injury process into three distinct phases—pre-injury, injury, and post-injury phase. The pre-injury phase is before energy transfer; and injury is the phase of energy transfer, which is the shortest of three, and post-injury phase is the phase of recovery and rehabilitation after energy transfer. Combining these three injury phases with the causal model of injury helps to identify the preventive strategy for injuries. This simple yet effective matrix is known as "Haddon Matrix" developed by Dr. William Haddon in the United States in 1972. Using these three phases of injury, Haddon categorized the preventive strategies into four components—Host, Vehicle and Vector, Physical environment, and Sociocultural environment. This matrix has been the base for road safety measures since decades now. An example of its application in road traffic accidents is shown in Table 1.1. The example shows preventive opportunities and possible interventions at four distinct factors—human, vehicle, physical environment, and sociocultural environments in each of the three phases of injury. The interventions in phase of pre-injury include the controlling the risk factors, interventions in injury phase

Table 1.1 Haddon matrix with illustration of road traffic injuries example

	Factor			
Phase of injury	Occupant	Motor vehicle	Physical environment	Socio-cultural environment
Pre-injury	Avoid psychoactive substance use, discourage road rage	Increase stability of vehicle, improve visibility	Road structure improvements and better traffic management	Increase awareness toward road safety
Injury	Use of seat belt and proper installment of child seats	Include safety features like airbags, head rests, ABS, TPMS systems	Install energy-absorbing guard rails on sides of roads	Policies to ensure safe vehicles with mandatory safety features
Post-injury	Control bleeding and stabilize injuries to prevent complications	Designing vehicle for easy extraction of passengers	Swift emergency medical systems and trained field care staff	Support trauma care and rehabilitation services

mainly target on mitigating effect of impact, and the post-injury interventions are focused on rescue and rehabilitative services.

1.9 Summary

For a surgeon, it is very important to understand the epidemiology of trauma as to shift the focus from curative part to preventive and rehabilitative components of health care. Globally the injuries contribute a major portion of the morbidities, mortality, and DALYs. The huge impact of injury in form of loss of productive workforce is due to its involvement of the most productive years of life. In India, the preventable injuries constitute around 98% of mortalities.

The burden of the problem visible from these statistics is huge, however, these figures are largely underestimate of the actual problem. This clearly demands immediate and concentrated actions toward triangulation of existing data and development of injury registries that include both hospital and community-based components.

Like any other disease, injuries also follow the epidemiological triad of agent-host-environment with energy transfer being the agent and the vehicle or vector playing the environment role. To understand the epidemiology of injuries, it is important to understand the basic concept of epidemiology in trauma and injury such as the causal model of injuries, model for risk factors, and the Haddon matrix which is being used for decades now for planning preventive strategies.

References

1. Robertson LS. Injury epidemiology. 4th ed. Morrisville: Lulu Books; 2015.
2. Langley J, Brenner R. What is an injury? Inj Prev. 2004;10:69–71. https://doi.org/10.1136/ip.2003.003715.
3. Hogarth J. Glossary of health care terminology. Copenhagen: Regional Office for Europe, World Health Organization; 1975.
4. WHO. The top 10 causes of death. Geneva: WHO; 2020. https://www.who.int/news-room/fact-sheets/detail/the-top-10-causes-of-death.
5. Vos T, Lim SS, Abbafati C, Abbas KM, Abbasi M, Abbasifard M, et al. Global burden of 369 diseases and injuries in 204 countries and territories, 1990–2019: a systematic analysis for the Global Burden of Disease Study 2019. Lancet. 2020;396:1204–22. https://doi.org/10.1016/S0140-6736(20)30925-9.
6. Traffic crash injuries and disabilities: the burden on Indian Society. Washington, DC: World Bank Group. http://documents.worldbank.org/curated/en/761181612392067411/Traffic-Crash-Injuries-and-Disabilities-The-Burden-on-Indian-Society.
7. Detels R, editor. Oxford textbook of global public health. 6th ed. Oxford: Oxford University Press; 2015.
8. Dahlberg L. Violence: a global public health problem. Ciênc Saúde Coletiva. 2006;11. https://doi.org/10.1590/S1413-81232006000200007.

9. Yang J, Campo S, Ramirez M, Krapfl J, Cheng G, Peek-Asa C. Family communication patterns and teen drivers' attitudes toward driving safety. J Pediatr Health Care. 2013;27(5):334–41. https://doi.org/10.1016/j.pedhc.2012.01.002.
10. Nyberg C, Schyllander J, Ekman D, Janson S. Socio-economic risk factors for injuries in Swedish children and adolescents: a national study over 15 years. Glob Public Health. 2012;7(10):1170–84. https://doi.org/10.1080/17441692.2012.736172.

Laboratory Investigation in Trauma Patients

2

Nidhi Prasad and Binay Kumar

2.1 Introduction

Trauma is a major public health issue globally and accounts for approximately one in ten deaths [1]. Reporting and management of which is neglected in many developing countries because there are no clear guidelines and record keeping of such incidents. There is a common misunderstanding that Trauma cases are only referred to road traffic accidents. Road traffic injuries comprise only 22.8% of all trauma-related injuries. Rest 77.2% includes other trauma incidents like [2]:

Falls from height (mostly pediatrics age group)
Agricultural related trauma
Fire arms
Assault
Fall of objects
Natural disasters
Terrorist attacks

Trauma-related injury leads to death of 5.8 million people each year accounting for 90% of deaths in low- and middle-income countries [3]. People affected by trauma face fatal or non-fatal injuries which may lead to hospital visits in emergency and further management. In Indian scenario, reports suggest that trauma-related injuries contribute to 13–18% of total deaths [4]. RTA cases are increasing at annual rate of 3%, and 10.1% of all deaths were due to accidents and injuries. A life is lost in every 2 min due to trauma-related injuries in India. Young adults

N. Prasad (✉)
Indira Gandhi Institute of Medical Sciences, Patna, Bihar, India

B. Kumar
Netaji Subhas Medical College and Hospital, Patna, Bihar, India

© The Author(s), under exclusive license to Springer Nature Singapore Pte Ltd. 2024
A. Agrawal et al. (eds.), *Special Considerations in Trauma Care*,
https://doi.org/10.1007/978-981-99-9662-9_2

(20–44 years) are the most common age group affected. In addition to such a high mortality, those who survived with permanent disability are the other aspect that needs to be addressed. This leads to gross loss of productivity and blow to economy. India loses approximately 2–2.5% of its GDP to only road traffic injuries. Many multicentric studies done across the globe shows mortality rate as high as 20% in trauma-related injuries and majority of these incidents are preventable, if the injured person was admitted and managed at hospital meticulously.

For active management of trauma cases, we need to develop dedicated emergency hospitals or trauma emergency sections and train the health care staffs who can deal with trauma cases with clinical acumen. Also, a standardized management and treatment protocol should be drafted and followed. So, early presentation at emergency, diagnosis, management and investigation can bring a lot of difference in the future outcome of the patient. In this section of this book, we are mainly concerned about and dealing with the basic laboratory investigation that is mainly needed in the management of trauma cases. But before we proceed, there are two different schools of thought for the need and the timing at which these investigations should be ordered during hospitalization of trauma patients. Mostly, it is seen that in order to reduce the cost of health care, there is a random reduction of the essential test, which should not happen. Also, these days the tests are automated and easily done, so it can be ordered easily, to get quick results. Our approach should be rationale and efficient use of test for correct and timely diagnosis. Both, over and underutilization of resources should be eliminated.

So, framing a standardized testing protocol is the need of the hour to save valuable lives of trauma patients. In India, the health system is already over-burdened and over strained, so we need to use the resources wisely. Primarily we need to categorize the patient into clinically stable, moderately severe and very severe at the time of presentation at trauma emergency in the hospital using ISS score or ATLS guidelines. The above-mentioned tests should be done on PoCT (Point of Care Testing) analyzer. However testing on PoCT analyzer is bit costlier as compared to central lab analyzer as the cost per test is high. But the early availability of test results within minutes helps in saving crucial time in making clinical decisions. This can make a huge impact on overall management and can also reduce the morbidity; shortened hospital stays or mortality in trauma patients. So, PoCT results can be considered potentially beneficial in the evaluation, treatment and final outcome of trauma patients, especially in critical cases where decisions need to be taken in minutes.

Based on the need we can suggest a primary set and a secondary set of investigation panel (trauma investigation panel).

Primary Panel consists of number of tests that are commonly written to all patients irrespective of severity. It consists of CBC, serum electrolytes, renal function test (BUN, Sr creatinine), coagulation profile (PT, aPTT), blood grouping and Rh typing, cross-matching, routine urine analysis, and arterial blood gas analysis.

2.2 Complete Blood Count (CBC)

It is the most commonly written test, many studies suggested that full panel is not needed in every trauma patient. Hb% and Hct (hematocrit) can suffice the need and fluctuations in the level of both parameters can warrant the treating clinician about internal hemorrhage and need for blood transfusion. But there is conflicting data regarding the timings about ordering a CBC profile. As Hb% is not a real-time indicator of intravascular blood volume, changes are obvious after some time. One set of studies like Keller et al. reported that routine blood tests have little value in the management of injured patients [5].

While other sets of researchers advocated the use of CBC and its variations to predict significant hemorrhage [6]. Early Hb measurement is a meaningful parameter in predicting SH (significant hemorrhage). While POC-Hb estimation in hospitalized patients had a greater ability to predict SH when compared to shock index.

Some common conditions that should be ruled out before starting any blood transfusion:

(a) Prehospitalization IV fluid transfusion should be ruled out as this can erroneously lower the HB.
(b) Taking blood from the same side of infusion should be avoided to rule out any hemodilution.
(c) Using recommended gauge needle for phlebotomy, as small narrow needle such as butterfly leads to abnormal results due to cell lysis and clotting.

Hb <10 g/dL in females and <12 g/dL in males, WBC value $>15 \times 10^3/\text{mm}^3$ indicates serious illness. Elevated WBC count can be seen in stress. While platelet count can be of relative use in head injury, WBC count can be of help in acutely ill patients.

Secondary Panel consists of organ-specific tests panel which cover the organ-specific test requisitions like serum amylase and lipase, urinary amylase and lipase, FDP, serum lactate, etc., and will be dealt in detail later in the book.

2.3 Hematocrit (Hct)

When there is trauma and blood loss, as a compensatory mechanism body fluid shift from interstitial space to vasculature is low and hematocrit is not affected. But in case of patient requiring emergency surgery, hematocrit correlates with shock as there is a rapid shift from interstitial space to vasculature. In occult injury, serial estimation of hematocrit has limited role. In clinical settings where CT scan availability is limited or absent, monitoring through serial HCT estimation is a reliable indicator of ongoing blood loss. Also, a Hct fall of 6 or greater during initial resuscitation is highly suspicious for ongoing blood loss, but even lesser changes have its predictive value in patient outcome [7, 8]. Other studies have shown that hematocrit though having diagnostic utility (due to high specificity), if its level is not falling on serial estimation, the possibility of major trauma cannot be entirely ruled out.

2.4 WBC

In initial assessment of trauma, WBC is one of the first tests that is asked for and the results are quickly available if done in emergency. It is an important predictor of abdominal injury and its severity. Raised WBC count is an important guide in absence of obvious clinical signs and symptoms and can suggest occult injury. While in absence of penetrating abdominal trauma, leucocytosis can be due to marked inflammatory response resulting from injury. Raised WBC count can be stress induced arising from increased release of stress hormones like catecholamine and cortisol. The injury or pain due to injury can result in stress, which induces stress hormones to release in response. Therefore, the severity of the trauma can be predicted by assessing the level of these hormones. Studies have shown that its predictive ability increases on combining with transaminases or hematocrit level. Bowel injury prediction score, a new score for bowel injury score, also has increased WBC as a component, others being mesenteric injury high grade on CT scan and abdominal tenderness [9].

2.5 Glucose

Increase in glucose level in trauma may be a stress response, mediated by glucagon, promoting oxidative stress and insulin resistance. This can further aggravate in presence of underlying diabetes. At the time of admission blood glucose level can predict mortality in trauma cases timely action in maintaining the strict glycemic control can reduce the risk of progression in post-trauma phase. Recent study has found, relative hyperglycemia defined by stress hyperglycemia ratio (SHR) [10], that is glucose at time of admission divided by the estimated average glucose derived from glycosylated hemoglobin can be tool in finding out stress hyperglycemia, this can be marker of trauma or other conditions apart from full blown diabetes. Cardiac arrest is seen in pre-hospital trauma cases with hypoglycemic and hyperglycemic. The association is significant with rising blood glucose concentration [11].

In case of severe traumatic brain injury (TBI), the serum glucose level is significantly higher than mild TBI. Glucose level of more than 151 mg/dL will probably develop coagulopathy, leading to increased morbidity and mortality.

2.6 Coagulation in Trauma

In trauma patients, coagulation and fibrinolytic cascade get activated very early within 1–2 h of incident. This leads to uncontrolled hemorrhage and shock if not attended, though it is most preventable causes of death. Trauma-induced coagulopathy (TIC) leads to the usual complications like shock, hemorrhage and associated injuries acute renal injury, acute lung injury, increased transfusion requirements and longer hospital stays [12, 13]. TIC is a hypercoagulable state commonly presenting with venous thromboembolic episodes and multiple organ failure.

In patients with significant coagulopathy, chances of death increase to 8 times within 24 h of injury. PT, aPTT and TT levels are significantly prolonged along with the reduction of mean platelet count. Coagulopathy in trauma patients can be defined as PT value >18 s (or INR >1.2) and/or aPTT value >36 s [14, 15]. Out of these parameters raised, PT level is the strongest predictor of mortality and fatality.

2.7 Pathophysiology of Coagulation

Tissue trauma is the key stimulus for coagulopathy causing activation of coagulation cycle. Primary source of most coagulation proteins is liver. So, severe liver injury and/or significant shock result in compromised liver function which further jeopardize the compensation of coagulation factors by body [16]. The reasons of coagulopathy in people presenting as trauma cases are loss of blood, colloid interference, low calcium level, functional impairment, hypothermia as well as dilution and consumption of platelet and coagulation factors [1]. Normally hemostasis is terminated when platelet fibrin complex plugs the area of breach that stops bleeding and forms a physical barrier making an impermeable surface preventing the loss of activated factors and helping in speedy healing processes. So, coagulopathy can occur when procoagulants are consumed or diluted or when one or more of normal control mechanisms are disrupted. Trauma-induced coagulopathy is a fibrinolytic type DIC and is markedly different from thrombotic subtype seen commonly in sepsis-induced coagulopathy [17, 18]. Although sepsis-induced DIC is frequent incident in critical care settings and is marked by microcapillary thrombosis leading to organ hypoperfusion injury [19–21]. Whereas, TIC-induced DIC increases the fibrinolytic activity. Both subtypes of DIC gets activated in trauma. Plasma PAI suppresses fibrinolysis in thrombotic phenotype, whereas fibrinolysis is activated by tissue-plasminogen activator (t-PA) in DIC with the fibrinolytic phenotype. In severe trauma, hypercoagulable state and fibrinolysis cascade can occur simultaneously. Severity of injury can be assessed by high ISS and low GCS score. This vicious cycle decreases plasma fibrinogen more rapidly and can be the earliest parameter to measure even before other routinely measured parameters like PT, aPTT, TT and Platelet. In judicious use of I.V fluid infusion or blood transfusion leads to dilution of clotting factors. This decreased level of factors affects the normal hemostasis leading to acute blood loss and poor outcome. So, although sepsis-induced DIC cannot be so serious, trauma-induced DIC can lead to massive blood loss, especially in the acute phase of trauma contributes to massive bleeding and death [22–24].

2.8 Electrolyte in Trauma Patient

Electrolyte imbalance is not so significantly altered in trauma cases only exception is the cases of TBI. Normally body fluid and electrolyte levels are continuously under the control of CNS, hormones and organs like heart and kidney. Major electrolyte imbalance is hyponatremia with serum sodium level falling below 135 mmol/L, commonly presenting within 7 days of trauma. Impaired function of hypothalamic pituitary adrenal axis with secondary adrenal insufficiency leads to hyponatremia, common causes are cerebral salt wasting syndrome, syndrome of inappropriate antidiuretic hormone (SIADH) and drugs like mannitol, thiazide and furosemide. Other contributing risk factors are severity of head injury, any associated comorbidity like kidney and heart failure, elderly and hyperventilation [25–28]. Hypernatremia is the most common electrolyte imbalance followed by hyponatremia and hypokalemia which is a disorder called as syndrome of inappropriate antidiuretic hormone (SIADH) [29].

Longer stay in ICU and existing nutritional status of patient further aggravate hypoalbuminemia resulting from protein break down, and as calcium circulates in body bound to albumin, estimated serum calcium level can be falsely low. Stress provoked catecholamine release further led to hypokalemia and increased leucocyte count. Commonly used drugs like thiazide also results in decreased magnesium and phosphate level.

Few other studies also tell us about the most common, electrolyte imbalance and acidosis due to hypokalemia. Though hypernatremia is less common than hypokalemia, it has higher odds of death in post operative period in first 24 h after head injury. Acidosis and level of glucose in blood being other important predictors of death in TBI cases.

As a consequence of this imbalance, sign and symptoms seen are as follows. Low calcium and sodium levels result in altered cognition, ranging from depression to confusion and precipitation of seizures. Very low calcium level results in spasm of airways, whereas low phosphate interferes with diaphragm contraction leading to difficulty in weaning from mechanical ventilation. Further, adding to this, low magnesium has cardiac manifestation like arrythmias. Hence, continuous monitoring and evaluation of the electrolyte levels will not only halt the deleterious effects on organs but also shorten the hospital stay.

2.9 Urine Analysis in Trauma Patient

The utility of urinalysis (UA) by dipstick or routine microscopy to rule out any intra-abdominal (IA) or genitourinary (GU) injury after blunt trauma remains controversial. The test has low sensitivity and specificity in diagnosing blunt abdominal or genitourinary injuries and is subjected to bias. Study by Isaacman et al. showed its only utility as screening test in excluding pediatric renal injury [30]. But for sure, if a negative UA should be evaluated prospectively with other clinical findings and vital signs assessment. It suggests low risk for GU and IA injury after blunt abdominal trauma while in penetrating injury its use is recommended to rule out any obvious hematuria. A negative UA with normal vitals and physical assessment helps to rule out any unwarranted-unnecessary radiation exposure from CT/X-Ray particularly in children [31].

2.10 Amylase

Pre-admission estimation of serum amylase and lipase value in victims of blunt trauma as an indicator of intra-abdominal injury especially pancreas. Although serum amylase and lipase can be raised in pancreatic injury, brain injury, salivary, gland and gastrointestinal tract involvement, but its raised level is more specific for pancreatic trauma and timely estimation of its value in suspected pancreatic injury is important because of high rate of mortality in pancreatic injury. Study showed serum amylase >2-fold and lipase >4-fold from its normal level warrants the need of CT scan examination and found reliable in diagnosing missed blunt trauma injury [32]. Other than the pancreatic injury, serum amylase and lipase; urinary amylase-lipase, liver enzyme level, routine urine, CBC count, etc. also help to predict other intra-abdominal injuries.

2.11 Alanine Transaminase (ALT) and Aspartate Transaminase (AST)

Alanine transaminase (ALT) and aspartate transaminase (AST) are mitochondrial and cytoplasmic enzymes found in liver cells, neurons, muscle and pancreatic cells, blood, and many tissues. Transaminase levels rise in injuries of the heart, liver, skeletal muscle, kidneys, pancreas, spleen and lungs. Elevated serum transaminase level above its normal cut off ($\leq$50 IU/L) indicates liver injury and a normal level excludes the possibility of liver injury, which does not require any treatment. So, liver enzymes level can be used as a screening tool for blunt liver injury and as a guide to avoid CT scan in pediatric blunt trauma cases [33].

2.12 Myoglobin and CK

Estimation of two important parameters myoglobin, an iron-containing protein along with CK level, which is released due to muscular injury in trauma helps in diagnosis. Myoglobin does not bound to any protein and is freely excreted in urine if plasma level rises above 1.5 mg/dL, causing brown or red-colored urine. Myoglobin can be detected in urine dipstick at levels of 0.5–1 mg/dL. Half-life of myoglobin is 2–3 h which is shorter than CK (1.5 days) and is quickly metabolized resulting in normal level in serum in 6–8 h. The serum CK after injury begins to rise in 2–12 h and reaches to maximum 72 h after which it declines to normal within 3–5 days of cessation of muscle injury. Therefore, in rhabdomyolysis, myoglobin appears and disappears before CK, so dipstick may be negative in half of the patients. So, for initial assessment, myoglobin is preferred to predict AKI (acute kidney injury) and assess severity of rhabdomyolysis at the time of admission. Its prognostic value is better than CK in critically ill patients [34]. The CK has three isotypes CK-MM, MB, and BB. MM fraction arises from skeletal muscle fraction and a small portion may be of myocardial fraction. In case of high myoglobin, baseline troponin is also high but level is not clinically significant for acute myocardial injury. Urine in myoglobin suggests propensity of AKI in high injury severity score and is a guide for further management of extensive fluid hydration [35].

2.13 Arterial Blood Gas and Lactate

The arterial blood gas (ABG) is a bedside analyzer and it is a must routine assessment for initial risk assessment, also helps in the diagnosis guide us about the clinical condition of heart, kidney and lung's function. The value obtained like (pH, pCO2, pO2), base excess, oxygenation, hemoglobin, electrolytes, (K, Na, HCO3, Ca), glucose and lactate during the diagnostic process aids in initial and targeted management of trauma patients. VBG are relied to guide clinical decision-making. Continuous monitoring of acid-base (pH, HCO3, and BD) status is an important guide to resuscitation or indicating occult ongoing blood loss. (Acidosis correction, fluid administration, intubation.) Though ABG is gold standard but routinely VBG is adopted as screening tool as it is non-invasive, feasibility in critically ill, when pulse is non-palpable. There are many controversies regarding the differences in the values but VBG can guide in clinical decision-making. In case of clinical concern with normal VBG, ABG can be measured. In any trauma case, serial measurement of ABG base deficit and lactate is a useful indicator of hemorrhagic shock and serial marker of response to treatment. Similarly, Davis et al. [36] and Rutherford et al. [37] mention BD as useful guide to fluid replacement in the resuscitation and a marker for significant risk of mortality respectively in trauma cases. Commonly, it is seen that patient receive only one sample within 4 h i.e., VBG, lactate and base deficit are commonly used to diagnose shock. Lactate in favored in non-trauma cases but base excess is used since ages in trauma cases. Base deficit is inadequately related in ABG and VBG samples, so lactate is a consistent marker of shock. The value of BD is greater than or equal to 15 mmol/L in a patient younger than 55 years of age without a head injury; or greater than or equal to 8 mmol/L in elderly patients (55 years or older) without a head injury or a young patient with a head injury. The finding concluded by studies is continuous check on base deficit is the guide for prompt resuscitation and management in trauma patients [38, 39].

Special Cases:

(a) **Children and Adolescent** is a vulnerable age group predisposed to various traumas including fall from height, violence, physical abuse, neglect and injury from road traffic accidents. Apart from the routine test, we have to evaluate them for coagulopathy and factors (8 and 9) assay in these cases especially when presented with bruise and petechiae and intracranial bleeding. Newborns and toddlers lack vitamin K-dependent factor, and liver not mature enough to produce clotting factors and hence have a higher coagulopathy. PT-INR is used to make assessment for coagulopathy. The International Society for Thrombosis and Haemostasis (ISTH) has a score with INR, plasma fibrinogen, D-dimer, and thrombocytes to diagnose DIC [20]. In cases of systemic inflammatory response, the inflammatory markers identify high risk and are of prognostic value. CRP and CBC are widely used. CRP can be a diagnostic and prognostic marker as well. In motor vehicle crashes, burns can also result and interleukin, IL-6 and IL-10 values are reduced in children as compared to adults. Here, we have to be cautious in interpretation as neither CRP nor PCT correlated with the increase mortality. Base deficit and lactate level are still debated prognostic markers. In soft tissue injury, specific test for organ involved should be done as measured above and evaluation of hemodynamic in abuse should be done. Diagnostic peritoneal lavage can also be done when needed.

(b) **Pregnancy**

Apart from the routine test, if a pregnant lady comes with trauma, evaluation of mother and fetus should be done. The test can be CBC, urinalysis, urine pregnancy test (if applicable) blood glucose, serum electrolyte, blood grouping and Rh typing, coagulation profile. Coagulation profile should be assessed, keeping in mind that most coagulation factor rise throughout pregnancy, but value of fibrinogen that remain the same. Kleihauer-Betke test (Rh incompatibility) is to be specially prescribed in mother with Rh-ve blood group. In some cases of placental abruption, D-dimer testing is advocated to determine the course of action.

(c) **Geriatric Cases**

In elderly, blood grouping and cross-matching. ABG/VBG, CBC, KFT, serum electrolyte and PT INR should be done. In impending rhabdomyolysis, serum lactate and base deficit must be done. In polytrauma cases, initial lactate level and blood gas analysis suggest abnormal values due to hypoperfusion or hemodynamic instability even if the patient is normotensive. In such cases repeat testing and 2 h follow up, serum lactate (greater than 2.4 mmol/L) suggest hypo perfusion and resuscitation and admission to ICU is suggested.

Toxicology screening is mandatory in few cases depending on the history as it may worsen successful recovery. Alcohol level estimation in blood is of utmost important, breath analyzer test is at point of care testing more reliable and done often.

2.14 Conclusion

It is very important to recognize and choose wisely among the wide battery of laboratory tests available. Tests are conducted for initial assessment of the trauma (screening tools), diagnosis and prognosis. Minor, major and occult trauma must not be missed out due to omitting certain tests nor do we want to conduct tests that are not necessary. Carefully chalking out the test according to clinical sign and symptom, type of trauma, organ involvement, age, gender and type of facility will always be a challenge. Other issues may be institutional policy, physician decision, legal issue, financial concern on patient behalf and optimum resource utilization. For triaging patient with minor trauma and those who are stable, tests should be carried after initial assessment clinically. There is certain test, despite being a part of CBC are never ordered, utility of these has to be identified. Therefore, we must develop protocol and standardized criteria in special conditions for systematic approach, so that we don't sacrifice the urgent test in further management. Time is precious in emergency and clarity on the diagnostic accuracy is a guide in saving time and delivering best to and for the patient need, good clinical acumen with judicious choice of test lead to further planning of steps in trauma management and a step toward decreasing morbidity and mortality.

References

1. Ganapathy N. Coagulopathy in trauma. Ind J Trauma Anaesth Crit Care. 2007;8(2):621–6.
2. https://traumaindia.org/trauma-india-factfile.php. Accessed Apr 2022.
3. WHO. Global status report on road safety, 2018. 2018. https://www.who.int/publications-detail-redirect/9789241565684.
4. Gururaj G. Road traffic deaths, injuries and disabilities in India: current scenario. Natl Med J India. 2008;21(1):14.
5. Keller MS, Eric Coln C, Trimble JA, Christine Green M, Weber TR. The utility of routine trauma laboratories in pediatric trauma resuscitations. Am J Surg. 2004;188(6):671–6.
6. Figueiredo S, Taconet C, Harrois A, Hamada S, Gauss T, Raux M, Duranteau J. How useful are hemoglobin concentration and its variations to predict significant hemorrhage in the early phase of trauma? A multicentric cohort study. Ann Intensive Care. 2018;8(1):1–10.
7. Thorson CM, Ryan ML, Van Haren RM, Pereira R, Olloqui J, Otero CA, Schulman CI, Livingstone AS, Proctor KG. Change in hematocrit during trauma assessment predicts bleeding even with ongoing fluid resuscitation. Am Surg. 2013;79(4):398–406.
8. Zehtabchi S, Sinert R, Goldman M, Kapitanyan R, Ballas J. Diagnostic performance of serial haematocrit measurements in identifying major injury in adult trauma patients. Injury. 2006;37(1):46–52.
9. McNutt MK, Chinapuvvula NR, Beckmann NM, Camp EA, Pommerening MJ, Laney RW, Clark West O, et al. Early surgical intervention for blunt bowel injury: the Bowel Injury Prediction Score (BIPS). J Trauma Acute Care Surg. 2015;78(1):105–11.
10. Roberts GW, Quinn SJ, Valentine N, Alhawassi T, O'Dea H, Stranks SN, Burt MG, Doogue MP. Relative hyperglycemia, a marker of critical illness: introducing the stress hyperglycemia ratio. J Clin Endocrinol Metabol. 2015;100(12):4490–7.
11. Kreutziger J, Schmid S, Umlauf N, Ulmer H, Nijsten MW, Werner D, Schlechtriemen T, Lederer W. Association between blood glucose and cardiac rhythms during pre-hospital care of trauma patients—a retrospective analysis. Scand J Trauma Resusc Emerg Med. 2018;26(1):1–10.
12. Puranik GN, Verma TYP, Pandit GA. The study of coagulation parameters in polytrauma patients and their effects on outcome. J Hematol. 2018;7(3):107.
13. Mujuni E, Wangoda R, Ongom P, Galukande M. Acute traumatic coagulopathy among major trauma patients in an urban tertiary hospital in sub Saharan Africa. BMC Emerg Med. 2012;12(1):1–7.
14. Gando S, Wada H, Kim HK, Kurosawa S, Nielsen JD, Thachil J, Toh C-H, Scientific and Standardization Committee on DIC of the ISTH. Comparison of disseminated intravascular

coagulation in trauma with coagulopathy of trauma/acute coagulopathy of trauma-shock. J Thromb Haemost. 2012;10(12):2593–5.
15. Johansson PI, Sørensen AM, Perner A, Welling KL, Wanscher M, Larsen CF, Ostrowski SR. Disseminated intravascular coagulation or acute coagulopathy of trauma shock early after trauma? An observational study. Crit Care. 2011;15(6):1–10.
16. DeLoughery TG. Coagulation defects in trauma patients: etiology, recognition, and therapy. Crit Care Clin. 2004;20(1):13–24.
17. Gando S, Hayakawa M. Pathophysiology of trauma-induced coagulopathy and management of critical bleeding requiring massive transfusion. Semin Thromb Hemost. 2016;42(2):155–65.
18. Gando S, Otomo Y. Local hemostasis, immunothrombosis, and systemic disseminated intravascular coagulation in trauma and traumatic shock. Crit Care. 2015;19(1):1–11.
19. Asakura H. Classifying types of disseminated intravascular coagulation: clinical and animal models. J Intensive Care. 2014;2(1):1–7.
20. Taylor FB Jr, Toh C-H, Hoots KW, Wada H, Levi M. Towards definition, clinical and laboratory criteria, and a scoring system for disseminated intravascular coagulation. Thromb Haemost. 2001;86(11):1327–30.
21. Hayakawa M, Gando S, Ono Y, Wada T, Yanagida Y, Sawamura A. Fibrinogen level deteriorates before other routine coagulation parameters and massive transfusion in the early phase of severe trauma: a retrospective observational study. Semin Thromb Hemost. 2015;41(1):35–42.
22. Yanagida Y, Gando S, Sawamura A, Hayakawa M, Uegaki S, Kubota N, Homma T, et al. Normal prothrombinase activity, increased systemic thrombin activity, and lower antithrombin levels in patients with disseminated intravascular coagulation at an early phase of trauma: comparison with acute coagulopathy of trauma-shock. Surgery. 2013;154(1):48–57.
23. Sawamura A, Hayakawa M, Gando S, Kubota N, Sugano M, Wada T, Katabami K-i. Disseminated intravascular coagulation with a fibrinolytic phenotype at an early phase of trauma predicts mortality. Thromb Res. 2009;124(5):608–13.
24. Hayakawa M, Sawamura A, Gando S, Kubota N, Uegaki S, Shimojima H, Sugano M, Ieko M. Disseminated intravascular coagulation at an early phase of trauma is associated with consumption coagulopathy and excessive fibrinolysis both by plasmin and neutrophil elastase. Surgery. 2011;149(2):221–30.
25. Rhoney DH, Parker D Jr. Considerations in fluids and electrolytes after traumatic brain injury. Nutr Clin Pract. 2006;21(5):462–78.
26. Krishnamoorthy V, Distelhorst JT, Vavilala MS, Thompson H. Traumatic brain injury in the elderly: burden, risk factors, and prevention. J Trauma Nurs. 2015;22(4):204–8.
27. Fu WW, Fu TS, Jing R, McFaull SR, Cusimano MD. Predictors of falls and mortality among elderly adults with traumatic brain injury: a nationwide, population-based study. PLoS One. 2017;12(4):e0175868.
28. Carney N, Totten AM, O'Reilly C, Ullman JS, Hawryluk GWJ, Bell MJ, Bratton SL, et al. Guidelines for the management of severe traumatic brain injury. Neurosurgery. 2017;80(1):6–15.
29. Rafiq MFA. Hyponatremia still remains largely undiagnosed and untreated. Anaesth Pain Intensive Care. 2019;21(1):1–3.
30. Isaacman DJ, Scarfone RJ, Kost SI, Gochman RF, Davis HW, Bernardo LM, Nakayama DK. Utility of routine laboratory testing for detecting intra-abdominal injury in the pediatric trauma patient. Pediatrics. 1993;92(5):691–4.
31. Jones TS, Stovall RT, Jones EL, Knepper B, Pieracci FM, Fox CJ, Moore EE, Burlew CC. A negative urinalysis is associated with a low likelihood of intra-abdominal injury after blunt abdominal trauma. Am J Surg. 2017;213(1):69–72.
32. Hosseininejad SM, Bozorgi F, Assadi T, Montazar SH, Jahanian F, Hoseini V, Shamsaee M, Tabarestani M. The predictive role of amylase and lipase levels on pancreas injury diagnosis in patients with blunt abdominal trauma. Horm Mol Biol Clin Invest. 2020;41(3).
33. Bruhn PJ, Østerballe L, Hillingsø J, Svendsen LB, Helgstrand F. Posttraumatic levels of liver enzymes can reduce the need for CT in children: a retrospective cohort study. Scand J Trauma Resusc Emerg Med. 2016;24(1):1–5.

34. Mikkelsen TS, Toft P. Prognostic value, kinetics and effect of CVVHDF on serum of the myoglobin and creatine kinase in critically ill patients with rhabdomyolysis. Acta Anaesthesiol Scand. 2005;49(6):859–64.
35. Wasfie T, DeLeu B, Roberts A, Hille J, Knisley T, McCullough J, Yapchai R, Barber KR, Shapiro B. Impact of raising serum myoglobin on resuscitation of trauma patients with high injury severity score (ISS). Surg Open Sci. 2020;2(2):81–4.
36. Davis JW, Shackford SR, Mackersie RC, Hoyt DB. Base deficit as a guide to volume resuscitation. In: 50 landmark papers every trauma surgeon should know. Boca Raton: CRC Press; 2019. p. 35–8.
37. Rutherford EJ, Morris Jr JA, Reed GW, Hall KS. Base deficit stratifies mortality and determines therapy. J Trauma. 1992;33(3):417–23.
38. Sauaia A, Moore FA, Moore EE, Haenel JB, Read RA, Lezotte DC. Early predictors of postinjury multiple organ failure. Arch Surg. 1994;129(1):39–45.
39. Siegel JH, Rivkind AI, Dalal S, Goodarzi S. Early physiologic predictors of injury severity and death in blunt multiple trauma. Arch Surg. 1990;125(4):498–508.

Radiology and Imaging in Neurotrauma 3

Deep Yadav, Krishan K. Yadav, and M. S. Sridhar

The nervous system is almost entirely inaccessible to revolutionary development in medical science and direct examination.

The exceptions to this are trifling.

Sir William Gowers, 1886

3.1 Introduction

Trauma can be said to be the most rapidly progressing epidemic of our times contributing to almost 10% of all deaths. Neurotrauma is the largest cause with an annual incidence of 200–600 cases/100,000 population [1].

In any case of trauma, it is imperative that there are set protocols and guidelines to maximize efficiency and minimize the risk of overlooking some important aspects. Immediate assessment and management of any such patient should be quick, methodical, and effective and it is best to follow the ATLS guidelines.

Once the patient has been stabilized, the next step is imaging to document the extent of injuries and decide the best line of management.

3.2 Historical Aspects

Injuries and wars have fascinated us through the ages and the study of distribution and mechanism of trauma has contributed vastly to our understanding of the history of civilizations as well as provided the building blocks for advancements in medicine, forensics, and public health. The earliest evidence of head trauma has been found in Tanzania and points toward a likely crocodile bite that took place approx. 2,000,000–1,800,000 years BCE [2].

D. Yadav
Radiodiagnosis, Command Hospital Air Force Bangalore, Bangalore, Karnataka, India

K. K. Yadav (✉) · M. S. Sridhar
Neurosurgery, Command Hospital Air Force Bangalore, Bangalore, Karnataka, India

© The Author(s), under exclusive license to Springer Nature Singapore Pte Ltd. 2024

A. Agrawal et al. (eds.), *Special Considerations in Trauma Care*,
https://doi.org/10.1007/978-981-99-9662-9_3

Trepanation or the process of making a hole in the skull is among the oldest surgical procedures documented and skulls with evidence of trepanation have been found dating back to at least 10,000 BC. In ancient Egypt, one of the earliest recorded documentations on trauma is in the form of Edwin Smith Papyrus (1600 BC), which records symptoms and management of various diseases including traumatic brain injury and spinal injury. The fact that ancient Egyptians recognized the significance of neurotrauma is evidenced by the fact that it records 48 cases of trauma by anatomy, out of which 28 concern the head [2]. Sushruta, the famous Indian surgeon (800–600 BC), has described multiple surgical procedures for battle head injuries and trepanation [3].

Humans have always strived to visualize what was within the skull but were constantly frustrated by the skull. Sir William Macewen described the brain as a "Dark Continent". The first success in this attempt was with the invention of the ophthalmoscope by Helmholtz in 1851.

The discovery of X-rays in 1895 by Wilhelm Conrad Roentgen provided for the first time a chance to peer into the skull. In 1897, Oppenheim radiologically confirmed the diagnosis of a pituitary tumor. Capabilities to discern pathologies in the head improved with techniques like cisternography and angiography but were still seriously limited till the invention of CT scan in 1971.

However, the most important quantum leap in our ability to image the brain occurred with the invention of MRI. The first successful MRI image of the brain was produced in the early 1980s. Since then there have been rapid strides in both hardware and software with newer sequences providing ever-improved visualization of the nervous system and its pathologies.

3.3 Indication for Imaging

Almost 50 million cases of TBI are reported every year and estimates have shown that the associated mortality and morbidity is probably more than that of Alzheimer's disease and CVAs [1]. Neuroimaging, from radiographs to CT scans and MR Imaging technology has been playing a significant role in the management of these craniospinal trauma which in turn has led to better outcomes.

The most important and overriding indication for imaging in a case of trauma is clinical. However, since imaging is a limited resource (expenses, time, and availability factors), there have been attempts to devise guidelines and scoring systems to help decide escalation along the imaging pathway.

The most popular of these for imaging of head are the "American College of Radiology Appropriateness criteria" and the "NICE guidelines" [4–6].

According to the NICE guidelines, there are separate algorithms for imaging the head for adults and children with Head Injuries:

A. Adults:

Noncontrast CT head is recommended within 60 min of **any of the** risk factors mentioned below:

- GCS <13 (initial assessment).
- GCS <15 (at 120 min after injury).
- Suspicion of skull fracture (depressed or open).
- Suspicion of fracture skull base.
- Any post-trauma seizure.
- Post-traumatic focal neurological deficit.
- Vomiting (>1 episode).

Noncontrast CT head is recommended within 8 h if

- Presently taking anticoagulants (without any of indications mentioned above).
- H/O unconsciousness or memory loss after injury AND age more than 65 years or H/O bleeding dyscrasia or suggestion of high energy impact or memory loss of more than half an hour.

B. Children:

Noncontrast CT head is recommended within 60 min of **any** of the risk factors mentioned below:

- If NAI (nonaccidental injury) is suspected.
- Post-trauma seizure (without any previous H/O epilepsy).
- GCS <14 (Initial assessment), or GCS (pediatric) <15 (if age <1 year).
- GCS <15 (120 min post-injury).
- Tense fontanelle or suspicion of skull fracture (depressed or open).
- Suspicion of fracture skull base.
- Post-traumatic focal neurological deficit.
- <1 year age with swelling, bruise, or laceration on the head (>5 cm).

C. Children:

Noncontrast CT head is recommended within 60 min of **more than 01** of the risk factors mentioned below (and none of those in the list "B" above):

- Witnessed Unconsciousness for >5 min.
- Abnormal drowsiness.
- Vomiting (03 or more discrete episodes).
- Injury due to dangerous mechanisms (high-speed RTA, fall from a height >3 m).
- Memory loss lasting >5 min.

D. Children with injury to the head and have **only one** of the risk factors in "C" (and none of those in "B") are recommended to be observed for at least 4 h post the said injury. Obtain a NCCT head scan within 60 min if any under-mentioned risk factors are observed.

- GCS <15.
- Additional episodes of vomiting.
- Another observed drowsiness.

E. Any patient on anticoagulants who has a head injury (and no other risk factor) should undergo a NCCT head within 8 h of the injury.

NICE guidelines suggest that in a case of Head Injury, a NCCT of cervical spine is recommended within 60 min of identification of any of the following risk factor:

A. Adults: Head injury with initial GCS <13 AND

(a) The patient required intubation.
(b) Technically inadequate radiography.
(c) Radiography—Abnormal (definite or suspected).
(d) Requirement of definite cervical spine injury rule out.
(e) CT being performed for other body areas, e.g., for head injury or polytrauma.
(f) Alert and stable patient with clinically suspected cervical spine injury AND at least one of the following:
  - Age >65 years.
  - Dangerous mechanism of injury (fall from a height >01 m or five stairs; axial loading to the head (e.g., dive injury); high-speed RTA).
  - Focal neurological deficit (peripheral) post-injury or paresthesia in any extremity.

B. Children with head injury, require a NCCT cervical spine scan in limited situations (because of generally lower risk of significant spinal injury and to avoid thyroid irradiation) *only if* any one of the following conditions:

(a) GCS <13 (initial assessment).
(b) Intubated.
(c) Focal peripheral neurological signs.
(d) Paresthesia in any extremity.
(e) Requirement of definite cervical spine injury rule out.
(f) CT being performed for other body areas, e.g., for head injury or polytrauma.
(g) Strong clinical suspicion of injury despite normal X-rays.
(h) Technically inadequate or difficult radiography.
(i) Significant bony injury on radiography.

In a suspected case of spinal cord or cervical column injury (without head injury), the NICE guidelines recommend that imaging be done in the following settings:

A. Children:

(a) MRI cervical spine is recommended for children (<16) in the setting of strong suspicion of Injury of cervical spinal cord **or** cervical spinal column.
(b) Consider Radiography in children (<16) not meeting the criteria for MRI, however if even after repeated clinical assessment, clinical suspicion remains.

B. Adults: NCCT of cervical spine is recommended in adults if

(a) Indicated by the Canadian C-spine rule.
(b) There is a strong suspicion of thoracic or lumbosacral spine injury associated with abnormal neurological signs or symptoms.

C. MRI of the spinal cord is recommended (regardless of whether or not the abnormality is evident on CT) in the presence of a neurological finding that could be attributable to spinal cord injury.

In case of suspicion of isolated thoracic/lumbosacral column injury, NICE guidelines recommend the following:

(a) Radiography is preferred as the first-line investigation in the absence of abnormal neurological signs or symptoms.
(b) CT is recommended if the X-ray is abnormal or in the presence of clinical signs/symptoms of injury to the spinal column.
(c) The entire spinal column is to be imaged if a new spinal column fracture is found.

Whole body CT scan (consisting of a vertex-to-toes scanogram followed by CT from vertex to mid-thigh) is indicated in the following settings:

(a) Adults with suspected polytrauma. Such patients should not be repositioned while performing the whole-body CT.
(b) In adults (16 or over) with limb trauma, it is suggested that clinical findings and the scanogram be used to direct CT of the limbs.
(c) In children, clinical judgment should be used to limit CT to those body areas which need detailed assessment, rather than routinely using whole-body CT.

3.4 Imaging Protocols

3.4.1 NCCT Head Adults

Axial Scan with head/gantry angulation to reduce lens radiation exposure with standard brain and bone reconstructions in all three planes. Axial images at submillimeter sections can be used to make 3D reconstructions of the calvarium and skull base when necessary.

However, a helical scan has the advantage of being faster and being able to cover the head and cervical scan in a single run. The images should be reviewed in multiple window settings, i.e., brain, bone, and liver windows to detect small bleeds and fractures that may otherwise be missed.

While MRI is widely recognized as being more sensitive at demonstrating epidural hematoma (EDH), subdural hematoma (SDH), nonhemorrhagic cortical contusions, brainstem injuries, and white matter axonal injuries, it is also more sensitive for the detection of hemorrhagic parenchymal contusions, all stages of SAH [7].

Although there is a clear indication of MRI of the brain in traumatic brain injury with no significant findings on NCCT, its widespread use as primary modality of imaging is not in vogue due to multiple factors including potential unknown contraindications (e.g., metallic foreign body, cost, time taken and requirement of specialized equipment for monitoring/ventilation) and may be better suited for a delayed evaluation, if required.

The recommended MRI protocol includes diffusion-weighted and susceptibility-weighted imaging and 2D/3D T1 and fat-suppressed T2-weighted and fluid-attenuated inversion-recovery (FLAIR) sequences.

There are very limited indications for CECT or CEMRI in the setting of acute trauma. CT Angiogram or MR angiography is recommended in fractures involving the carotid canal, penetrating injury, and when the intracranial hemorrhage pattern is atypical for trauma (e.g., isolated SAH in the basilar cisterns, in the anterior interhemispheric fissure or isolated large-volume SAH in the Sylvian fissure—conditions when intracranial aneurysm need to be ruled out). AVMs should be suspected if there are large draining veins, if calcification is seen or if the large intraparenchymal bleed is not commensurate with site. And severity of trauma and in such cases CT/MR angiogram is imperative. CT/MR venograms are also useful in cases where fractures cross dural venous sinuses as they may be associated with venous extravasation/venous thrombosis [8].

3.5 Imaging Findings in Traumatic Brain Injury

3.5.1 Skull Fractures

The bony calvarium is often fractured in both blunt and penetrating injuries. These fractures may be linear, comminuted, or depressed. Fractures involving the anterior cranial fossa may be complicated by CSF leak, communication with frontal sinus and involvement of the orbits. Fractures involving carotid canal or dural sinus attachment may be associated with EDH or occlusion of the involved vessels. Fractures involving the skull base may be associated with cranial nerve injury and require high-resolution imaging in addition to routine scans.

3.5.2 Epidural Hematoma

Epidural hematomas are contained between the inner table of the calvarium and the outer layer of the dura. As the dura is tightly attached to the skull at the sutures, EDH is typically limited by sutures and also has a biconvex lentiform shape. However, it is important to remember that especially in children, when the fracture travels along and across the sutures, EDH can be seen crossing the suture lines [9]. The epidural hematoma may be due to a venous bleed (dural sinus is injured) or arterial (if meningeal artery is injured). EDH can be treated by surgical decompression (if large enough to cause significant mass effect), or by middle meningeal artery embolization/follow-up. A representative case image is shown in Figs. 3.1 and 3.2.

3.5.3 Subdural Hematoma

Blood is contained between the dura and the arachnoid layer of the meninges. This bleed is commonly due to rupture of the bridging cortical veins. These bleeds are concavo-convex in shape, cross sutures, but are limited by dural reflections like tentorium and falx.

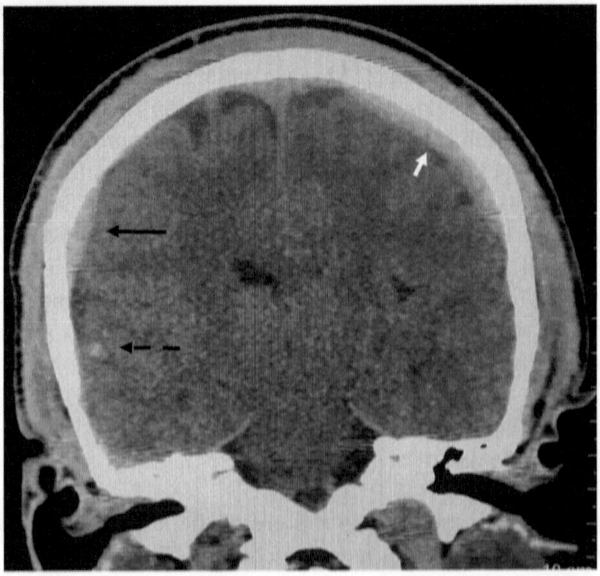

Fig. 3.1 A 45-year-old male. Case of RTA. NCCT head, coronal reformatted image shows hyperdense biconvex collection in the right parietal region (black arrow) suggestive of extradural hemorrhage and a concavo-convex hyperdense extra-axial collection in the left parietal region (white arrowhead) suggestive of subdural hemorrhage. Notice the focal parenchymal hyperdensities in the right temporal lobe suggestive of hemorrhagic contusions (black dashed arrow)

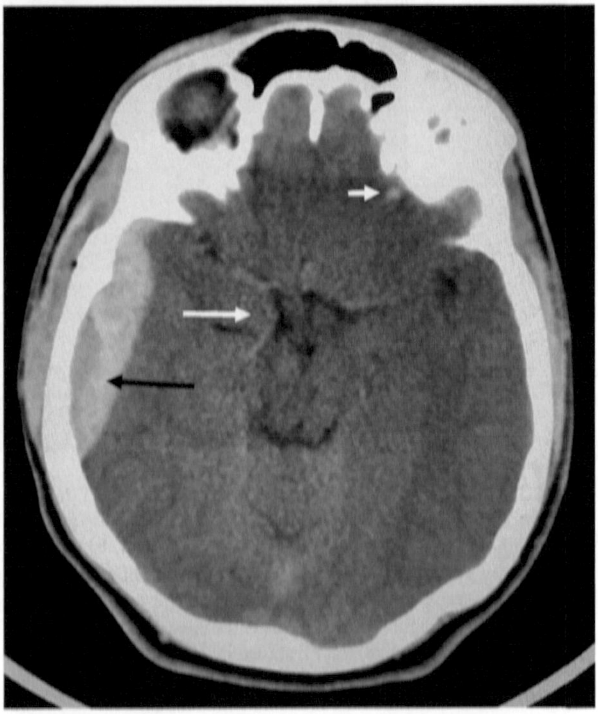

Fig. 3.2 A 16-year-old male, case of RTA. NCCT head, axial section shows a hyperdense extra-axial collection in the right temporal region with differential density within (black arrow) suggestive of extradural hematoma with ongoing bleed. The white arrow annotates right uncal herniation. Note the punctate hyperdensity in the left basifrontal region (white arrowhead) representing a hemorrhagic contusion

Acute SDH can show heterogeneous appearances on CT especially in cases of ongoing bleeding (esp. if patient is on anticoagulants or has a bleeding disorder). The density of the hematoma may also be lower in patients with decreased hematocrit. As the hematoma ages, multiple membranes of granulation can form within it resulting in enhancing septae which cause loculation. These septae are friable, can bleed, and cause recurrent bleed. Chronic SDH can show evidence of wall calcification [10].

Because of increased potential subdural space, especially in elderly, SDH can slowly accumulate over a period of hours to days and cause delayed clinical presentation. Smaller SDH are managed conservatively, whereas the ones causing mass effect are treated by burr hole evacuation, evacuation by craniotomy, subdural evacuation port system, or middle meningeal artery embolization. A representative case image is shown in Figs. 3.3b and 3.4.

3.5.4 Subdural Hygroma

Subdural hygroma are formed due to rupture of the arachnoid membrane causing collection of CSF between the dura and arachnoid. These are slowly accumulating

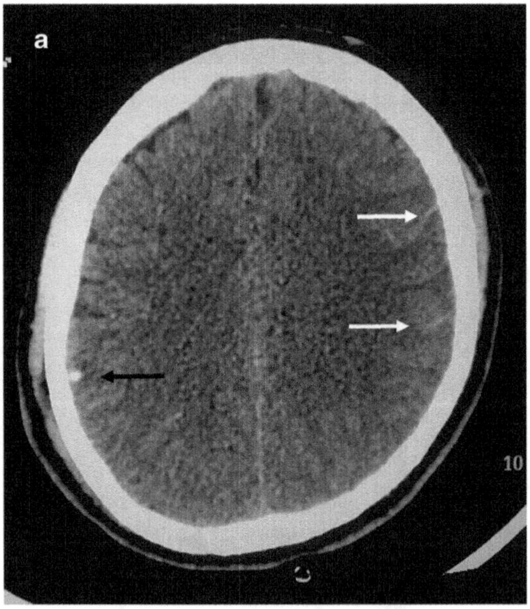

Fig. 3.3 (**a**) A 32-year-old male, case of RTA. NCCT head, axial section shows small hemorrhagic contusion in the right parietal lobe (black arrow) with mild associated perilesional edema. Thin feathery hyperdensity in the sulcal spaces on the left represents subarachnoid hemorrhage (white arrows). (**b**) A 32-year-old male, case of RTA. NCCT head, axial section shows concavo-convex extra-axial hyperdense collection in the left temporal region (black arrow) suggestive of subdural hemorrhage. (**c**) A 32-year-old male, case of RTA. NCCT head, axial section shows longitudinal, linear, nondisplaced fracture involving the right petrous temporal bone

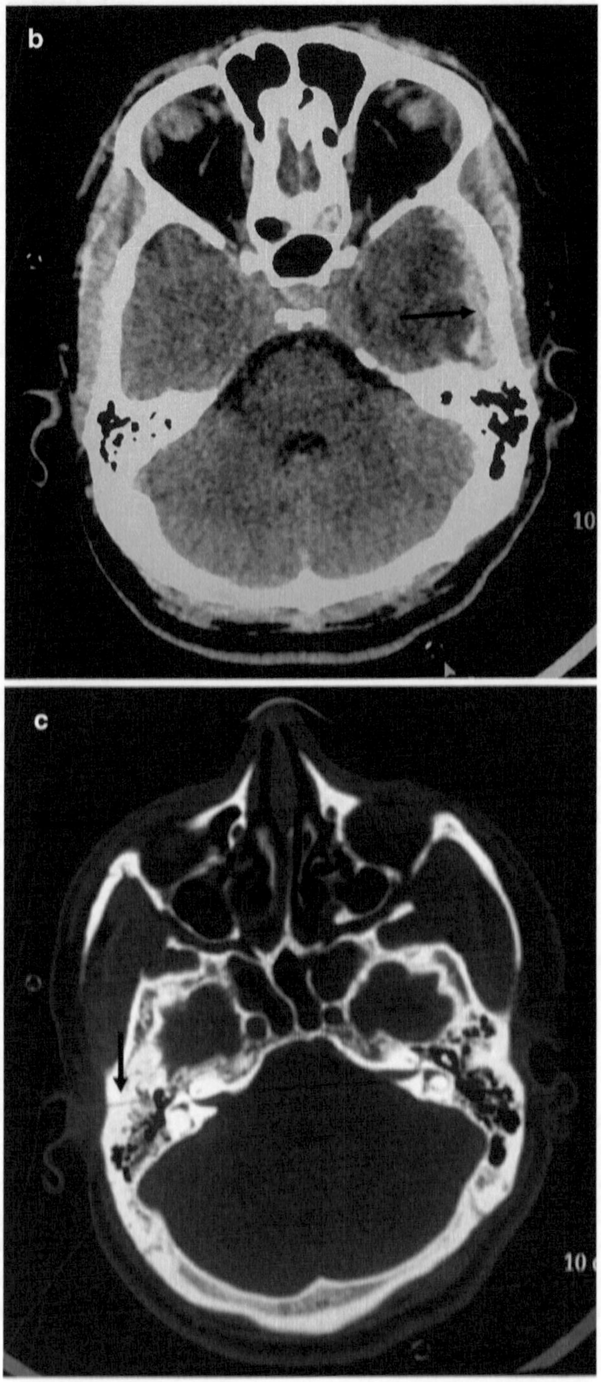

Fig. 3.3 (continued)

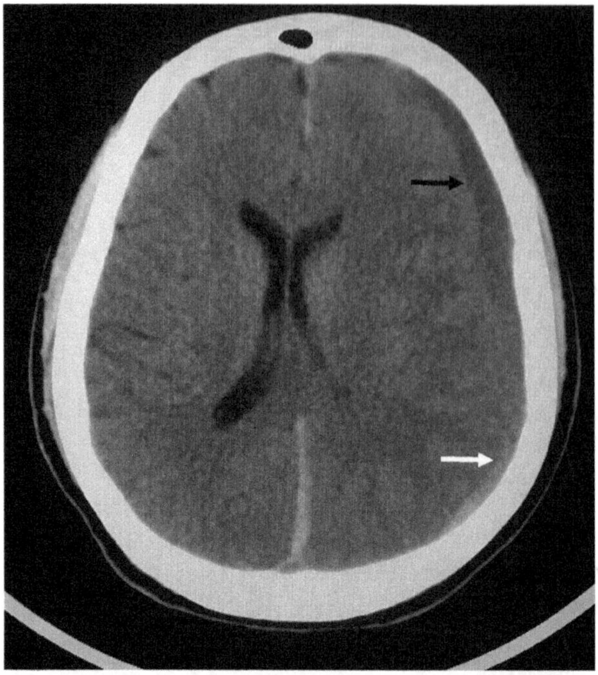

Fig. 3.4 A 38-year-old male. Case of AML with thrombocytopenia, history of trivial trauma 2 days back. NCCT head, axial section shows concavo-convex extra-axial collection in the left frontoparietal region suggestive of subdural hematoma. Notice the predominant hypodensity (black arrow) and dependent hyperdense layering (white arrow) consistent with acute on chronic bleed in a case of bleeding disorder. Significant mass effect is seen in the form of buckling of the underlying cortex, narrowing of the ipsilateral lateral ventricle, and a midline shift of 8 mm to the right and mild subfalcine herniation. The hyperdensity along the falx represents falcine subdural hemorrhage

CSF attenuation (sometimes minimally increased HU compared to CSF) collections with concavo–convex shapes similar to SDH. Often these are admixed with blood, giving rise to hematohygromas.

3.5.5 Traumatic Subarachnoid Hemorrhage

SAH refers to bleeding between the arachnoid and pia mater. Morphologically it is seen as feathery areas of hyper-attenuation (on NCCT) within the sulcal spaces. Traumatic SAHs are usually localized to the site of coup or contrecoup injury. Isolated SAH in locations typical for ruptured aneurysms, e.g., basal cisterns, Sylvian fissure, and anterior interhemispheric SAH should prompt CT/MR angiography even in the setting of trauma.

3.5.6 Intraventricular Hemorrhage

Intraventricular hemorrhage (IVH) in trauma is most commonly an extension of bleeding from parenchymal or subarachnoid hemorrhage. Rarely it can be seen due to rupture of the sub-ependymal veins. Small IVHs are seen as hyper-attenuating fluid levels in the dependent part of the occipital horns, and these should be carefully looked for.

3.5.7 Brain Contusion

Traumatic impact to the brain parenchyma can cause bruises to the brain that occur at the site of impact as well as at the contrecoup location. These are related to both direct impact as well as shear injuries. They are most common at the basifrontal and basitemporal locations where the brain parenchyma is intimately related to the contours of the skull base. They can also be commonly seen at the point of impact with the falx. MRI is much more sensitive than CT scan for detection of contusions, the superiority being even more pronounced in case of nonhemorrhagic contusions. On NCCT, the hemorrhagic contusions are seen as areas of hyperdensity surrounded by ill-defined hypodensity (edema).

Nonhemorrhagic contusions on NCCT are seen as hypodense ill-defined lesions at the points of coup or contrecoup impact. On MRI contusions are seen as hyperintensities on T2/FLAIR images that show blood products (hyperintense on T1 and blooming on GRE) in case of hemorrhagic contusions. Contusions need to be closely followed up on imaging as they often show increased hemorrhagic areas as well as increasing mass effect on the subsequent scans. If the mass effect increases significantly, surgical intervention may be warranted. A representative case image is shown in Fig. 3.3a.

3.5.8 Axonal Injuries

Axons in the brain are arranged in long tracts and may be injured by stretching as well as shear stress. These may be single or multiple, hemorrhagic, or nonhemorrhagic. MRI is much more sensitive than CT in the detection of both hemorrhagic and nonhemorrhagic foci of axonal injuries. These lesions are seen as foci of T2/FLAIR hyperintensity at the points most vulnerable to shear injury i.e. the gray-white junction of the cerebral lobes (esp. frontal lobe), corpus callosum (esp. splenium), internal capsules, and dorsal midbrain and/or pons. These lesions often show restriction of diffusion esp. in the acute phases.

Diffuse axonal injury (DAI) is graded in order of increasing severity—Grade 1 involves the subcortical white matter, grade 2 the corpus callosum, and grade 3 the brainstem [8]. Patients with DAI are often clinically much worse off than what the imaging would suggest. A representative case image is shown in Fig. 3.5.

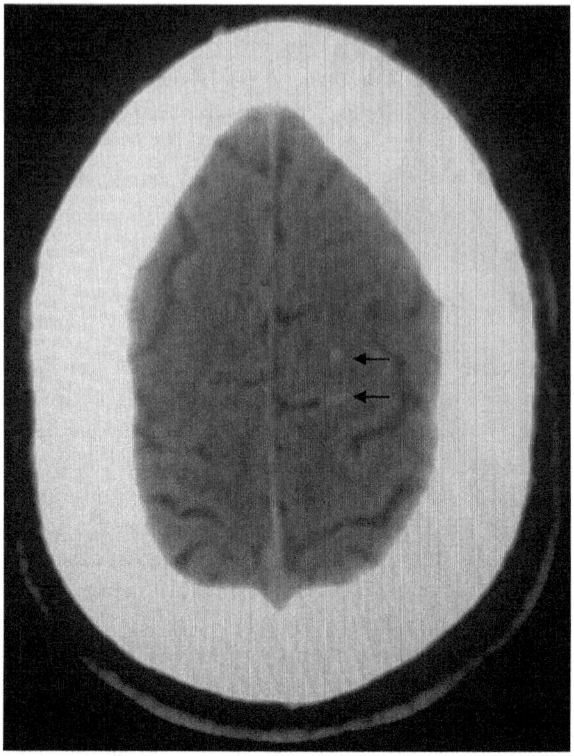

Fig. 3.5 A 26-year-old male who fell from a horse. NCCT head, axial section reveals few, small, punctate hyperdensities in the grey-white matter interface in the left high frontal lobe (black arrows) suggestive of hemorrhagic foci of diffuse axonal injury (DAI)

3.5.9 Diffuse Edema

Head injury can cause dysfunction of cerebral vascular auto-regulation resulting in diffuse nonspecific cerebral edema. The edema may be both vasogenic and cytotoxic and may be related to release of various inflammatory mediators that may increase vascular permeability [8].

3.5.10 Vascular Injury

Injury to the head and cervical spine is sometimes associated with vascular injury that may manifest itself in the form of spasm, extravasation, pseudoaneurysm, caroticocavernous fistula, dissection, or occlusion. Any fracture that is closely related to the ICA or vertebral arteries needs to be further imaged by angiography (CT, MR, or conventional). A representative case image is shown in Fig. 3.6.

Secondary Brain Injuries and Herniations—These are injuries that occur not due to the trauma itself but are a result of the changes that take place due to the injury. Mass effects associated with extradural/subdural hemorrhage, contusions, axonal injury, or post-traumatic edema can cause significant shift of the brain across dural folds and compartments. These movements can cause perfusion reduction, not

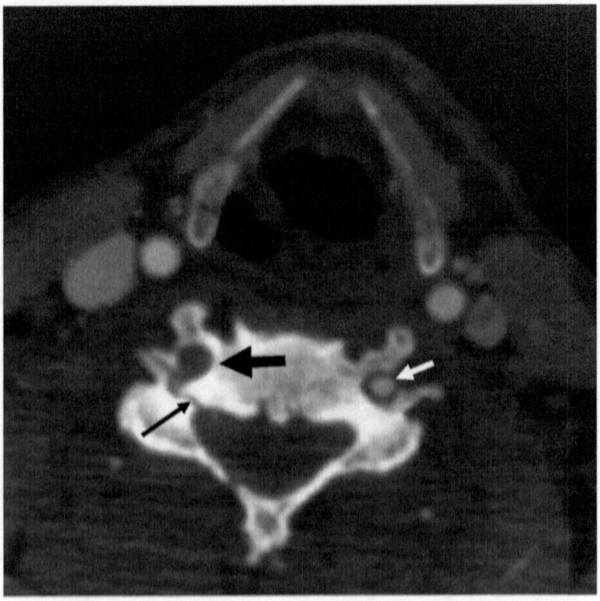

Fig. 3.6 A 69-year-old male. Case of fall from height (8 ft). CT angiogram, oblique axial reformatted images shows a fracture involving the right foramen transvarium of C5 vertebra (black arrow). Note the nonopacification of the right vertebral artery (black arrow head) due to dissection. The left vertebral artery is well opacified (white arrow)

only of the part that is herniated and thus trapped in these dural passages, but compression of the larger vessels passing through these locations can also cause infarcts in locations remote to the herniation sites.

The common herniations are ascending or descending trans-tentorial herniations, uncal herniations, sub-falcine herniations, and tonsillar herniation.

3.6 Imaging Findings in Traumatic Spinal Injury

Worldwide 2.5–5 lac new cases of Spinal cord Injury are reported. In India, the number of new cases added per year is between 15,000 and 20,000 [11]. To explain the mechanism and severity of spinal trauma, Dennis proposed a three-column classification for spine with anterior column consisting of anterior 2/3rd of vertebral body and ALL, middle column consisting of posterior 1/3rd of vertebral body, and PLL and posterior column consisting of posterior elements and ligaments around them [12]. Ligamentum flavum connects laminae interspinous spine ligaments connect spinous processes and supra-spinous ligament connects tip of spinous processes.

The three basic mechanisms of spinal trauma are hyperflexion, hyper-extension, and axial loading. Cord injury can occur at the time of impact known as primary injury or can occur later (k/a secondary injury). Mechanism of secondary injury is not clear; however, it is thought to involve both systemic and local factors that further worsen the injury. These secondary factors include hypoxia, shock, hemorrhage, endothelial injury, cytokine release, and electrolyte shift [13]. Clinical presentation and description are beyond the scope of this chapter however patients with spinal injury can present with pain, dyspnea, loss of sensations, and paresis/plegia.

The cord injury level is roughly related to the vertebral injury level as per the following paradigm: cervical cord—same level, upper dorsal—02 segments, lower dorsal—03 segments, DV11—LV3–4 segments, DV12—LV5 segments and LV1—SV1–5 and Co1 segments. Quadriplegia happens at a level from vertebral CV1 to DV1. Paraplegia usually happens at a level below DV2.

Spinal injuries can be evaluated by plain radiography, CT, and MRI. Plain radiography has a limited role in evaluation of vertebral injuries in the acute setting. They may be done in stable patients with low index of suspicion of spinal trauma or in settings where CT is not available. In such settings, the plain radiography should include AP and lateral views and open-mouth view (where applicable).

The initial assessment on the NCCT spine is best done following the rules that have been designed for plain radiography. It is therefore quickest to evaluate the sagittal reformatted images as these provide the most valuable surgical information.

Evaluation of the three lines, i.e., anterior longitudinal line, posterior longitudinal line, and spino-lamellar line is the fastest way to get an overview of the state of the spine. The facet joint integrity is also best evaluated by the far lateral sagittal views. This is also the best view for evaluating atlantoaxial integrity, prevertebral soft tissues, and the space available for the cord.

Radiological signs of instability include more than one vertebral column involvement, increased or reduced intervertebral disc space height, increased interspinous distance, facet joint widening, and vertebral compression greater than 25% [14].

Rather than a pure axial view, the axial view at each vertebral level should be angled along the orientation of the vertebra on the sagittal view. This angle's axial view is the best to evaluate injuries to the pedicles, lamellae, and the vertebral artery foramen. The coronal views are best for evaluation of the transverse processes and the orientation of occipito-axial and atlantoaxial joints.

Spinal cord injury without radiographic abnormality (SCIWORA) may be an indication for MRI if there is persistent and objective myelopathy after trauma with normal radiograph/CT.

Hyperflexion injuries are the most common and include flexion teardrop fracture, clay-shoveler fracture, facet dislocation, and anterior subluxation. Flexion-teardrop fracture is commonly caused by flexion and compression and is a sagittal fracture through the antero-inferior vertebral body. Facetal dislocation occurs when the inferior articular process of the cranial vertebra moves anterior to the superior articular process of the caudal vertebra and may be unilateral (stable) or bilateral (unstable). A representative case image is shown in Fig. 3.7.

Hyperextension cervical spine fractures include hangman fracture and extension teardrop fracture. Hangman fracture is a traumatic spondylolisthesis of axis vertebra (bilateral lamina and pedicle fracture at C2) and is commonly seen in judicial hanging and high-speed motor vehicle accident (MVA). It is usually associated with anterolisthesis of C2 on C3 and an additional risk of vertebral artery injury if the fracture extends to transverse foramina. Extension teardrop fracture is an avulsion fracture of the attachment of the anterior longitudinal ligament. The fragment is

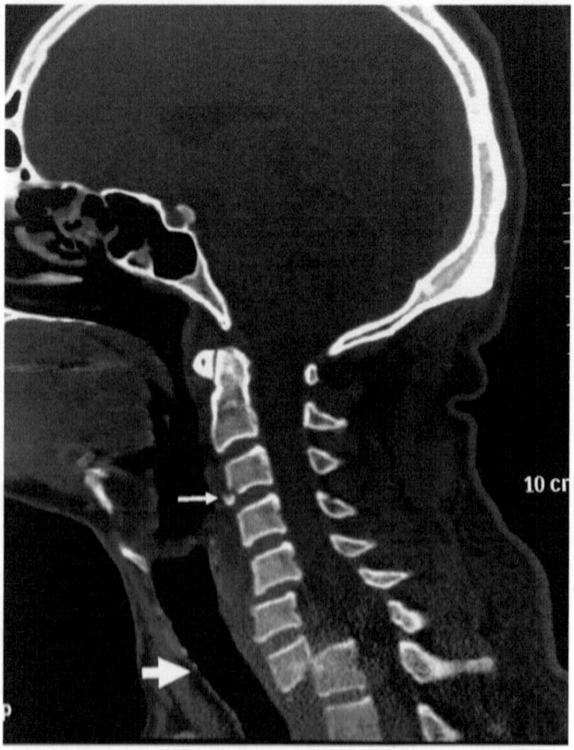

Fig. 3.7 A 32-year-old male. Fell during military training. NCCT cervical spine, sagittal reformatted image shows Grade 4 anterolisthesis of C7 over D1 vertebra (large arrow) with widening of the spinal canal. Fortunately, in spite of the severe injury the patient had preserved power in all limbs. Also note the flexion teardrop fracture at antero-inferior margin of C3 vertebral body (small arrow)

triangular in shape and the vertical height of the fragment is equal or greater than width.

Axial loading fractures include Jefferson's fracture and burst (compression) fracture. Jefferson's fracture is a burst fracture of C1 vertebral and involves fractures through the anterior and posterior arches. In addition, complex mechanisms of cervical spine injury can cause fractures of the dens and atlantoaxial dislocations. Traumatic atlantoaxial dislocations and subluxations are a sign of significant ligamentous injury. These are unstable injuries, with significant risk of being fatal. They are more common in children because of relatively larger heads.

MRI of the spine is invaluable in the evaluation of injuries to the cord as well as extent of ligamentous injuries. However, as discussed MRI examination is constrained by multiple factors including availability, possibility of metal shrapnel, time taken, and limited options of patient monitoring. Cord injuries can range from normal-looking cord, to cord indentation/compression without signal change, cord contusion, and cord transection. Appearances of the cord must be noted on T1, T2 sequences on sagittal and axial images for complete evaluation. The bony-ligamentous complexes are best evaluated on STIR, gradient, and T1 images.

Multiple scoring systems have been devised to help in the grading of spinal trauma. The most popular of these are the Subaxial Injury Classification and Severity

Table 3.1 Subaxial injury classification and severity scoring system for decision-making in subaxial cervical spine injuries

Subaxial injury classification and severity score (SLIC)			
Injury characteristic	Type	Score	Modality
Morphology	• Compression • Burst • Distraction • Translation-rotation	1 2 3 4	CT
Disco-ligamentous complex	• Intact • Suspected-indeterminate • Disrupted	0 1 2	MRI
Neurologic status	• Intact • Nerve root injury • Complete cord injury • Incomplete cord injury • Incomplete cord injury with ongoing cord compression	0 1 2 3 4	Clinical
Score		**Management**	
0–3		Nonoperative	
4		Surgeon's choice	
5 and above		Surgical	

Table 3.2 Thoracolumbar injury classification and severity scoring system for decision-making in thoracolumbar spine trauma

Thoracolumbar injury classification and severity score			
Injury characteristic	Type	Score	Modality
Morphology	• Compression • Burst • Translation-rotation • Distraction	1 2 3 4	CT
PLC integrity	• Intact • Suspected-indeterminate • Injured	0 2 3	MRI
Neurologic status	• Intact • Nerve root-complete cord • Incomplete cord • Cauda equina	0 2 3 3	Clinical
Score		**Management**	
0–3		Nonoperative	
4		Surgeon's choice	
5 and above		Surgical	

Score and the Thoracolumbar Injury Classification and Severity Score as shown in Tables 3.1 and 3.2, respectively. These are numerical radiological-clinical evaluation tools that can help stratify patients into surgical and nonsurgical groups.

3.7 Conclusion

Patients of trauma are often critical and it is therefore important to have a protocol-based approach to prioritize the various assessment and management actions that need to be performed near simultaneously. Imaging is an essential tool in the evaluation of patients with suspected neurological injuries, both for severity assessment as well as to determine the next line of management. All radiological modalities, i.e., X-rays, ultrasound, CT, and MRI have their own advantages and limitations. A thorough knowledge and methodical approach toward imaging of such patients is invaluable in emergency treatment and also long-term recovery.

Conflict of Interest None.

References

1. Rubiano A, Carney N, Chesnut R, et al. Global neurotrauma research challenges and opportunities. Nature. 2015;527:S193–7.
2. Muresanu D, Dobran SA, Cretoiu D. The birth of neurotrauma: a historical perspective from the Academy of Multidisciplinary Neurotraumatology (AMN). J Med Life. 2021;14(6):737–9. https://doi.org/10.25122/jml-2021-1006.
3. Singh V. Sushruta: the father of surgery. Natl J Maxillofac Surg. 2017;8(1):1–3. https://doi.org/10.4103/njms.NJMS_33_17.
4. Expert Panel on Neurological Imaging, Shih RY, Burns J, Ajam AA, Broder JS, Chakraborty S, Kendi AT, Lacy ME, Ledbetter LN, Lee RK, Liebeskind DS, Pollock JM, Prall JA, Ptak T, Raksin PB, Shaines MD, Tsiouris AJ, Utukuri PS, Wang LL, Corey AS. ACR Appropriateness Criteria® head trauma: 2021 update. J Am Coll Radiol. 2021;18(5S):S13–36. https://doi.org/10.1016/j.jacr.2021.01.006.
5. National Institute for Health and Care Excellence. Head injury: assessment and early management. London: NICE; 2014. https://www.nice.org.uk/guidance/cg176.
6. National Institute for Health and Care Excellence. Spinal injury: assessment and initial management. London: NICE; 2016. Clinical guideline [NG41]. https://www.nice.org.uk/guidance/ng41.
7. Mutch CA, Talbott JF, Gean A. Imaging evaluation of acute traumatic brain injury. Neurosurg Clin N Am. 2016;27(4):409–39. https://doi.org/10.1016/j.nec.2016.05.011.
8. Schweitzer AD, Niogi SN, Whitlow CT, Tsiouris AJ. Traumatic brain injury: imaging patterns and complications. Radiographics. 2019;39(6):1571–95. https://doi.org/10.1148/rg.2019190076.
9. Huisman TA, Tschirch FT. Epidural hematoma in children: do cranial sutures act as a barrier? J Neuroradiol. 2009;36(2):93–7. https://doi.org/10.1016/j.neurad.2008.06.003.
10. Yadav YR, Parihar V, Namdev H, Bajaj J. Chronic subdural hematoma. Asian. J Neurosurg. 2016;11(4):330–42. https://doi.org/10.4103/1793-5482.145102.
11. Hagen EM. How to prevent early mortality due to spinal cord injuries? New evidence & update. Indian J Med Res. 2014;140(1):5–7.
12. Denis F. Updated classification of thoracolumbar fractures. Orthop Trans. 1982;6(8):41–8.
13. Alizadeh A, Dyck SM, Karimi-Abdolrezaee S. Traumatic spinal cord injury: an overview of pathophysiology, models and acute injury mechanisms. Front Neurol. 2019;10:282. https://doi.org/10.3389/fneur.2019.00282.
14. White AA, Panjabi MM. Clinical biomechanics of the spine. 2nd ed. Philadelphia: Lippincott Williams & Wilkins; 1990.

Neuroimaging and Its Application in the Diagnosis and Early Prognostication of Traumatic Brain Injury (TBI)

4

Hardik Siroya and Anil Kumar Sharma

4.1 Evolution of Neuroimaging

Neuroimaging in traumatic brain injury dates to not more than half a century ago. Although attempts to appraise and gauge the contents of the skull have been in situ since 300 BC, when Aristotle attached brain with a secondary role of just being a medium of heat dissipation. He stressed heart to be the seat of all actions. However, progress to gander this mystique entity continued, albeit at a lackadaisical pace. Not until 1664 when Oxford physiologist Thomas Willis promulgated the first diagram of brain that it was considered a hollow space filled with humorous fluid. Guesstimating the skull contents was constrained due to a lack of imaging and autopsies. The archetypal anecdote of Phineas Gage's impalement injury to brain in 1848 provides some clues into this realm and cannot be underestimated. Theoretical Neuroimaging (Phrenology) proposed by Franz Joseph Gall by estimating the attributes or virtues based on contours of skull although termed ersatz by many, formed one of the earliest bases for functional organisation in brain. It was in 1880 that the world saw its first realistic attempt at neuroimaging by Italian physiologist Angelo Mosso of which few transcripts and drawings remain. It was an endeavour proposing that parts of the brain during functional load draw increased blood supply, which forms the bases of modern-day functional MRI (fMRI). Pursuit for better neuroimaging continued after the invention of X-rays by William Roentgen, a physicist in 1895 with Walter Dandy introducing Pneumoencephalography in 1918, Egas Moniz inventing cerebral angiography in 1920, Hans Berger devising EEG in 1924, Gordon Brownell and colleagues developing positron emission tomography (PET) in the 1950s. The groundbreaking discovery of computerised tomography (CT) conceived by William Oldendorf and applied by Hounsfield in 1973 opened new vistas into those parts of brain that remained unwitnessed till date. It was followed by the most

H. Siroya · A. K. Sharma (✉)
Neurosurgery, AIIMS, Raipur, Raipur, India

© The Author(s), under exclusive license to Springer Nature Singapore Pte Ltd. 2024
A. Agrawal et al. (eds.), *Special Considerations in Trauma Care*,
https://doi.org/10.1007/978-981-99-9662-9_4

promising discovery of current human imaging research by Paul Lauterbur in 1971. He developed magnetic resonance imaging (MRI), which would not only provide intricate anatomic details but also form the basis of molecular imaging in brain giving insights into functional, physiological and electrical roleplay. In the same year, clinical application of MRI in diagnosing brain cancer by Raymond Damadian would lay the foundation of diagnostic and prognostic neuroimaging.

4.2 Introduction

Traumatic brain injury is a complex anatomico-patho-physiologic occurrence after a violent external force produces a jolt on the skull/brain causing temporary or permanent anatomical or functional impairment. It can lead to primary injury (usually manifested within 1–2 h when the patient has still not reached emergency services) or secondary injury (as a temporal and distant result of primary injury usually in form or hypoxia, oedema, hyper-/hypocarbia, etc. occurring after few hours of trauma). The culmination could be a stage of irreversible damage if not intervened timely. Over 70 million cases are reported from all over the world every year. In America every 21 s, someone sustains TBI [1]. In 2020, US reported 223,135 TBI-related hospitalisations and 64,362 TBI-related deaths [2]. Among these, the American Indians formed the largest share of about 71.5 per 100,000 hospitalisations [2, 3]. People older than 75 years old were highest and formed 32% of TBI-related hospitalisations and 28% of deaths [2]. Children (<17 years) had 16,070 TBI-related hospitalisations and 2774 TBI-related deaths [2]. Males are two times more likely to be hospitalised and three times more likely to die from a TBI as compared to females [2]. India has the highest incidence of TBI in the world reporting 25 times more cases [4]. In total, 60% are contributed by RTA (Road traffic accidents) with fatality being 70 per 10,000 vehicles [4]. In US however, the major share is from suicides (35.5%) whereas RTA contributes just under 20% [2]. Moreover, for every 3 min, a person dies due to TBI and every 1.9 min due to trauma in India [4]. Additionally, contrary to United States and Europe, most of the people in India belong to 20–40 years age group which are the sole breadwinners of the family of which 78% are male [4]. Causes of TBI can be varied likewise: RTA, falls (paediatric age group), agricultural-related trauma, fire arms, intentional self-harm/suicides, assault, fall of objects, natural disasters, terrorist attacks. CDC divides these categories into unintentional motor vehicle traffic crashes (17%), unintentional falls (29.9%), unintentionally struck by or against an object, other unspecified unintentional injuries, suicides (35.5%), homicides and others. In order to adjudge the type and extent of TBI, multiple radiological investigations exist [2]. Each has its own advantages and are described herewith.

4.3 Screening Imaging

Glasgow Coma Scale (GCS) as a screening tool is undervalued in many studies with only 40–60% of patients having a complete score [5]. Thus, multiple other criteria along with GCS have been elucidated in various studies. Most of these criteria have common points. Moreover, it is proven without doubt that NCCT (plain CT) is the gold standard and investigation of choice for screening evaluation in all cases of trauma. Who requires CT? Multiple screening tools or criteria exist in the literature with varied sensitivity and specificity. Initial evaluation pertains to classifying the TBI into mild/concussion (MI), moderate (MOI) and severe injury (SI). Major debacle exists related to MI injuries. Criteria have been defined for their screening as well. However, none of these are flawless, and clinical acumen of the physician seems unavoidable in these circumstances. NICE [6], CCHR [7], Scotland SIGN [8], New Orleans NOC [9], CHALICE [10], MACE guidelines [11], NEXUS II [12], CATCH, CHIP [13], EFNS [14], NCWFNS [15], Scandinavian Strict Criteria [16], Scandinavian lenient Criteria [16], UCD [17], PECARN [18], and RCS [19] are some of the few recent approved criteria for assessing MI (GCS-13-15) especially with risk factors of age (>60 years).

Diagnostic Imaging Both CT and MRI form the cornerstones of diagnostic imaging. MRI is usually used for negative MI's with less than full GCS or with cognitive deficits. In cases of MOI and SI, it has more of a role of prognostic than diagnostic utility. Nonetheless, patients with grade I diffuse axonal injury (DAI) can be diagnosed with good accuracy on MRI. Diagnostic imaging usually occurs in the secondary phase of injury. The primary event principally dismantles elongated and lengthy structures like white matter tracts and blood vessels due to rotational shear strain causing either diffuse axonal injury or hematomas respectively. In the event of continued insult, secondary phase progresses to cellular mitochondrial failure, disruption of blood-brain barrier (BBB) and trigger of neuroinflammatory response leading to either apoptosis (reversible) or necrosis (irreversible). For all practical purposes, TBI is broadly classified depending on the mode of injury into open/penetrating and closed/non-penetrating injuries.

NCCT has a high sensitivity and specificity for demonstrating intracranial haemorrhage, extra-axial collections, oedema, swelling, midline shift, herniation, brain stem petechiae, diffuse axonal injuries (especially grade 2 to grade 4) fractures and hydrocephalus. As per the fourth edition of Brain Trauma Foundation (BTF) [20] guidelines, Table 4.1 represents evidence synthesis of prognosis in various brain findings as seen on CT. CT scans which are ubiquitous and abundant with round the clock availability make them invaluable tools for not only therapeutic decisions, intracranial pressure (ICP) but also predict prognosis. It forms a pertinent and indispensable tool for continuous inpatient and outpatient follow-up assessment for both preoperative/medically managed and postoperative patients. Prognosis in mild head has a different approach and will be discussed later. Let us draw our attention to

Table 4.1 Prognosis of findings based on CT scan as per fourth edition of brain trauma foundation guidelines

	CT finding	Type of head injury	Class of evidence	PPV	Outcome
1	Any abnormality	Severe (GCS ≤8)	I, II	77–78%	Unfavourable (severe, disabled)
2	No abnormality	Severe (GCS ≤8)	I, II	60–80%	Favourable (moderate disability/good recovery)
3	TCDB (Traumatic Coma Data Bank) [21] classification (grade I)	Severe (GCS ≤8)	II	75%	Favourable
4	AIS [22] (0–3)	Severe (GCS ≤8)	I	95%	Favourable
5	Compressed to absent basal cisterns	Severe (GCS ≤8)	I, II, III	73–97%	Unfavourable
6	tSAH (basal cisterns)	Severe (GCS ≤8)	I	72%	Unfavourable
7	Midline shift	Severe (GCS ≤8)			
	>5 mm, >45 years		I	78%	Unfavourable
	>1.5 cm		II	70%	Poor (dead/vegetative)
8	Intracranial lesions:	Severe (GCS ≤8)			
	High-density intra- and extracerebral lesions		I	67%	Unfavourable
	>15 mL, >45 years		I	79%	Poor (dead/vegetative)
	Evacuated		II	77%	Unfavourable
	Not evacuated		II	89%	Unfavourable

					Sensitivity	Specificity
AIS (0–3)	Severe (GCS < =8)	I	95%	Favourable	40%	98%
TCDB Classification I–IV		I, II	75%	Favourable	51%	86%
GCS score 6–8		I	59%	Favourable	57%	69%
Fisher grades III and IV		I	62–78%	Unfavourable		

various early radiological prognostic markers in the setting of moderate to severe TBI.

(a) ***Absence of abnormality on CT scan***: A CT brain with no findings is very common especially in patients with GCS >13 and MI. Overall negative scans are seen in 60–95% of the patients [21, 23–25]. Among these patients with GCS 15 show approximately 6–13% positivity, GCS 14 shows 25% positivity, and GCS 13 shows 38% positive scans [5, 26, 27]. For GCS ≤8, the rate of positivity is more than 85% with GCS 9–12 lying in between [27–30]. In fact as per EBIC survey, GCS ≤12 showed 87% positive scans [31]. Thus negative predictive value (absence of abnormality) in severe injuries is a much better predictor of prognosis (favourable outcome) as compared to the presence of an abnormality. Likewise, prognosis in mild head injuries correlates well with positive CT. As most MI have negative CT, other imaging modalities like MRI are indicated as discussed later. In the patients of severe head injury, an initial negative scan does not rule out the possibility of a new finding in second consecutive scan. It has been shown that a repeat CT may show positivity in 30–50% of severe head injuries, 20–30% of moderate and approximately 10% patients of mild head injuries [5, 25, 26, 32]. Outcomes at 6 months get affected significantly in case of SI with new findings and drop to almost to 2/3rd to ½ depending on the type of lesion—acute subdural hematoma (SDH) < diffuse axonal injury (DAI) < epidural hematoma (EDH)—with increased in-hospital mortality [33–35]. Moreover, 40–80% of patients with negative scans showed persistently raised ICP during hospital stay with 1/3rd requiring CSF diversion and ICP monitoring [36, 37]. Thus, consecutive scans are indicated every 12 h unless the ICP stabilises or at 24 h there is nil new finding on radiology whichever occurs later.

(b) ***Partial or complete obliteration of basal cisterns and third ventricle***: Presence or absence of basal cisterns is done at the level of midbrain whereas third ventricle is done just above the suprasellar cistern and below foramen of Monroe. Although validity, reliability, and reproducibility of basal cisterns are proven, validity and reliability of third ventricle remain questioned and of dubious value with conflicting results [38–41]. Nonetheless, interobserver variability for both remains highly acceptable and less than 5%. Liu et al. (Class III) in a retrospective study of 334 patients proposed a grading system for obliteration of basal cisterns with outcomes at 12 months with a good correlation [42]. Multiple Class I and II studies have divided this entity into three basic groups of open, partially obliterated/compressed (visualisation of hypodense slits in one of the hemispheres), complete obliteration and absence and have found a very good correlation with outcomes at 3 months. Although the third and lateral ventricle progressively get effaced → slit-like → obliterated usually does not add much to prognosis, they do predict increased mortality in presence of absent basal cisterns. In fact addition of above two can increase the mortality from 33% to 77% in cases of absent basal cisterns to almost 66–99% if above ventricles are progressively obliterated additionally [29, 38, 43–45]. Values of other cisterns like Sylvian cistern have also been described but with conflicting evidences and weak studies. *Correlation with other parameters*: (a) *GCS score*—mortality increases progressively as GCS falls in patients with compressed cisterns by almost 50% for every two-point fall [43, 45]. (b) *Pupillary reactivity*—it was seen that in case of open cisterns, pupillary reactivity was maintained in bilateral pupils in 30–80% of patients, in partial compression, unilateral or bilateral reactive pupils were maintained for 15–60% cases, whereas in cases of complete absence, pupillary reactivity was noticed in less than 30% of the cases [23, 40]. (c) *Hypotension/hypoxia*—a definite correlation exists between a single episode of hypoxia/hypotension in the prehospital period with compressed cisterns (diffuse brain swelling). A patient with no hypoxia had a 30% chance of brain swelling, about 45% with suspected hypoxia and it doubles to 60% with established blood gas parameters suggestive of hypoxia [21]. Similarly, there was almost 15% rise in brain swelling in patients with a single episode of hypotension in prehospital stage [21]. (d) *Focal lesion*—in a Class III retrospective study by Yanaka et al., it was seen that acute subdural hematoma was associated with most unfavourable to poor outcomes in presence absent cisterns [43, 46]. (e) *Raised ICP*—raised ICP was seen three times more in patients with complete obliteration whereas more than half of the patients demonstrated raised pressure [21, 36, 38, 40, 47].

(c) ***Traumatic Subarachnoid haemorrhage (tSAH)***: The incidence of tSAH is between 20% and 50% with SI reaching incidence of almost 50% [27, 39, 48–52]. Multiple grading systems exist to grade tSAH, of which two given by Fischer and modified for trauma by Greene have been used predominantly in TBI across literature [49]. Grades for Fisher remain the same as aneurysmal SAH, which were modified by Greene in 1995 into 4 grades in a retrospective study (Class III) of 252 patients. Whatever the classification, these grades could not be relied for PPV in view of significant interobserver variability (94%) [49] in computing the grade of SAH barring grade 4 and severe head injuries which had PPV of 70–80% [33, 49–51, 53]. Hence their use is limited. However, there is confirmatory evidence in multiple Class I studies regarding poor/unfavourable outcomes with 72% PPV in patients with SI for suprasellar/ambient/mesencephalic/basal cisternal SAH (least common) [53]. It was also highly associated with vasospasm and delayed ischaemic deficits (DCI). Although Sylvian fissure SAH is second most common, it is most commonly associated with breach in pia leading to localised contusions in 50–80% of patients [48, 51, 54]. The significance of convexity SAH (cSAH) which is most common is equivocal [48]. Nonetheless, SAH in any compartment signifies a diffuse injury with a poorer prognosis especially in severe TBI. It is seen in multiple Class I and II studies that mortality and poor outcomes increase twofold from 30% to 60% in patients with tSAH, especially basal cisternal SAH, and also a good predictor of raised ICP [21, 53]. There is a 60% correlation with focal lesions and 40–50% with acute SDH of tSAH with mortality in later reaching almost 90% in case of SI [21, 35, 48, 49, 53]. tSAH is considered only second to obliteration of basal cisterns and adds to other CT prognostic markers for accurately predicting poor outcomes in patients with severe head injury. However, their role in MOI and MI is less ascertained. In a Class III study by Gaetani et al. in 1995, it was reported that almost 25–35% of convexity tSAH had unfavourable outcomes, whereas basal showed 45–55% having unfavourable outcomes [48]. The mixed (basal + convexity) variant showed more than 85% with unfavourable outcomes [48]. Lang et al. (Class III) showed similar outcomes with intraventricular haemorrhage [39].

(d) ***Midline shift***: It is measured at the level of septum pellucidum and its displacement in relation to midline. Although it can also be measured by shift of aqueduct or pineal gland [43, 44, 55]. Many authors have given varied measurements of midline shifts for predicting prognosis ranging from any form of shift to a shift of more than 6 mm to call it of any prognostic value. However, only one Class I study and two Class II studies exist for predicting prognosis for midline shifts. All three studies predict prognosis in patients with SI. Eisenberg et al. in 1990 (Class II) reported a shift of 1.5 mm (PPV-70%) to 3 mm (PPV-78%) as being statically significant in SI to predict prognosis leading to an increase in mortality by almost 70%, whereas it was 76% in a study by Kotwica and Brzezinski [21, 50, 53, 56]. Whereas Vollmer et al. in their study of 661 patients reported a shift of 5 mm in more than 45 years age group to have a PPV of 75–80% in predicting poor outcomes [57]. In younger patients, however, they found that reliability of only measuring midline shift for prognosis to be conflicting. Nonetheless, in presence of other factors like effaced mesencephalic cisterns, basal cisternal SAH and poor GCS it showed more reliability and increased poor outcomes to twofold [57]. This difference may be partly due to the more space in elderly brain with more chances of midline shift, whereas younger patients manifest with diffuse oedema or diffuse injury or bilateral lesions causing injury to erroneously evade shift of midline. Thus, midline shift correlates better with type of pathology like diffuse injury or intracerebral lesions and severity of injury. For example, midline shift in acute subdural hematoma even if it's less having a poorer prognosis than extradural hematoma with much greater blood volume and midline shift. This is a result of diffuse axonal injury or diffuse cerebral oedema and mode of injury which usually is usually more dangerous in acute subdural [43]. The greatest significance of midline shift is seen in GCS <5 and ≥ 8 with maximum PPV in predicting poor and favourable outcomes respectively [55, 58]. Recently the importance and value of midline shift and its correlation with outcomes has been questioned, and a novel concept of mid-surface shift (MSS) has been proposed which appears more apt in view of variations in head position during CT, single slice measurements affecting the measurement of true shift. It was seen that MSS correlated better in predicting prognosis as compared to MLS [59]. *Correlation with other parameters*: (a) *GCS score*—Conflicting results exist for association between GCS score and midline shift. No Class I study could establish a good association. Although midline shift >5 mm in presence of GCS ≤ 5 had the highest predicted value for poor outcomes across studies varying between 70% and 80% only in first 24 h, beyond which this PPV is not reliable [55, 60]. (b) *Pupillary reactivity*—The association between pupillary reactivity and midline shift is dubious. In fact no correlation was established between the two in a Class II study for moderate and severe SI [21]. Only effacement of basal cisterns was associated with a clear strong association with pupillary reactivity [21, 60]. Nonetheless, most studies testing their role together in prognosis have met with conflicting results enforcing the need to consider other additive parameters. (c) *Focal lesions*—Focal lesions are associated to cause raised ICP in cases of SI in almost 80% of the patients. Focal lesions affect prognosis in the following order [43, 61, 62]: Acute subdural hematoma > contusion/intracerebral haemorrhage > extradural hematoma in the presence of midline shift of >1.5 mm in GCS <8 especially when the shift is more than the thickness of hematoma and an urgent evacuation with decompression is warranted [63]. Shift out of proportion to thickness with poor GCS was predicted of poor outcomes in 70% of the patient (PPV-70% for mortality) [21, 25, 57, 58, 61]. Only one study (Class III) did not report any difference in outcomes in acute subdural vs. epidural vs. contusion in patients with GCS ≤8 [62]. (e) *Raised ICP*—Eisenberg et al. and Lobato et al. showed a significant correlation between raised ICP and midline shift of more than 3–5 mm in poor GCS patients (SI) [21, 37].

(e) ***Intracranial lesions***: Intracranial lesions are grouped into extradural, subdural, intracerebral, intraventricular, or small bleeds in subcortical white matter/brainstem (DAI). All the above are known to affect prognosis in varying extent. Overall the prognosis in MOI to SI is affected for these types in the following order of most poor to favourable likewise; acute subdural > contusions > diffuse axonal injury > extradural hematoma [56, 61, 64, 65]. They are usually additive in already disposed brain with oedema, tSAH, basal cisternal effacement, and midline shift with MOI and SI. Any lesions that can be decompressed or evacuated affect the prognosis significantly. Volume/mass/thickness of the lesion not only influences therapeutic decisions but also correlates well with other prognostic parameters. *Extradural*: Extradural hematomas had the best prognosis of all when found in a pure state for comparable GCS across other lesions with least mortality (10–20% in SI and MOI) [66–69]. However, localisation of epidural hematoma in brain is not associated with prognostic significance [33, 66, 67]. Overall the mortality associated with other single lesion (indicative of diffuse injury) increases twofold from approximately 30–55% in severe head injuries [65–69]. The most significant association is with age for which elderly patients seem more prone for diffuse injuries with poorer outcomes as compared to young. Moreover, the incidence of epidural hematoma rises fourfold from young to elderly population [67]. Volume of epidural hematoma requiring intervention is usually kept at a cut-off of 30 cc for MI. For MOI and SI, even 15 cc (Class I) is considered a threshold and associated with poor outcomes if not evacuated [70]. In MI the usual amount causing poor outcomes is hyperdense lesion with clot volume of more than 150 cc (50–60% poor outcomes) if not evacuated timely [66, 68–70]. *Acute subdural*: Pure acute subdural without associated injuries is very rarely seen. They are witnessed most commonly in elderly patients with atrophic brain and trivial falls with already predisposing comorbidities. Thus multiple studies have found no association between acute subdural hematoma and other lesions in brain to additively affect prognosis. This is commensurate with the fact that patients with acute subdural hematomas already have diffuse injury and other prognostic parameters (tSAH, effaced basal cisterns, etc.) which cause unfavourable outcomes [34, 46, 56, 63, 65]. However, other studies report a threefold to fourfold increase in mortality if an additional intracerebral lesion coexists with acute subdural [56, 65]. Nonetheless, a Class I study by Narayan et al. could find a less impressive PPV of 64% for intracerebral lesions affecting outcomes [70]. Volume of acute subdural in SI causing unfavourable outcomes is as low as 15 cc if not evacuated whereas in MI, the cut-off is usually 100 cc beyond which prognosis deteriorates if not evacuated in absence of midline shift or shift <3 mm [46, 57, 63]. Thickness of acute subdural lesser than the midline shift has a PPV of 70–80% for unfavourable outcomes, whereas mortality increases for more than 1 cm thickness in SI and MOI and is between 30% and 50% which doubles for more than 2 cm [63, 65, 67]. Additionally H (thickness)/MS (midline shift) ratio has recently been shown to be a better predictor of GCS at admission and thus prognosis as compared to measuring singly [71, 72]. Any ratio score less than 1 portends poorer GCS at admission and poor outcomes, whereas score of more than 1 portends better outcomes. *Contusions/intracerebral haemorrhage*: Pure haemorrhagic high-density contusions usually have a good prognosis, although multiple lesions decrease the outcomes progressively. With each lesion prognosis drops 1/3rd starting from 60% favourable outcomes for single lesion, 20% for two, and so on [21, 29, 61, 70, 73, 74]. Moreover development of every new lesion in consecutive scans is associated with drop in outcomes by almost 20% for each. Approximately 10–35% of patients develop new lesions within a span of 12 h from the trauma whereas 25–45% increase in size in first 6–9 h after trauma [29, 75–80]. Furthermore, addition of intraventricular haemorrhage decreases the outcomes further [81, 82]. On the other hand, lower-density lesions tend to have a better prognosis [29]. Such patients usually present with GCS >8 and further prognosis depends on associated factors like tSAH, status of mesencephalic cisterns, midline shift, etc. Overall prognosis depends on timely intervention with evacuation. Class I and Class II evidence suggest that any lesion more than 15 mL in age >45 years with GCS <12 needs intervention for favourable outcomes and in case of non-evacuation had PPV of 75–85% for poor outcomes [28, 70, 83]. In case of GCS ≤8, the PPV increases to almost 90% (Class II) in case of non-evacuation [28, 83]. *Diffuse axonal injury*: IMPACT study showed that diffuse injuries of grade III/IV as per Marshall criteria had the poorest outcomes for comparable GCS with acute SDH [84]. It was placed second after acute SDH in BTF-4 (brain trauma foundation) prognostic review [20]. This discrepancy may be due to the fact that most studies in BTF had acute SDH with diffuse injuries or rather it is very difficult to separate pure acute SDH from diffuse injuries which was carried out in IMPACT study. *Intraventricular haemorrhage (tIVH)*: It can occur either due to rupture of subependymal vein/venule or retrograde backflow of blood from subarachnoid space or rupture of Liliequist's membrane causing retribution of subarachnoid blood in a gravity-dependent manner. In a multicentre study published in 2006, prevalence of traumatic IVH was less than 2% with majority associated with other injuries and 70% having poor outcomes while 76% had combined outcomes [81]. Poor outcomes were usually associated with SI and MOI and involvement of third or fourth ventricle but not related to age. Isolated tIVH without other injuries had good outcomes in more than 95% of cases. However multiple recent studies have shown this prevalence to be much higher to about

5–25% [84–86]. This difference may be due to the time period when first CT was performed. In a study by Laleva et al. delayed tIVH was seen in almost 12% of the cases within first 48 h [85]. Most of these patients were elderly above 60 years of age and associated with SI or MOI and poor outcomes (p <0.001) (30–50%). About 40–50% in this age group showed intracerebral lesion which increased in size whereas 100% patients with new lesions had tIVH over time. In fact higher IVH scores correlated very well with DAI stages II (p = 0.0025) and III (p <0.0003) [85, 87]. In-house mortality ranges from 10% to 20% depending on other additive parameters and GCS. The Traumatic Graeb Score can also be used for predicting functional outcomes associated with tIVH, comprising the sum of GCS scores, age ≥65 years and Graeb score [88, 89]. A Traumatic Graeb Score ≥4 is the cut-off for poor outcomes.

(f) ***CT classification systems***: Multiple classification systems exist. Amongst these, the Marshall/modified Marshall and Rotterdam criteria have been used for prognostication. Marshal score was introduced in 1991 Traumatic Coma Data Bank (TCDB) study [21]. This study published a classification given by Marshall et al. for predicting the prognosis in TBI. It proved to be a valuable tool in predicting outcomes. It had a PPV-75% with overall 51% sensitivity and 86% specificity for grades I–IV. An Abbreviated Injury Scale (AIS) was introduced by American Association for Automotive Medicine in 1990 and used by Walder et al. in 1995 to compare it with Marshall score [22]. It was noted that good outcomes associated with AIS scores ≤3 had positive predictive value 95%, specificity 98%, and sensitivity 40%. However for higher AIS scores the PPV progressively decreased with prediction of poor outcomes by an AIS of 4 or 5 had 100% sensitivity, 35% specificity and PPV of 58%. Maas et al. introduced Rotterdam score in 2006 in a study comparing it with Marshall score [84]. They found the usual AUC = 0.67 significantly improved on rearranging the variables (AUC = 0.71) which further improved to AUC = 0.77 when categories of tSAH and intraventricular haemorrhage were added along with detailed differentiation of mass lesions and basal cisterns. Mahadewa et al. in 2018 gave a modification of Marshall score (MCTC—Marshall CT classification) for predicting outcomes in MOI and SI combining Revised trauma score (RTS), a physiologic score with Marshall score, an anatomico-pathological score [90]. The RTS–Marshall combination had higher sensitivity with risk ratio of 4.5 (CI 95% = 2.55–8.0; P = 0.001) for predicting of unfavourable outcomes. All patients had GCS ≤12. Mortality was about 37% and favourable outcomes were seen in 61%. A formula was generated to form one score for predicting outcomes in SI and MOI = (0.56 × RTS) + (0.6 × MCTC) − 4.1. In a study by Katsnelson et al., they compared various physiological, clinical, and radiological score for predicting outcomes [91]. Only APACHE II (Acute Physiology and Chronic Health Evaluation II) (P = 0.003), APACHE-non-GCS (P = 0.004), Marshall (P <0.001), and Rotterdam scores (P <0.001) were associated with mortality whereas GCS on arrival was not associated with mortality. No relationship between GCS, ISS (Injury severity score), Marshall, or Rotterdam scores and subsequent ICP or PbtO2 (brain tissue oxygen tension) was observed. Only APACHE II score had a stronger correlation with inverse relation to amount of time of reduced PbtO2. In an annual meeting of The Radiological Society of North America in Chicago it was reported that Marshall score was a slightly better predictor of outcomes and early deaths among patients with MI, MOI and SI (p <0.0001) in a study of 245 patients presented by Mbemba et al., although both scores were shown comparable (AUC = 0.85) for both early and long-term outcomes [86]. Mohammaddifard et al. reported that the Rotterdam criteria was more accurate for predicting mortality at 2 weeks, 1 month and 3 months than Marshall CT score [92]. However, Asim et al. conclude that Marshall (74.3% sensitivity and 76.3% specificity for cut-off of 2.5) and Rotterdam (sensitivity, 61.2%; specificity, 85.6% for cut-off of 3.5) scoring systems were independent predictors of mortality [93]. Deepika et al. report that both these scores have a good correlation (r = 0.68) for GSC ≤12 [94]. In essence, both scores are comparable and have a good correlation in predicting early and long-term outcomes.

Mild Head Injury It's a different spectrum altogether and forms more than 70% of the cases of head injury [9, 95]. Much of the CT classifications and CT characteristics are not adept to prognosticate MI with accuracy. This is because 60% and 90% of patients with head injury do not have any detectable abnormality on CT brain scans [13]. In the remnant, CT proves valuable as a gold standard for neurosurgical clinical decision-making. For non-neurosurgical negative CT scans, MRI although has potential to prognosticate, is still in early stages. Nonetheless 10–20% of patients with concussions suffer from long-term cognitive deficits (miserable minority) [96]. Newer advances in MRI sequences have brought in new spectra of findings that are able to predict and prognosticate such patients with certain accuracy. However, these dispositions are still in their infancy and further research in this regard is pertinent.

Need for CT Brain Plain As already stated, multiple criteria exist. However Canadian CT head rule (CCHR) [7] and New Orleans Criteria (NOC) [9] have the highest sensitivity and acceptable specificity in adults. For high risk criteria, CCHR has sensitivity of 99–100% and specificity of 37–48% [97, 98], whereas NOC matches with similar sensitivity and poor specificity (3–33%) [9, 97, 99, 100]. In medium risk criteria, it is 80–100% sensitivity for CCHR with slightly better specificity (40–50%) [99, 100]. Mata-Mbemba et al., however, found CCHR to be a better predictor of positive CT findings in mild head injuries [86]. In a multicentre validation study by Smits et al., only EFNS (European Federation of Neurological Sciences) guidelines proved to be most reliable with 100% sensitivity, although with extremely poor specificity (0–0.5%) [13]. In children however, no rule is better than other. The sensitivities and specificities are described in tables herewith. Nonetheless, CHALICE and NEXUS II rules have the highest reliability for intracranial injury in children.

Consensus does exist on the signs and symptoms associated with positive CT findings. These include abnormal GCS (relative risk [RR] −5.58), old age (3.70), post-traumatic seizure (PTS) (3.24), severe headache (RR-2.44), nausea (2.16), vomiting (2.13), loss of consciousness (LOC) (2.29), focal neurological deficits (1.80), pedestrian crash victim (1.70), alcohol intake (1.62), fall from a height (1.61), amnesia (1.32), and male gender (1.26). In children, focal neurological deficit (9.43), abnormal GCS (5.51), and LOC (2.23) were associated with positive CT findings [101]. In spite of the above, more than 70% of patients are associated with negative CT findings. We review the roles of various MRI sequences and their role in prognosis in patients with all grades of head injury.

MRI versus CT Conventional MRI and CT suffer from significantly low sensitivity (MI) and low specificity (SI) [102]. However in cases of negative CT, a T2 fast spin echo sequence termed as Quick brain MRI taking 1–3 min is very valuable [103].

Conventional MRI: Detecting focal lesion is easy on T1 and T2 weighed imaging. The burden and location of DAI lesions is an acceptable prognostication tool. However, prognosticating is difficult as it depends on changes in transitional area of grey/white matter junction which blurs depending on stage of blood between the usual contrast imaging provided by T1 and T2 [104]. This takes into account only the contrast differences in T1 and T2 in a specific voxel. Thus, prognostication is impractical and non-sensical as a complete 3D representation of brain with volumetric and morphometric analyses gives a more accurate picture. Combination of T_2, fluid-attenuated inversion recovery (FLAIR), and susceptibility-weighted imaging (SWI)could provide a more accurate assessment of white matter injury and hence help prognosticate [104]. Moenninghoff et al. demonstrated that UHF (ultra-high-field) SWI MRI detects an average of 41% more microbleeds than does 3 T SWI; also these appear larger on UHF SWI MRI [105].

Newer Domains of MRI They include structural, functional, connectomical and molecular imaging. Classical 1.5 and 3 T MRIs usually were implied to detect focal lesions with increasing sensitivity. Their usefulness in quantitatively measuring volumetric and morphometric data for predicting future functional outcomes although promising in still in its infancy. However, their role in prognostication and poor sensitivity demands newer vistas in MRI armamentarium. This led to exploration of connectomical pathways on MRI along with their structural, anatomical, biochemical, volumetric and morphometric analysis for prognostication. CT/MRI alone suffers from acceptable sensitivity and specificity. Thus, spectrum of multimodality imaging like FLAIR, SWI, diffusion imaging techniques (HARDI, DTI, DSI) and functional imaging (fMRI) has provided new caveats into less explored realm of prognostic imaging in mild TBI.

Structural Imaging It involves volumetric and morphometric calculation of 3D model of brain in time and space [106–110]. Efforts to predict prognosis are extremely poor and variable in multiple studies due to laborious manual segmentation and inter-observer differences thus causing attrition and inadequate sample size. Computational algorithms [111–113] are unsuccessful in this regard due to distorted brain in view of trauma and inefficient standard trauma models for comparison. Additional MR sequences like FLAIR, gradient-recalled echo (GRE) T2-weighted imaging, and SWI can increase the predictive power of MRI to distinguish different lesions likewise; FLAIR (nullifies CSF signal)—oedema, GRE and SWI—haemorrhages which appear hypointense. A combination of T_1, T_2, FLAIR and SWI imaging allows proper segmentation and 3D model construction for brain, oedema and haemorrhage [104]. Nonetheless, volumetrics (cortical thickness, GM and WM volume, etc.) [114] and morphometrics (curvature, folding index) in TBI have suffered from major topological defects, failure to fit cortical surfaces and subcortical segmentation errors [115–118]. The major segmentation error includes differentiating between grey/white matter junction when both sides are injured leading to underestimation in short-term/acute and overestimation in long term for volume measurements. Additionally, morphometric calculation of local curvature and the folding index of the cortical surface are also erred. Niethammer et al. have introduced geometric metamorphosis method to counteract this geometric deformation for accurate estimation of volumetric data [119].

4.4 Connectomical Imaging

DTI DTI is used to construct tractography for qualitatively and quantitively assessing connectivity algorithms like fibre track length and fibreconnection density. They are highly sensitive in diagnosing injury to white matter tracts and structures. Coup/contrecoup, acceleration/deceleration injuries are better detected on DTI than structural imaging due to effects on distant structures from the site of primary pathology affected by diffusion/fractional anisotropy (FA) and mean diffusivity (MD) of axoplamic flow across axoplasmic membrane [120–122]. They quantify uni- and multivoxel-based restriction of water molecules helping differentiate between vasogenic (diffuses) and cytotoxic oedema (restricted) oedema and thus extent of axonal injury [123–125]. Severity and timing of DTI imaging play a significant role in predicting prognosis. In MI, cytotoxic-induced oedema causing restricted diffusion usually normalises over time [126]. Additionally, grossly affected FA correlates significantly with worse 3- and 6-month GOS-E [127]. In moderate-to-severe TBI, DTI time-dependent changes increase up to 18 months postinjury and correlate with functional outcomes [128]. However, such time-dependent changes were not noted in a metanalyses conducted by Wallace et al. [129–131]. Moreover in moderate to severe TBI, an increase in FA on the initial postinjury DTI is associated with a favourable outcomes assumed to be secondary to axonal regrowth [132]. Also, another recent meta-analysis reported a high FA that correlated well with better cognitive outcomes [131]. Diffusion spectrum imaging (DSI) allows to map complex fiber diagrams by analysing 3D spectra of tissues [133]. Above imaging is capable of identifying DAI which cannot be diagnosed on T_2 Spin Echo, T_2* GRE or FLAIR sequences. Additionally, a patient-oriented personalised connectogram (circle of radially aligned elements) by linking the each fibre tract extremity can be obtained at two-time points (acute and chronic stages respectively) from which change in density of fibres in white matter can be calculated [134–136]. This can estimate the amount of atrophy in particular brain region signifying the effect of TBI on clinical status and help improve and tailor patient rehabilitation protocols [137–139]. However, the quantitative tools of this brain network disruption are still in their early stages and require honing. There is a shift towards time-dependent network theoretic models to overcome shortcomings from an objective eye visualisation and prediction of probable network involvement which although affirmative is not reproducible due to lack of quantitative tools [134, 139–141]. This circumvents the problem of comparison with scans of other diseases and provides a personalised data for comparison over a period of time. Major recovery mechanisms include resilience to injury, cortical re-organisation, hierarchical reorganisation, large or small-scale rewiring or permanent loss of function [140–143]. It is valuable to note that certain areas of brain are particularly sensitive to acceleration/deceleration and coup/contrecoup injuries in face of negative CT and MRI scans. These areas have been studied to be particularly helpful in predicting long-term prognosis for certain functions of the brain. The network topography of these fibres is either in vertical direction or passing through bottleneck connectomes. These include interhemispheric white matter [144], cingulate cortex [145, 146], splenium [147], brainstem fibres, supra-callosal [148] and callosal fibres [145, 149, 150], anterior corona radiata [121, 150], supratentorial projection fiber bundles [121], fronto-temporo-occipital association bundles [121], uncinate fasciculus [150], genu of the CC [121, 150], inferior longitudinal fasciculus [121, 150], and cingulum bundle [145, 150] etc. Multiple studies have shown that patients with mild TBI having diffusion restriction objectively show cognitive deficits/decline in the form of executive dysfunction, slower processing speed, defective working memory, behavioural dysfunctioning, motor speed, decline in academic skills, etc., due to affection of these fibres in both adults and children [120, 145, 148–150]. However, Bendlin et al. report improvement in few of these functions at first year follow-up on neuropsychological testing [145]. Thus, DTI can prove to be very useful tool to predict recovery in patients with recovering/restoring white matter organisation and form a bridge between structural and functional imaging for predicting outcomes.

Functional Imaging Future trends in TBI support the use of multimodality approaches involving structural as well as functional imaging in order to increase prediction, validation and specificity of prognostic imaging. Not only fMRI gives a real-time picture of affected functional areas in brain and its correlation to structural damage but also help document the takeover of function by surrounding undamaged areas by developing newer network fibres or redistribution of functions in already existing fibres. Disorders of consciousness (DOC) can be diagnosed and their prognosis predicted by evaluating fMRI data on default mode network correction post-injury as seen by Threlkeld et al. Patients with severe head injury and suffering from DOC are known to have covert consciousness which is being studied in a prospective trial [151–153]. It takes the help of blood oxygen-level dependent (BOLD) signals coming from brain signifying the amount of oxygen extracted by a working tissue while resting or in reponse to stress. Although its use in acute stages is questionable in view of non-cooperative patients and presence of blood affecting signalling, its utility for long-term prognostication and rehabilitation is quite promising. Many authors have reported improved task performance, redistribution to frontal lobes, right hemisphere, precuneus, posterior cingulate cortex, lateral prefrontal cortex, hyper or hypoactivation of functions, having residual cognition in vegetative states, for individuals with severe TBI in acute stages signifying activation of default mode networks and even in long-term follow-up of neuropsychological testing years post-injury [154–160].

CT and MRI Perfusion Multiple modalities can assess cerebral perfusion likewise: perfusion CT (CTP), dynamic susceptibility-weighted contrast-enhanced perfusion MRI (DSC-MRI), and MRI arterial spin labelling (ASL). Perfusion imaging involves the mean transit time of blood flow through a defined volume of tissues based on the relationship between a defined tissue volume, the mean transit time through that tissue, and flow of blood through that tissue. While ASL (labels endogenous H_2O) is devoid of contrast injection; the other modalities require non-diffusible intravenous contrast. These modalities help detect the amount of cerebral ischaemia which is a major cause of poor outcomes especially in acute settings. Thus it can identify areas of brain at impending risk of hypoperfusion and ischaemic damage. Soustiel et al. demonstrated diagnosis of certain contusions within 48 h of injury on CTP which otherwise revealed after 7 days on normal CT plain [161]. Many studies have highlighted the role of CTP in moderate and severe injury, wherein hyperperfusion in acute stages is associated with good long-term outcomes [129, 162–164]. Not only it helps predict prognosis, but it can also help as a therapeutic option by reducing perfusion pressure of the brain in case of raised ICP secondary to increased perfusion pressure or increase perfusion in certain areas of hypoxia with help of measuring local O_2 saturation. Metting et al. could predict 6 month functional outcomes in cases of MI with negative CT by observing correlation between post-traumatic amnesia and frontal lobe perfusion defects [165]. MRI perfusion plays a role where CTP cannot be performed due to varied contraindication or contradiction to contrast agents (in which case ASL is done).

MR Spectroscopy Magnetic resonance spectroscopy (MRS) can help in prognosis by detecting early reduction in *N*-acetyl aspartate (NAA) levels, reduced NAA/choline ratios, reduced NAA/creatine ratios signifying acute brain injury and also help predict long-term cognitive outcomes from subcortical white matter regions in the brain [166–168]. Gardener et al. in their meta-analysis of MI reported persistent and progressive metabolic derangements in MR spectra even after concussion symptoms abated [167]. In future, MRS could prove to be a valuable tool for classification and severity-based prognostication especially in MI and MOI.

MR Elastography Magnetic resonance elastography (MRE) measures tissue displacement in response to a propagated MRI acoustic pulse sequence [169]. This displacement gives information about the inherent viscoelasticity of part of brain [170]. Post-traumatic brain has changed viscoelasticity as demonstrated in rat models [171, 172]. Although this technique hold promise, the developments are only in pre-clinical stages and much work is expected in coming time which would help us in better prognostication of brain injuries.

Convolutional Neural Networks Convolutional neural networks (CNNs) are machine learning methods, based on biological neural systems, which divide and break complex brain images into simple continuous hierarchical structures helping pattern recognition. It role in prognostication was explained by Chartrand et al. where CNNs have been explored for medical image analysis [173]. Liu et al. reported the utility of CNNs for diagnosing cerebral microbleeds, with comparable accuracy to that of an experienced radiologist [174]. Albeit premature, this technology holds great promise to decode complex brain networks in patients with TBI for predicting short and long-term outcomes and to tailor personalised approaches for specific connectomes.

References

1. Brain Injury Facts & Statistics | Brain Injury Alliance of Connecticut. http://www.biact.org/understanding-brain-injury/brain-injury-facts-statistics. Accessed 14 Jul 2022.
2. TBI Data | Concussion | Traumatic Brain Injury | CDC Injury Center. 2022. https://www.cdc.gov/traumaticbraininjury/data/index.html. Accessed 16 May 2022.
3. Rutland-Brown W, Wallace LJD, Faul MD, Langlois JA. Traumatic brain injury hospitalizations among American Indians/Alaska Natives. J Head Trauma Rehabil. 2005;20(3):205–14.
4. Traumatic Brain Injury | Indian Head Injury Foundation. https://indianheadinjuryfoundation.org/traumatic-brain-injury/. Accessed 14 Jul 2022.
5. Currie S, Saleem N, Straiton JA, Macmullen-Price J, Warren DJ, Craven IJ. Imaging assessment of traumatic brain injury. Postgrad Med J. 2016;92(1083):41–50.
6. Overview | Head injury: assessment and early management | Guidance | NICE. https://www.nice.org.uk/guidance/cg176. Accessed 21 Jul 2022.
7. Stiell IG, Wells GA, Vandemheen K, et al. The Canadian CT Head Rule for patients with minor head injury. Lancet. 2001;357(9266):1391–6.
8. Early management of patients with a head injury: a national clinical guideline—digital collections—National Library of Medicine. https://collections.nlm.nih.gov/catalog/nlm:nlmuid-101124501-pdf. Accessed 21 Jul 2022.
9. Haydel MJ, Preston CA, Mills TJ, Luber S, Blaudeau E, DeBlieux PM. Indications for computed tomography in patients with minor head injury. N Engl J Med. 2000;343(2):100–5.

10. Dunning J, Daly JP, Lomas J-P, Lecky F, Batchelor J, Mackway-Jones K, Children's head injury algorithm for the prediction of important clinical events study group. Derivation of the children's head injury algorithm for the prediction of important clinical events decision rule for head injury in children. Arch Dis Child. 2006;91(11):885–91.
11. Stone MEJ, Safadjou S, Farber B, Velazco N, Man J, Reddy SH, Todor R, Teperman S. Utility of the Military Acute Concussion Evaluation as a screening tool for mild traumatic brain injury in a civilian trauma population. J Trauma Acute Care Surg. 2015;79(1):147–51.
12. Mower WR, Hoffman JR, Herbert M, Wolfson AB, Pollack CV, Zucker MI, NEXUS II Investigators. Developing a decision instrument to guide computed tomographic imaging of blunt head injury patients. J Trauma. 2005;59(4):954–9.
13. Smits M, Hunink MGM, Nederkoorn PJ, et al. A history of loss of consciousness or post-traumatic amnesia in minor head injury: "conditio sine qua non" or one of the risk factors? J Neurol Neurosurg Psychiatry. 2007;78(12):1359–64.
14. Vos PE, Battistin L, Birbamer G, et al. EFNS guideline on mild traumatic brain injury: report of an EFNS task force. Eur J Neurol. 2002;9(3):207–19.
15. Servadei F, Teasdale G, Merry G, Neurotraumatology Committee of the World Federation of Neurosurgical Societies. Defining acute mild head injury in adults: a proposal based on prognostic factors, diagnosis, and management. J Neurotrauma. 2001;18(7):657–64.
16. Ingebrigtsen T, Romner B, Kock-Jensen C. Scandinavian guidelines for initial management of minimal, mild, and moderate head injuries. The Scandinavian Neurotrauma Committee. J Trauma. 2000;48(4):760–6.
17. Palchak MJ, Holmes JF, Vance CW, Gelber RE, Schauer BA, Harrison MJ, Willis-Shore J, Wootton-Gorges SL, Derlet RW, Kuppermann N. A decision rule for identifying children at low risk for brain injuries after blunt head trauma. Ann Emerg Med. 2003;42(4):492–506.
18. Kuppermann N, Holmes JF, Dayan PS, et al. Identification of children at very low risk of clinically-important brain injuries after head trauma: a prospective cohort study. Lancet. 2009;374(9696):1160–70.
19. sitecore \lduncan@rcseng.ac.uk. The Royal College of Surgeons of England. In: Royal College of Surgeons. https://www.rcseng.ac.uk/. Accessed 21 Jul 2022.
20. Brain Trauma Foundation. https://www.braintrauma.org/coma/guidelines. Accessed 21 Jul 2022.
21. Eisenberg HM, Gary HE, Aldrich EF, Saydjari C, Turner B, Foulkes MA, Jane JA, Marmarou A, Marshall LF, Young HF. Initial CT findings in 753 patients with severe head injury. A report from the NIH Traumatic Coma Data Bank. J Neurosurg. 1990;73(5):688–98.
22. Walder AD, Yeoman PM, Turnbull A. The abbreviated injury scale as a predictor of outcome of severe head injury. Intensive Care Med. 1995;21(7):606–9.
23. van Dongen KJ, Braakman R, Gelpke GJ. The prognostic value of computerized tomography in comatose head-injured patients. J Neurosurg. 1983;59(6):951–7.
24. Lee H, Wintermark M, Gean AD, Ghajar J, Manley GT, Mukherjee P. Focal lesions in acute mild traumatic brain injury and neurocognitive outcome: CT versus 3T MRI. J Neurotrauma. 2008;25(9):1049–56.
25. Lobato RD, Rivas JJ, Gomez PA, Castañeda M, Cañizal JM, Sarabia R, Cabrera A, Muñoz MJ. Head-injured patients who talk and deteriorate into coma. Analysis of 211 cases studied with computerized tomography. J Neurosurg. 1991;75(2):256–61.
26. Clement MO. Imaging of brain trauma. Radiol Clin North Am. 2019;57(4):733–44.
27. Rincon S, Gupta R, Ptak T. Imaging of head trauma. Handb Clin Neurol. 2016;135:447–77.
28. Marshall L, Gautille T, Klauber M, Eisenberg H, Jane J, Luerssen T, Marmarou A, Foulkes M. The outcome of severe closed head injury. J Neurosurg. 1991;75:S28–36. https://doi.org/10.3171/SUP.1991.75.1S.0S28.
29. Sweet RC, Miller JD, Lipper M, Kishore PR, Becker DP. Significance of bilateral abnormalities on the CT scan in patients with severe head injury. Neurosurgery. 1978;3(1):16–21.
30. A multicenter trial of the efficacy of nimodipine on outcome after severe head injury. The European Study Group on Nimodipine in Severe Head Injury. J Neurosurg. 1994;80(5):797–804.

31. Murray GD, Teasdale GM, Braakman R, et al. The European Brain Injury Consortium survey of head injuries. Acta Neurochir. 1999;141(3):223–36.
32. Lobato RD, Cordobes F, Rivas JJ, de la Fuente M, Montero A, Barcena A, Perez C, Cabrera A, Lamas E. Outcome from severe head injury related to the type of intracranial lesion. A computerized tomography study. J Neurosurg. 1983;59(5):762–74.
33. Domenicucci M, Strzelecki JW, Delfini R. Acute posttraumatic subdural hematomas: "intradural" computed tomographic appearance as a favorable prognostic factor. Neurosurgery. 1998;42(1):51–5.
34. Haselsberger K, Pucher R, Auer LM. Prognosis after acute subdural or epidural haemorrhage. Acta Neurochir. 1988;90(3–4):111–6.
35. Hatashita S, Koga N, Hosaka Y, Takagi S. Acute subdural hematoma: severity of injury, surgical intervention, and mortality. Neurol Med Chir (Tokyo). 1993;33(1):13–8.
36. Holliday PO, Kelly DL, Ball M. Normal computed tomograms in acute head injury: correlation of intracranial pressure, ventricular size, and outcome. Neurosurgery. 1982;10(1):25–8.
37. Lobato RD, Sarabia R, Cordobes F, Rivas JJ, Adrados A, Cabrera A, Gomez P, Madera A, Lamas E. Posttraumatic cerebral hemispheric swelling. Analysis of 55 cases studied with computerized tomography. J Neurosurg. 1988;68(3):417–23.
38. Colquhoun IR, Burrows EH. The prognostic significance of the third ventricle and basal cisterns in severe closed head injury. Clin Radiol. 1989;40(1):13–6.
39. Lang DA, Teasdale GM, Macpherson P, Lawrence A. Diffuse brain swelling after head injury: more often malignant in adults than children? J Neurosurg. 1994;80(4):675–80.
40. Teasdale E, Cardoso E, Galbraith S, Teasdale G. CT scan in severe diffuse head injury: physiological and clinical correlations. J Neurol Neurosurg Psychiatry. 1984;47(6):600–3.
41. Teasdale G, Teasdale E, Hadley D. Computed tomographic and magnetic resonance imaging classification of head injury. J Neurotrauma. 1992;9(Suppl 1):S249–57.
42. Liu HM, Tu YK, Su CT. Changes of brainstem and perimesencephalic cistern: dynamic predictor of outcome in severe head injury. J Trauma. 1995;38(3):330–3.
43. Athiappan S, Muthukumar N, Srinivasan US. Influence of basal cisterns, midline shift and pathology on outcome in head injury. Ann Acad Med Singap. 1993;22(3 Suppl):452–5.
44. Tóth A, Schmalfuss I, Heaton SC, et al. Lateral ventricle volume asymmetry predicts midline shift in severe traumatic brain injury. J Neurotrauma. 2015;32(17):1307–11.
45. Toutant SM, Klauber MR, Marshall LF, Toole BM, Bowers SA, Seelig JM, Varnell JB. Absent or compressed basal cisterns on first CT scan: ominous predictors of outcome in severe head injury. J Neurosurg. 1984;61(4):691–4.
46. Yanaka K, Kamezaki T, Yamada T, Takano S, Meguro K, Nose T. Acute subdural hematoma—prediction of outcome with a linear discriminant function. Neurol Med Chir (Tokyo). 1993;33(8):552–8.
47. Miller JD, Gudeman SK, Kishore PR, Becker DP. CT scan, ICP and early neurological evaluation in the prognosis of severe head injury. Acta Neurochir Suppl (Wien). 1979;28(1):86–8.
48. Gaetani P, Tancioni F, Tartara F, Carnevale L, Brambilla G, Mille T, Rodriguez y Baena R. Prognostic value of the amount of post-traumatic subarachnoid haemorrhage in a six month follow up period. J Neurol Neurosurg Psychiatry. 1995;59(6):635–7.
49. Greene KA, Marciano FF, Johnson BA, Jacobowitz R, Spetzler RF, Harrington TR. Impact of traumatic subarachnoid hemorrhage on outcome in nonpenetrating head injury. Part I: a proposed computerized tomography grading scale. J Neurosurg. 1995;83(3):445–52.
50. Harders A, Kakarieka A, Braakman R. Traumatic subarachnoid hemorrhage and its treatment with nimodipine. German tSAH Study Group. J Neurosurg. 1996;85(1):82–9.
51. Kakarieka A. Traumatic subarachnoid haemorrhage. 1st ed. Berlin: Springer; 1996.
52. Marshall LF, Maas AI, Marshall SB, et al. A multicenter trial on the efficacy of using tirilazad mesylate in cases of head injury. J Neurosurg. 1998;89(4):519–25.
53. Kakarieka A, Braakman R, Schakel EH. Clinical significance of the finding of subarachnoid blood on CT scan after head injury. Acta Neurochir. 1994;129(1–2):1–5.
54. Shigemori M, Tokutomi T, Hirohata M, Maruiwa H, Kaku N, Kuramoto S. Clinical significance of traumatic subarachnoid hemorrhage. Neurol Med Chir (Tokyo). 1990;30(6):396–400.

55. Ross DA, Olsen WL, Ross AM, Andrews BT, Pitts LH. Brain shift, level of consciousness, and restoration of consciousness in patients with acute intracranial hematoma. J Neurosurg. 1989;71(4):498–502.
56. Kotwica Z, Brzeziński J. Acute subdural haematoma in adults: an analysis of outcome in comatose patients. Acta Neurochir. 1993;121(3–4):95–9.
57. Vollmer D, Torner J, Jane J, Sadovnic B, Charlebois DB, Eisenberg H, Foulkes M, Marmarou A, Marshall L. Age and outcome following traumatic coma: why do older patients fare worse? J Neurosurg. 1991;75:S37–49. https://doi.org/10.3171/SUP.1991.75.1S.0S37.
58. Young B, Rapp RP, Norton JA, Haack D, Tibbs PA, Bean JR. Early prediction of outcome in head-injured patients. J Neurosurg. 1981;54(3):300–3.
59. Jiang C, Cao J, Williamson C, Farzaneh N, Rajajee V, Gryak J, Najarian K, Soroushmehr SMR. Midline shift vs. mid-surface shift: correlation with outcome of traumatic brain injuries. Proc (IEEE Int Conf Bioinform Biomed). 2019;2019:1083–6.
60. Fearnside MR, Cook RJ, McDougall P, McNeil RJ. The Westmead Head Injury Project outcome in severe head injury. A comparative analysis of pre-hospital, clinical and CT variables. Br J Neurosurg. 1993;7(3):267–79.
61. Quattrocchi KB, Prasad P, Willits NH, Wagner FC. Quantification of midline shift as a predictor of poor outcome following head injury. Surg Neurol. 1991;35(3):183–8.
62. Seelig JM, Marshall LF, Toutant SM, Toole BM, Klauber MR, Bowers SA, Varnell JA. Traumatic acute epidural hematoma: unrecognized high lethality in comatose patients. Neurosurgery. 1984;15(5):617–20.
63. Zumkeller M, Behrmann R, Heissler HE, Dietz H. Computed tomographic criteria and survival rate for patients with acute subdural hematoma. Neurosurgery. 1996;39(4):708–12; discussion 712–713.
64. Gennarelli TA, Champion HR, Copes WS, Sacco WJ. Comparison of mortality, morbidity, and severity of 59,713 head injured patients with 114,447 patients with extracranial injuries. J Trauma. 1994;37(6):962–8.
65. Wilberger JE, Harris M, Diamond DL. Acute subdural hematoma: morbidity, mortality, and operative timing. J Neurosurg. 1991;74(2):212–8.
66. Bricolo AP, Pasut LM. Extradural hematoma: toward zero mortality. A prospective study. Neurosurgery. 1984;14(1):8–12.
67. Jamjoom A. The influence of concomitant intradural pathology on the presentation and outcome of patients with acute traumatic extradural haematoma. Acta Neurochir. 1992;115(3–4):86–9.
68. Jones NR, Molloy CJ, Kloeden CN, North JB, Simpson DA. Extradural haematoma: trends in outcome over 35 years. Br J Neurosurg. 1993;7(5):465–71.
69. Kuday C, Uzan M, Hanci M. Statistical analysis of the factors affecting the outcome of extradural haematomas: 115 cases. Acta Neurochir. 1994;131(3–4):203–6.
70. Narayan RK, Greenberg RP, Miller JD, Enas GG, Choi SC, Kishore PR, Selhorst JB, Lutz HA, Becker DP. Improved confidence of outcome prediction in severe head injury. A comparative analysis of the clinical examination, multimodality evoked potentials, CT scanning, and intracranial pressure. J Neurosurg. 1981;54(6):751–62.
71. Bartels RH, Meijer FJ, van der Hoeven H, Edwards M, Prokop M. Midline shift in relation to thickness of traumatic acute subdural hematoma predicts mortality. BMC Neurol. 2015;15:220.
72. Moussa WMM, Khedr WM, Elwany AH. Prognostic significance of hematoma thickness to midline shift ratio in patients with acute intracranial subdural hematoma: a retrospective study. Neurosurg Rev. 2018;41(2):483–8.
73. Choksey M, Crockard HA, Sandilands M. Acute traumatic intracerebral haematomas: determinants of outcome in a retrospective series of 202 cases. Br J Neurosurg. 1993;7(6):611–22.
74. Eide PK, Tysnes OB. Early and late outcome in head injury patients with radiological evidence of brain damage. Acta Neurol Scand. 1992;86(2):194–8.
75. Kobayashi S, Nakazawa S, Otsuka T. Clinical value of serial computed tomography with severe head injury. Surg Neurol. 1983;20(1):25–9.

76. Servadei F, Piazza G, Seracchioli A, Acciarri N, Pozzati E, Gaist G. Extradural haematomas: an analysis of the changing characteristics of patients admitted from 1980 to 1986. Diagnostic and therapeutic implications in 158 cases. Brain Inj. 1988;2(2):87–100.
77. Soloniuk D, Pitts LH, Lovely M, Bartkowski H. Traumatic intracerebral hematomas: timing of appearance and indications for operative removal. J Trauma. 1986;26(9):787–94.
78. Stein SC, Spettell C, Young G, Ross SE. Delayed and progressive brain injury in closed-head trauma: radiological demonstration. Neurosurgery. 1993;32(1):25–30; discussion 30–31.
79. Tseng SH. Delayed traumatic intracerebral hemorrhage: a study of prognostic factors. J Formos Med Assoc. 1992;91(6):585–9.
80. Yamaki T, Hirakawa K, Ueguchi T, Tenjin H, Kuboyama T, Nakagawa Y. Chronological evaluation of acute traumatic intracerebral haematoma. Acta Neurochir. 1990;103(3–4):112–5.
81. Atzema C, Mower WR, Hoffman JR, Holmes JF, Killian AJ, Wolfson AB, National Emergency X-Radiography Utilization Study (NEXUS) II Group. Prevalence and prognosis of traumatic intraventricular hemorrhage in patients with blunt head trauma. J Trauma. 2006;60(5):1010–7; discussion 1017.
82. Cordobés F, Lobato RD, Rivas JJ, Cabrera A, Sarabia M, Castro S, Cisneros C, Torres ID, Lamas E. Post-traumatic diffuse axonal brain injury. Analysis of 78 patients studied with computed tomography. Acta Neurochir. 1986;81(1–2):27–35.
83. Lipper MH, Kishore PR, Enas GG, Domingues da Silva AA, Choi SC, Becker DP. Computed tomography in the prediction of outcome in head injury. AJR Am J Roentgenol. 1985;144(3):483–6.
84. Maas AIR, Steyerberg EW, Butcher I, Dammers R, Lu J, Marmarou A, Mushkudiani NA, McHugh GS, Murray GD. Prognostic value of computerized tomography scan characteristics in traumatic brain injury: results from the IMPACT study. J Neurotrauma. 2007;24(2):303–14.
85. Laleva M, Gabrovsky N, Naseva E, Velinov N, Gabrovsky S. Delayed intraventricular hemorrhage in moderate-to-severe traumatic brain injury: prevalence, associated risk factors, and prognosis. Acta Neurochir. 2016;158(8):1465–72.
86. Mata-Mbemba D, Mugikura S, Nakagawa A, et al. Intraventricular hemorrhage on initial computed tomography as marker of diffuse axonal injury after traumatic brain injury. J Neurotrauma. 2015;32(5):359–65.
87. Hallevi H, Dar NS, Barreto AD, et al. The IVH score: a novel tool for estimating intraventricular hemorrhage volume: clinical and research implications. Crit Care Med. 2009;37(3):969.e1.
88. Morgan TC, Dawson J, Spengler D, et al. The modified Graeb score. Stroke. 2013;44(3):635–41.
89. The Modified Graeb Score | Stroke. https://www.ahajournals.org/doi/10.1161/STROKEAHA.112.670653. Accessed 21 Jul 2022.
90. Mahadewa TGB, Golden N, Saputra A, Ryalino C. Modified revised trauma–Marshall score as a proposed tool in predicting the outcome of moderate and severe traumatic brain injury. Open Access Emerg Med. 2018;10:135–9.
91. Katsnelson M, Mackenzie L, Frangos S, Oddo M, Levine JM, Pukenas B, Faerber J, Dong C, Kofke WA, le Roux PD. Are initial radiographic and clinical scales associated with subsequent intracranial pressure and brain oxygen levels after severe traumatic brain injury? Neurosurgery. 2012;70(5):1095–105; discussion 1105.
92. Mohammadifard M, Ghaemi K, Hanif H, Sharifzadeh G, Haghparast M. Marshall and Rotterdam computed tomography scores in predicting early deaths after brain trauma. Eur J Transl Myol. 2018;28(3):7542.
93. Asim M, El-Menyar A, Parchani A, Nabir S, Ahmed MN, Ahmed Z, Ramzee AF, Al-Thani A, Al-Abdulmalek A, Al-Thani H. Rotterdam and Marshall scores for prediction of in-hospital mortality in patients with traumatic brain injury: an observational study. Brain Inj. 2021;35(7):803–11.
94. Deepika A, Prabhuraj AR, Saikia A, Shukla D. Comparison of predictability of Marshall and Rotterdam CT scan scoring system in determining early mortality after traumatic brain injury. Acta Neurochir. 2015;157(11):2033–8.

95. Swann I, Teasdale G. Current concepts in the management of patients with so-called 'minor' or 'mild' head injury. Trauma. 1999;1:143. https://doi.org/10.1177/146040869900100206.
96. Trifan G, Gattu R, Haacke EM, Kou Z, Benson RR. MR imaging findings in mild traumatic brain injury with persistent neurological impairment. Magn Reson Imaging. 2017;37:243–51.
97. Ibañez J, Arikan F, Pedraza S, Sánchez E, Poca MA, Rodriguez D, Rubio E. Reliability of clinical guidelines in the detection of patients at risk following mild head injury: results of a prospective study. J Neurosurg. 2004;100(5):825–34.
98. Stein SC, Fabbri A, Servadei F, Glick HA. A critical comparison of clinical decision instruments for computed tomographic scanning in mild closed traumatic brain injury in adolescents and adults. Ann Emerg Med. 2009;53(2):180–8.
99. Rosengren D, Rothwell S, Brown AFT, Chu K. The application of North American CT scan criteria to an Australian population with minor head injury. Emerg Med Australas. 2004;16(3):195–200.
100. Smits M, Dippel DWJ, de Haan GG, et al. External validation of the Canadian CT Head Rule and the New Orleans Criteria for CT scanning in patients with minor head injury. JAMA. 2005;294(12):1519–25.
101. Dunning J, Stratford-Smith P, Lecky F, Batchelor J, Hogg K, Browne J, Sharpin C, Mackway-Jones K, Emergency Medicine Research Group. A meta-analysis of clinical correlates that predict significant intracranial injury in adults with minor head trauma. J Neurotrauma. 2004;21(7):877–85.
102. van der Naalt J, Hew JM, van Zomeren AH, Sluiter WJ, Minderhoud JM. Computed tomography and magnetic resonance imaging in mild to moderate head injury: early and late imaging related to outcome. Ann Neurol. 1999;46(1):70–8.
103. Sheridan DC, Newgard CD, Selden NR, Jafri MA, Hansen ML. QuickBrain MRI for the detection of acute pediatric traumatic brain injury. J Neurosurg Pediatr. 2017;19(2):259–64.
104. Irimia A, Wang B, Aylward SR, Prastawa MW, Pace DF, Gerig G, Hovda DA, Kikinis R, Vespa PM, Van Horn JD. Neuroimaging of structural pathology and connectomics in traumatic brain injury: toward personalized outcome prediction. Neuroimage Clin. 2012;1(1):1–17.
105. Moenninghoff C, Kraff O, Maderwald S, et al. Diffuse axonal injury at ultra-high field MRI. PLoS One. 2015;10(3):e0122329.
106. Bigler ED. Quantitative magnetic resonance imaging in traumatic brain injury. J Head Trauma Rehabil. 2001;16(2):117–34.
107. Van Leemput K, Maes F, Vandermeulen D, Suetens P. Automated model-based tissue classification of MR images of the brain. IEEE Trans Med Imaging. 1999;18(10):897–908.
108. Wang B, Prastawa M, Irimia A, Chambers MC, Vespa PM, Van Horn JD, Gerig G. A patient-specific segmentation framework for longitudinal MR images of traumatic brain injury. Proc SPIE Int Soc Opt Eng. 2012;8314:831402.
109. Wu Y, Warfield SK, Tan IL, Wells WM, Meier DS, van Schijndel RA, Barkhof F, Guttmann CRG. Automated segmentation of multiple sclerosis lesion subtypes with multichannel MRI. NeuroImage. 2006;32(3):1205–15.
110. Zhang Y, Brady M, Smith S. Segmentation of brain MR images through a hidden Markov random field model and the expectation-maximization algorithm. IEEE Trans Med Imaging. 2001;20(1):45–57.
111. Dale AM, Fischl B, Sereno MI. Cortical surface-based analysis. I. Segmentation and surface reconstruction. NeuroImage. 1999;9(2):179–94.
112. Desikan RS, Ségonne F, Fischl B, et al. An automated labeling system for subdividing the human cerebral cortex on MRI scans into gyral based regions of interest. NeuroImage. 2006;31(3):968–80.
113. Destrieux C, Fischl B, Dale A, Halgren E. Automatic parcellation of human cortical gyri and sulci using standard anatomical nomenclature. NeuroImage. 2010;53(1):1–15.
114. Fischl B, Dale AM. Measuring the thickness of the human cerebral cortex from magnetic resonance images. Proc Natl Acad Sci U S A. 2000;97(20):11050–5.
115. Kuperberg GR, Broome MR, McGuire PK, et al. Regionally localized thinning of the cerebral cortex in schizophrenia. Arch Gen Psychiatry. 2003;60(9):878–88.

116. Rosas HD, Liu AK, Hersch S, Glessner M, Ferrante RJ, Salat DH, van der Kouwe A, Jenkins BG, Dale AM, Fischl B. Regional and progressive thinning of the cortical ribbon in Huntington's disease. Neurology. 2002;58(5):695–701.
117. Salat DH, Buckner RL, Snyder AZ, Greve DN, Desikan RSR, Busa E, Morris JC, Dale AM, Fischl B. Thinning of the cerebral cortex in aging. Cereb Cortex. 2004;14(7):721–30.
118. Strangman GE, O'Neil-Pirozzi TM, Supelana C, Goldstein R, Katz DI, Glenn MB. Regional brain morphometry predicts memory rehabilitation outcome after traumatic brain injury. Front Hum Neurosci. 2010;4:182.
119. Niethammer M, Hart GL, Pace DF, Vespa PM, Irimia A, Van Horn JD, Aylward SR. Geometric metamorphosis. Med Image Comput Comput Assist Interv. 2011;14(Pt 2):639–46.
120. Kraus MF, Susmaras T, Caughlin BP, Walker CJ, Sweeney JA, Little DM. White matter integrity and cognition in chronic traumatic brain injury: a diffusion tensor imaging study. Brain. 2007;130(Pt 10):2508–19.
121. Rutgers DR, Toulgoat F, Cazejust J, Fillard P, Lasjaunias P, Ducreux D. White matter abnormalities in mild traumatic brain injury: a diffusion tensor imaging study. AJNR Am J Neuroradiol. 2008;29(3):514–9.
122. Vos PE, Bigler ED. White matter in traumatic brain injury: dis- or dysconnection? Neurology. 2011;77(9):810–1.
123. Bazarian JJ, Zhong J, Blyth B, Zhu T, Kavcic V, Peterson D. Diffusion tensor imaging detects clinically important axonal damage after mild traumatic brain injury: a pilot study. J Neurotrauma. 2007;24(9):1447–59.
124. Kou Z, Wu Z, Tong KA, Holshouser B, Benson RR, Hu J, Haacke EM. The role of advanced MR imaging findings as biomarkers of traumatic brain injury. J Head Trauma Rehabil. 2010;25(4):267–82.
125. Wilde EA, McCauley SR, Hunter JV, et al. Diffusion tensor imaging of acute mild traumatic brain injury in adolescents. Neurology. 2008;70(12):948–55.
126. Arfanakis K, Haughton VM, Carew JD, Rogers BP, Dempsey RJ, Meyerand ME. Diffusion tensor MR imaging in diffuse axonal injury. AJNR Am J Neuroradiol. 2002;23(5):794–802.
127. Yuh EL, Cooper SR, Mukherjee P, et al. Diffusion tensor imaging for outcome prediction in mild traumatic brain injury: a TRACK-TBI study. J Neurotrauma. 2014;31(17):1457–77.
128. Wilde EA, Ayoub KW, Bigler ED, Chu ZD, Hunter JV, Wu TC, McCauley SR, Levin HS. Diffusion tensor imaging in moderate-to-severe pediatric traumatic brain injury: changes within an 18 month post-injury interval. Brain Imaging Behav. 2012;6(3):404–16.
129. Kim N, Branch CA, Kim M, Lipton ML. Whole brain approaches for identification of microstructural abnormalities in individual patients: comparison of techniques applied to mild traumatic brain injury. PLoS One. 2013;8(3):e59382.
130. Lipton ML, Gulko E, Zimmerman ME, Friedman BW, Kim M, Gellella E, Gold T, Shifteh K, Ardekani BA, Branch CA. Diffusion-tensor imaging implicates prefrontal axonal injury in executive function impairment following very mild traumatic brain injury. Radiology. 2009;252(3):816–24.
131. Wallace EJ, Mathias JL, Ward L. The relationship between diffusion tensor imaging findings and cognitive outcomes following adult traumatic brain injury: a meta-analysis. Neurosci Biobehav Rev. 2018;92:93–103.
132. Sidaros A, Engberg AW, Sidaros K, Liptrot MG, Herning M, Petersen P, Paulson OB, Jernigan TL, Rostrup E. Diffusion tensor imaging during recovery from severe traumatic brain injury and relation to clinical outcome: a longitudinal study. Brain. 2008;131(Pt 2):559–72.
133. Wedeen VJ, Hagmann P, Tseng W-YI, Reese TG, Weisskoff RM. Mapping complex tissue architecture with diffusion spectrum magnetic resonance imaging. Magn Reson Med. 2005;54(6):1377–86.
134. Irimia A, Chambers MC, Torgerson CM, et al. Patient-tailored connectomics visualization for the assessment of white matter atrophy in traumatic brain injury. Front Neurol. 2012;3:10.
135. Mac Donald CL, Dikranian K, Bayly P, Holtzman D, Brody D. Diffusion tensor imaging reliably detects experimental traumatic axonal injury and indicates approximate time of injury. J Neurosci. 2007;27(44):11869–76.

136. Sun TFD, Boet R, Poon WS. Non-surgical primary treatment of chronic subdural haematoma: preliminary results of using dexamethasone. Br J Neurosurg. 2005;19(4):327–33.
137. Beaulieu C, Does MD, Snyder RE, Allen PS. Changes in water diffusion due to Wallerian degeneration in peripheral nerve. Magn Reson Med. 1996;36(4):627–31.
138. Povlishock JT, Katz DI. Update of neuropathology and neurological recovery after traumatic brain injury. J Head Trauma Rehabil. 2005;20(1):76–94.
139. Sharp DJ, Ham TE. Investigating white matter injury after mild traumatic brain injury. Curr Opin Neurol. 2011;24(6):558–63.
140. Dimitriadis SI, Laskaris NA, Tsirka V, Vourkas M, Micheloyannis S, Fotopoulos S. Tracking brain dynamics via time-dependent network analysis. J Neurosci Methods. 2010;193(1):145–55.
141. Kuceyeski A, Maruta J, Niogi SN, Ghajar J, Raj A. The generation and validation of white matter connectivity importance maps. NeuroImage. 2011;58(1):109–21.
142. Kaiser M, Martin R, Andras P, Young MP. Simulation of robustness against lesions of cortical networks. Eur J Neurosci. 2007;25(10):3185–92.
143. Varier S, Kaiser M, Forsyth R. Establishing, versus maintaining, brain function: a neurocomputational model of cortical reorganization after injury to the immature brain. J Int Neuropsychol Soc. 2011;17(6):1030–8.
144. Alstott J, Breakspear M, Hagmann P, Cammoun L, Sporns O. Modeling the impact of lesions in the human brain. PLoS Comput Biol. 2009;5(6):e1000408.
145. Bendlin BB, Ries ML, Lazar M, Alexander AL, Dempsey RJ, Rowley HA, Sherman JE, Johnson SC. Longitudinal changes in patients with traumatic brain injury assessed with diffusion-tensor and volumetric imaging. NeuroImage. 2008;42(2):503–14.
146. Blumbergs PC, Scott G, Manavis J, Wainwright H, Simpson DA, McLean AJ. Topography of axonal injury as defined by amyloid precursor protein and the sector scoring method in mild and severe closed head injury. J Neurotrauma. 1995;12(4):565–72.
147. Nakayama N, Okumura A, Shinoda J, Yasokawa Y-T, Miwa K, Yoshimura S-I, Iwama T. Evidence for white matter disruption in traumatic brain injury without macroscopic lesions. J Neurol Neurosurg Psychiatry. 2006;77(7):850–5.
148. Wozniak JR, Krach L, Ward E, Mueller BA, Muetzel R, Schnoebelen S, Kiragu A, Lim KO. Neurocognitive and neuroimaging correlates of pediatric traumatic brain injury: a diffusion tensor imaging (DTI) study. Arch Clin Neuropsychol. 2007;22(5):555–68.
149. Ewing-Cobbs L, Prasad MR, Swank P, Kramer L, Cox CS, Fletcher JM, Barnes M, Zhang X, Hasan KM. Arrested development and disrupted callosal microstructure following pediatric traumatic brain injury: relation to neurobehavioral outcomes. NeuroImage. 2008;42(4):1305–15.
150. Niogi SN, Mukherjee P, Ghajar J, et al. Extent of microstructural white matter injury in postconcussive syndrome correlates with impaired cognitive reaction time: a 3T diffusion tensor imaging study of mild traumatic brain injury. AJNR Am J Neuroradiol. 2008;29(5):967–73.
151. Laureys S, Celesia GG, Cohadon F, et al. Unresponsive wakefulness syndrome: a new name for the vegetative state or apallic syndrome. BMC Med. 2010;8:68.
152. Mason MF, Norton MI, Van Horn JD, Wegner DM, Grafton ST, Macrae CN. Wandering minds: the default network and stimulus-independent thought. Science. 2007;315(5810):393–5.
153. Threlkeld ZD, Bodien YG, Rosenthal ES, Giacino JT, Nieto-Castanon A, Wu O, Whitfield-Gabrieli S, Edlow BL. Functional networks reemerge during recovery of consciousness after acute severe traumatic brain injury. Cortex. 2018;106:299–308.
154. Christodoulou C, DeLuca J, Ricker JH, et al. Functional magnetic resonance imaging of working memory impairment after traumatic brain injury. J Neurol Neurosurg Psychiatry. 2001;71(2):161–8.
155. Kramer ME, Chiu C-YP, Walz NC, Holland SK, Yuan W, Karunanayaka P, Wade SL. Long-term neural processing of attention following early childhood traumatic brain injury: fMRI and neurobehavioral outcomes. J Int Neuropsychol Soc. 2008;14(3):424–35.
156. Laatsch L, Krisky C. Changes in fMRI activation following rehabilitation of reading and visual processing deficits in subjects with traumatic brain injury. Brain Inj. 2006;20(13–14):1367–75.

157. Monti MM, Vanhaudenhuyse A, Coleman MR, Boly M, Pickard JD, Tshibanda L, Owen AM, Laureys S. Willful modulation of brain activity in disorders of consciousness. N Engl J Med. 2010;362(7):579–89.
158. Sánchez-Carrión R, Gómez PV, Junqué C, Fernández-Espejo D, Falcon C, Bargalló N, Roig-Rovira T, Enseñat-Cantallops A, Bernabeu M. Frontal hypoactivation on functional magnetic resonance imaging in working memory after severe diffuse traumatic brain injury. J Neurotrauma. 2008;25(5):479–94.
159. Scheibel RS, Pearson DA, Faria LP, Kotrla KJ, Aylward E, Bachevalier J, Levin HS. An fMRI study of executive functioning after severe diffuse TBI. Brain Inj. 2003;17(11):919–30.
160. Rehabilitation of persons with traumatic brain injury. NIH Consens Statement. 1998;16(1):1–41.
161. Soustiel JF, Mahamid E, Goldsher D, Zaaroor M. Perfusion-CT for early assessment of traumatic cerebral contusions. Neuroradiology. 2008;50(2):189–96.
162. Bendinelli C, Cooper S, Evans T, Bivard A, Pacey D, Parson M, Balogh ZJ. Perfusion abnormalities are frequently detected by early CT perfusion and predict unfavourable outcome following severe traumatic brain injury. World J Surg. 2017;41(10):2512–20.
163. Doshi H, Wiseman N, Liu J, et al. Cerebral hemodynamic changes of mild traumatic brain injury at the acute stage. PLoS One. 2015;10(2):e0118061.
164. Wintermark M, van Melle G, Schnyder P, Revelly J-P, Porchet F, Regli L, Meuli R, Maeder P, Chioléro R. Admission perfusion CT: prognostic value in patients with severe head trauma. Radiology. 2004;232(1):211–20.
165. Metting Z, Rödiger LA, Stewart RE, Oudkerk M, De Keyser J, van der Naalt J. Perfusion computed tomography in the acute phase of mild head injury: regional dysfunction and prognostic value. Ann Neurol. 2009;66(6):809–16.
166. Aaen GS, Holshouser BA, Sheridan C, Colbert C, McKenney M, Kido D, Ashwal S. Magnetic resonance spectroscopy predicts outcomes for children with nonaccidental trauma. Pediatrics. 2010;125(2):295–303.
167. Gardner A, Iverson GL, Stanwell P. A systematic review of proton magnetic resonance spectroscopy findings in sport-related concussion. J Neurotrauma. 2014;31(1):1–18.
168. Holshouser B, Pivonka-Jones J, Nichols JG, Oyoyo U, Tong K, Ghosh N, Ashwal S. Longitudinal metabolite changes after traumatic brain injury: a prospective pediatric magnetic resonance spectroscopic imaging study. J Neurotrauma. 2019;36(8):1352–60.
169. Muthupillai R, Ehman RL. Magnetic resonance elastography. Nat Med. 1996;2(5):601–3.
170. Hiscox LV, Johnson CL, Barnhill E, McGarry MDJ, Huston J, van Beek EJR, Starr JM, Roberts N. Magnetic resonance elastography (MRE) of the human brain: technique, findings and clinical applications. Phys Med Biol. 2016;61(24):R401–37.
171. Alfasi AM, Shulyakov AV, Del Bigio MR. Intracranial biomechanics following cortical contusion in live rats. J Neurosurg. 2013;119(5):1255–62.
172. Boulet T, Kelso ML, Othman SF. Long-term in vivo imaging of viscoelastic properties of the mouse brain after controlled cortical impact. J Neurotrauma. 2013;30(17):1512–20.
173. Chartrand G, Cheng PM, Vorontsov E, Drozdzal M, Turcotte S, Pal CJ, Kadoury S, Tang A. Deep learning: a primer for radiologists. Radiographics. 2017;37(7):2113–31.
174. Liu S, Utriainen D, Chai C, Chen Y, Wang L, Sethi SK, Xia S, Haacke EM. Cerebral microbleed detection using susceptibility weighted imaging and deep learning. NeuroImage. 2019;198:271–82.

Airway Management in Acute Trauma

5

B. D. Vaishnavi, Palak Gupta, Shilpa Goyal, and Amit Goyal

5.1 Introduction

Trauma to the airway presents a unique set of challenges to the attending clinician due to the distorted airway anatomy and the need to act quickly with limited history. A team approach, with a designated team leader who can make decisions and other members who have tasks assigned to them, can help events flow more smoothly and efficiently. The airway trauma incidence though is <1% but is rapidly increasing [1]. Blunt and penetrating injury to the face, neck, and upper chest can result in early or delayed airway compromise if not approached methodically. A rapid airway assessment, as well as good clinical knowledge and skills, will aid in the timely management of a traumatized airway.

Emergent or urgent airway management is always indicated in a patient with respiratory distress and in those patients with an anticipated airway compromise [2]. The clinician managing these patients should be well versed with advanced airway management techniques and surgical airway due to a high chance of complicated airways. The presence of other system injuries (cerebral, pulmonary, and vascular injuries), as well as blood, vomitus, and soft tissue edema obstructing the airway, can complicate matters further. The clinician must be aware that patients with the above injuries can appear stable but can deteriorate rapidly from a partially obstructed airway to completely obstructed airway. The need for manual in-line stabilization of the cervical spine in all trauma patients exacerbates airway difficulties.

B. D. Vaishnavi
Sheffield Teaching Hospital NHS Trust, Sheffield, UK

P. Gupta · A. Goyal
Department of Otorhinolaryngology, AIIMS Jodhpur, Jodhpur, India

S. Goyal (✉)
Department of Anesthesiology and Critical Care, AIIMS Jodhpur, Jodhpur, India

© The Author(s), under exclusive license to Springer Nature Singapore Pte Ltd. 2024
A. Agrawal et al. (eds.), *Special Considerations in Trauma Care*,
https://doi.org/10.1007/978-981-99-9662-9_5

5.2 Challenges in Trauma Patients [3]

At the Site of the Accident

1. Unfavorable situations (inadequate light and space, improper patient access).
2. Difficult patient position (unattended on the road or trapped inside cars).
3. Contamination of the wounds.
4. Assistance of unskilled and unknown personnels.
5. Absence of prompt response from the emergency team.
6. Uncertainty of available equipment.

At the Hospital

1. Massive bleeding.
2. Maxillofacial and neck injuries.
3. Agitated or comatose patient.
4. No confirmation of the right airway device insertion or displacement of the device that was placed correctly initially.
5. Inadequate ventilation.
6. Cervical spine injury with a rigid cervical collar.
7. Assumed full stomach and incorrect Sellick's maneuver applied.
8. Uncertain volume status precluding the incorporation of necessary pharmacological agents.
9. Quick desaturation of the patient adding on to the stress of the helpers and doctors.
10. Uncooperative, comatose patients, or combative attendants.

5.3 Airway Assessment in the Traumatized Airway

Careful airway assessment is required to determine acute or impending ventilation and oxygenation failure in airway trauma. The following signs should not be missed [2]:

- Dyspnea.
- Stridor.
- Loss of phonation.
- Drooling and painful swallowing.
- Trismus.
- Extensive oral and nasal bleeding.
- Laryngeal and tracheal anatomical abnormality.
- Subcutaneous emphysema in the neck and upper chest.
- Hoarseness of voice.
- Expanding hematoma in the neck.
- Nonsuperficial facial burn.

A brief history and physical examination should be combined with a rapid airway examination using the following mnemonics:

1. ***LEMONS*** to assess for difficult airway [4, 5]:
   L: *Look externally* for potential difficulties like short neck, obesity, buck teeth, facial trauma, etc.
   E: *Evaluate the 3-3-2 rule*, i.e., capability to accommodate 3 fingers in order to assess the oral opening, ability to fit 3 fingers between the mentum and the hyoid to determine whether the mandible can accommodate the tongue, ability to fit 2 fingers between the mandible (mouth floor) and thyroid cartilage to determine the presence of a high larynx.
   M: *Mallampati grading*—Grades 3 and 4 suggest difficult airway.
   O: *Obstruction*—Determine the location of the obstruction below, at, or above vocal cords.
   N: *Neck mobility*—Assess for neck extension and flexion. To be avoided it in patient with cervical spine injury.
2. ***1-2-3- Finger*** assessment test [4]:
   1-finger test—Index finger is placed in front of the tragus and when the patient opens the mouth, the index finger indents in its space, indicating good mandibular sliding.
   2-finger test—The ability to place the index and middle fingers in the open mouth, indicating a space of more than 3 cm, which is adequate for the 2 cm flange of a direct laryngoscope.
   3-finger test—The ability to fit three fingers in the submandibular space with an extended head indicates that there is enough space in front of the larynx for the tongue to be compressed.
3. ***BONES*** to assess difficult bag and mask ventilation [6]:
   B: Presence of beard.
   O: Obesity (BMI >26 kg/m^2)/Obstructed sleep apnea.
   N: No teeth.
   E: Elderly >55 years.
   S: Snorer.
4. ***RODS*** for difficult supraglottic insertion [7]:
   R: Restricted lungs.
   O: Obstruction.
   D: Distorted airway.
   S: Short thyromental distance.
5. ***SMART*** for difficult cricothyrotomy [5]:
   S: Surgery.
   M: Mass (hematoma, abscess, or other mass).
   A: Access or Anatomy (obesity, poor landmarks).
   R: Radiation.
   T: Tumor.

5.4 Management of Traumatized Airway

The traumatized airway is always considered difficult to manage due to the limited mouth opening, pooling of blood and secretions in the oropharynx, and the need to act immediately. It is critical that all airway equipment, including the difficult airway cart, be available, checked daily, and signed by a designated person. The availability of all airway equipment in a designated location with a labeled box or drawers aids in better difficult airway scenario management and providing the right equipment at the right time when in an emergency.

A difficult airway trolley with a label containing an illustration of contents (top surface with 4–5 drawers) (Fig. 5.1) should include [8]:

- The top surface contains a fiberoptic bronchoscope.
- Side of trolley: bougie, airway exchange catheter, Aintree intubating catheter.
- Drawer 1 (Plan A): Various laryngoscopes like Macintosh, Miller, and Mc Coy with blades of all sizes.
  Short laryngoscope handle.
  Video-laryngoscope.
- Drawer 2 (Plan B): second generation LMA size #3, 4, 5, fiberoptic adjuvants—Ovassapian airway, nasal sponge, lignocaine 4% and 10%, etc.
- Drawer 3 (Plan C): Various sizes of oropharyngeal, nasopharynx, facemask.
- Drawer 4 (Plan D): Surgical cricothyroidotomy—large-bore iv cannula, No 20, dilator or hook, size #6 and 7 cuffed tube.
  Cannula cricothyroidotomy—Kink resistant jet ventilation cannula, Manujet III.

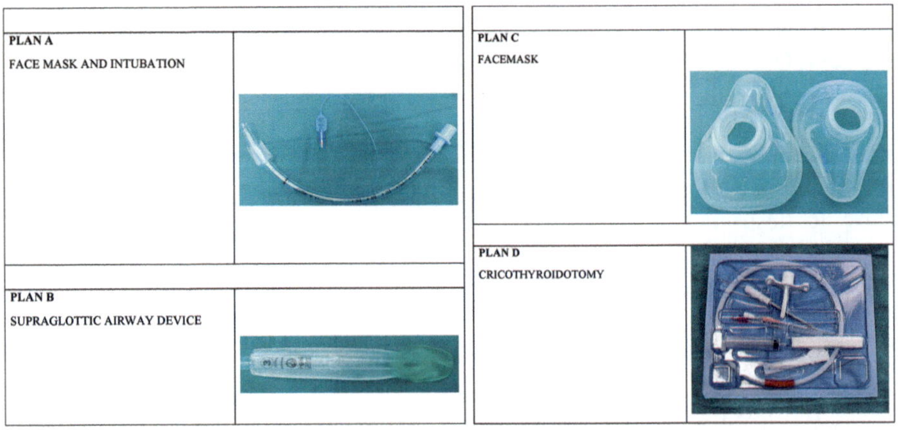

Fig. 5.1 Contents of different drawers of difficult airway trolley as per difficult airway plan

All trauma patients should be considered full stomach and with cervical spine injury unless ruled out, therefore, rapid sequence induction (RSI) with manual in-line stabilization (MILS) should be used for intubation. If time allows, adequate preoxygenation should be performed for 3–5 min before sedating the patient. Benzodiazepines and sedative-hypnotics such as propofol, etomidate, thiopental, ketamine, and opioids are all options, but etomidate and ketamine are preferred in trauma patients with hemodynamic instability. If there is no contradiction, succinylcholine is preferred for RSI as it has a short duration of action. Another alternative is an intubating dose of rocuronium can also be used.

Clinicians should be trained in national or international airway management guidelines in order to respond quickly and in a systematic way. A team approach with a team leader will aid in the formulation of a well-structured plan, for things to go smoothly. Prior to RSI, it is vital to check for suction, monitors, airway, and ancillary equipment along with proper positioning of the patient. End-tidal CO_2 should be used when available to confirm the endotracheal tube placement (ETT).

5.5 Airway Trauma Scenarios, Their Challenges, and Management

Direct airway trauma can be due to blunt or penetrating maxillofacial and neck trauma, burn injury, and caustic ingestion. All airway-related injuries have their own set of challenges in making airway management difficult. Airway trauma can be associated with other major trauma like neurological, pulmonary, and abdominal injuries requiring immediate action and should be managed simultaneously.

5.5.1 Maxillofacial Trauma

A facial fracture can affect the airway in many ways. A parasymphseal mandibular fracture can result in posterior displacement of the tongue and, as a result, obstruction of the airway, which is relieved in a sitting posture. A temporomandibular fracture can result in limited mouth opening. Lefort fractures I, II, and III (Fig. 5.2) can cause airway compromise due to posterior displacement of the fracture segment (especially in Lefort I and III) and extensive oral bleeding (especially in Lefort II), with the II and III types being further complicated by skull base fracture and CSF leak [9, 10].

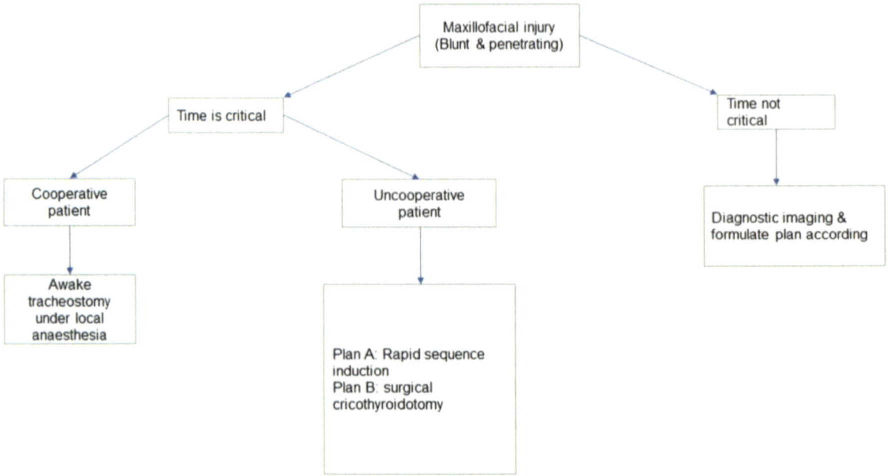

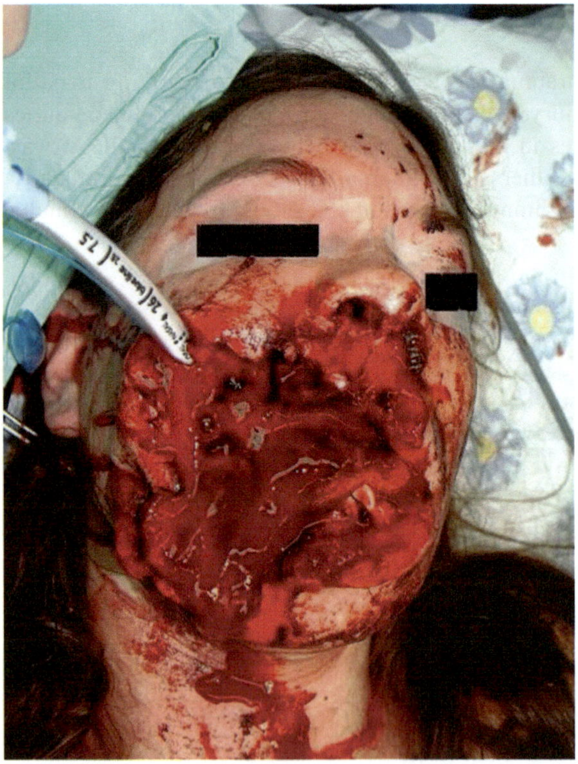

Fig. 5.2 Krausz AA, el-Naaj IA, Barak M. Maxillofacial trauma patient: coping with the difficult airway. *World Journal of Emergency Surgery* 2009;4:21. https://doi.org/10.1186/1749-7922-4-21

5.5.2 Neck Trauma

The neck can be divided into the following sections [10]:

Zone 1—extends from the clavicle to the cricoid cartilage and contains major arteries and veins such as the internal jugular vein, and carotid and subclavian arteries.
Zone 2—Extends from the cricoid cartilage to the angles of the mandible and contains vascular structures as well as the larynx, trachea, and esophagus.
Direct vascular injuries in zones 1 and 2 must be treated right away by securing the airway due to rapidly expanding hematoma with impending obstruction.
Zone 3—Area above the mandible's angles.

Subcutaneous emphysema indicates trauma to the air-filled structures of the neck. Bags and masks should be avoided as they can worsen the subcutaneous emphysema. Fatal traumas like a laryngeal fracture or tracheal resection (complete/incomplete) should be managed in the operating theatre with a tracheostomy performed distal to the resection due to the distorted anatomy and extensive bleeding hampering the vision. To avoid airway loss due to retraction of the distal end of the trachea, tracheal resection should be managed by intubating the distal resected end directly if visible in an emergency [9].

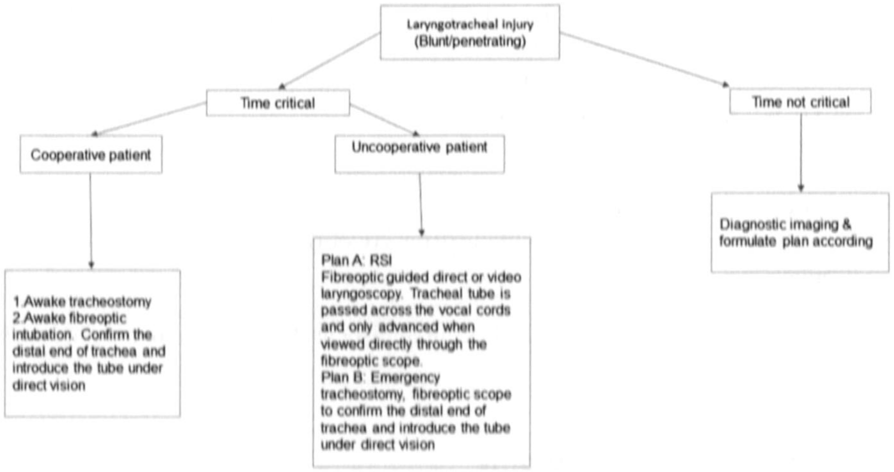

5.5.3 Burn and Corrosive Injury

Upper airway injury caused by direct heat and steam, as well as contact with corrosive agents, causes extensive swelling of the upper airway and tracheal mucosa. Swelling and edema can progress quickly, resulting in severe airway obstruction. To avoid difficult airway situations, these patients should be intubated as soon as possible.

Difficult airway drills and workshops should be done regularly to keep the clinicians updated and hands-on practice on mannequins should be conducted to train the personnel involved in acute airway trauma management. Video-laryngoscopes and fiberoptic bronchoscopes should be used routinely to familiarize ourselves with the equipment beforehand.

5.6 Need for Tracheostomy?

A surgical airway should be established in those patients in whom the initial adjuncts fail to provide an adequate airway access. It is also indicated in patients with severe facial or neck injuries that preclude an endotracheal tube insertion [11].

The maxillofacial trauma patient presents a problem of difficult mask ventilation and intubation. The trauma disrupts the normal anatomy causing edema and bleeding. Difficulty in performing the intubation arises mainly from a difficult visualization of the vocal cords with direct laryngoscopy [12].

Tracheostomy indications following facial trauma [13].

- Acute airway obstruction.
- Fracture of bilateral condyle with a symphyseal fracture that may affect the support of the tongue.
- Fractures involving the mid-face, Le Fort injuries with nose and mandible fractures, and basilar skull fracture.
- Severe edema of the oropharyngeal and glottic regions.
- Severe retropositioning of the maxilla.
- Cervical spine injury.
- Post maxilla-mandibular fixation patients requiring intubation.
- Floor of mouth and tongue lacerations.
- Patients were temporarily maintained on cricothyroidotomy on arrival at the hospital.

Securing the airway surgically has an indispensable role in managing such patients.

5.7 Role of Cricothyrotomy

Establishing an opening surgically through the cricothyroid membrane followed by placing a ventilation tube (Fig. 5.3). The membrane is present between the cricoid and thyroid cartilages and is separated from the skin only by the subcutaneous fat and cervical fascia [14].

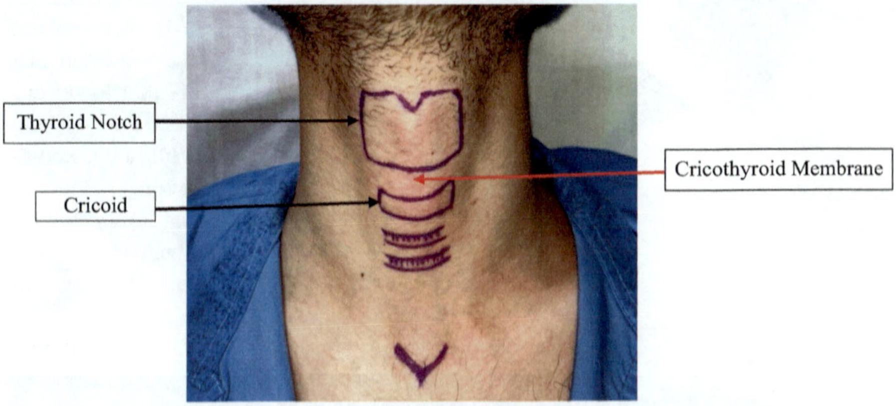

Fig. 5.3 Taken with consent, at ENT Department, AIIMS Jodhpur

5.7.1 Indications

The primary indication is the inability to intubate or do mask ventilation with an immediate need for definitive airway management. Often errors in the difficult airway management result from repeated unsuccessful intubation attempts. Once a "cannot intubate, cannot ventilate" situation is identified, an urgent consideration to a surgical airway should be given.

5.7.2 Contraindications

- Pediatric patients (<10 years).
- Trauma in the neck with difficulty in palpating landmarks.
- A diffuse neck hematoma.
- Pre-existing laryngeal malignancy.

A cricothyrotomy tube placed for emergency purposes should be converted to a tracheotomy tube within 72 h as the prolonged use of this airway access has been found to be associated with a risk of subglottic stenosis [11].

5.8 Transtracheal Needle Ventilation (Fig. 5.4a–e)

This can be used as a temporary option in a patient who cannot be ventilated or intubated. The airway can be established by puncturing the cricothyroid membrane or trachea with a syringe filled with saline and attached to the venflon (Fig. 5.4a–e). Oxygen can be delivered with this technique for 30–60 min, with hypercapnia acting as the limiting factor [15].

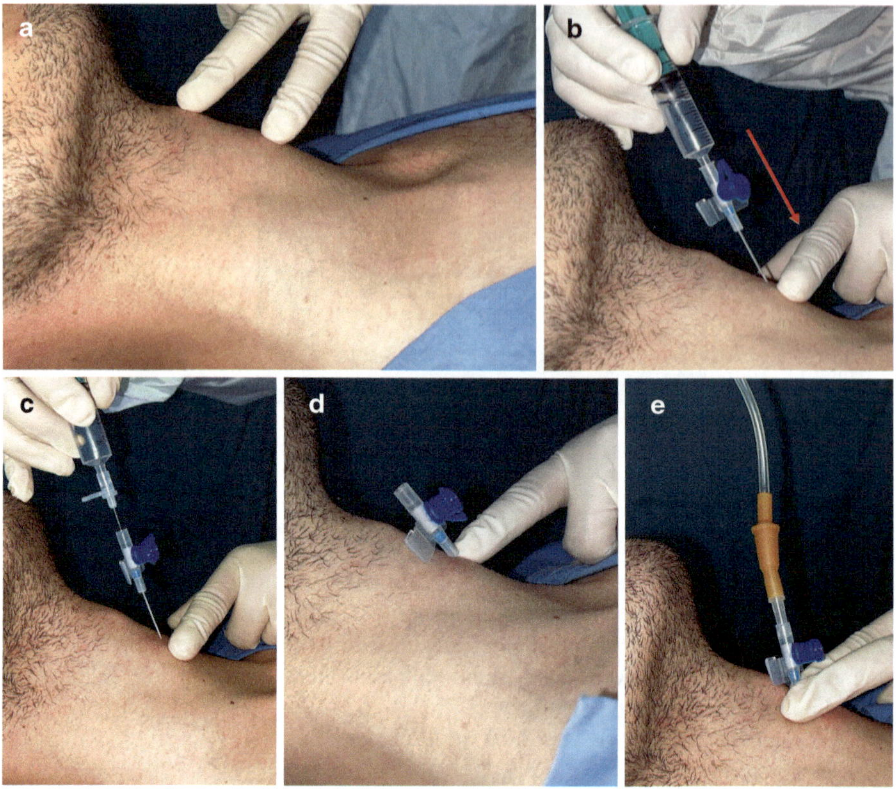

Fig. 5.4 (**a**) Hyperextend the neck if possible, palpate the cricothyroid membrane with your non-dominant hand. (Taken with consent, at ENT Department, AIIMS Jodhpur). (**b**) Attach a 14 gauge catheter attached with water-filled syringe. Insert it at an angle of 30–45° directed caudally. (Taken with consent, at ENT Department, AIIMS Jodhpur). (**c**) Once the trachea is entered, advance the catheter over the needle until the hub is flush with the skin. (Taken with consent, at ENT Department, AIIMS Jodhpur). (**d**) Remove the needle. (Taken with consent, at ENT Department, AIIMS Jodhpur). (**e**) Attach the oxygen supply and begin to ventilate the patient. (Taken with consent, at ENT Department, AIIMS Jodhpur)

5.9 Conclusion

A rapid airway assessment combined with a team approach to the trauma patient can help in timely management of the airway without any untoward incident. Airway management in trauma courses, simulations, and difficult airway drills can all aid in systematic management of traumatized airway.

References

1. Kummer C, Netto FS, Rizoli S, Yee D. A review of traumatic airway injuries: potential implications for airway assessment and management. Injury. 2007;38:27–33.
2. Mills TJ, Deblieux P. Emergency airway management in the adult with direct airway trauma. UpToDate, 2022.
3. Kumar A, Kohli A. Challenges in airway management of trauma patients: an update. Indian J Clin Anaesth. 2020;7:39–45.
4. Khan R. Airway management. 7th ed. Berlin: Springer; 2020.
5. Walls RM, Murphy MF. Manual of emergency airway management. 4th ed. Philadelphia: Wolters Kluwer/Lippincott Williams & Wilkins Heath; 2012.
6. O'Connor MF. Airway assessment of 25,000 patients in a preoperative clinic. Anaesth Analg. 2002;94:S113.
7. Hung O, Murphy M. Changing practice in airway management: are we there yet? Can J Anaesth. 2004;51:963–8.
8. Bjurström MF, Bodelsson M, Sturesson LW. The difficult airway trolley: a narrative review and practical guide. Anesthesiol Res Pract. 2019;2019:6780254.
9. Hammad YMHA, Shallik NA. Airway trauma: assessment and management. London: IntechOpen; 2021.
10. Raja A. The traumatized airway. In: Benumof and Hagberg's airway management: Third Edition. Amsterdam: Elsevier; 2012.
11. Talving P, DuBose J, Inaba K, Demetriades D. Conversion of emergent cricothyrotomy to tracheotomy in trauma patients. Arch Surg. 2010;145:87–91.
12. Krausz AA, el-Naaj IA, Barak M. Maxillofacial trauma patient: coping with the difficult airway. World J Emerg Surg. 2009;4:21.
13. Taicher S, Givol N, Peleg M, Ardekian L. Changing indications for tracheostomy in maxillofacial trauma. J Oral Maxillofac Surg. 1996;54:292–5.
14. Flint PW, Haughey BH, Lund VJ, Robbins KT, Thomas JR, Lesperance MM, et al., editors. Cummings otolaryngology-head and neck surgery. 7th ed. Philadelphia: Elsevier; 2020.
15. Roberts JR. Roberts and Hedges' Clinical procedures in emergency medicine and acute care. 7th ed. Amsterdam: Elsevier; 2017.

Anesthetic Considerations 6

Anuj Jain and Ashutosh Kaushal

6.1 Anesthetic Concerns in a Trauma Patient

Ever-growing mobility has led to a boom in the number of road traffic accidents (RTAs). Deaths due to RTAs have assumed colossal proportions, ever-growing speed of motor vehicles is making RTA more and more damaging. Many trauma patients require lifesaving emergency surgeries; providing anesthesia for trauma patients is challenging, not just due to its resource intensiveness but also due to the extreme perturbations of the normal physiology.

Although many major trauma patients do not make it to the healthcare services, but with ever-improving modes of communication, transport and increasing number of trauma centers, more and more patients with major trauma are getting benefitted.

This chapter intends to apprise the readers with the anesthesia considerations in patients with major trauma arising out of RTAs. This chapter encompasses anesthetic management of a trauma patient beyond the emergency room (ER). Details on resuscitation of a trauma patient are beyond the scope of this chapter.

The anesthesia concerns are closely related to the mechanism of accidents. The most serious concerns arise from injury to the central nervous system (CNS), neck and chest, abdomen, and pelvis. While trauma to the limbs is more obvious and dramatic in its presentation, it is comparatively easier to stabilize.

In order to achieve an optimal surgical outcome, a customized anesthesia approach needs to be formulated. In this chapter, we shall cover anesthesia considerations in patients with head injury, spinal cord injury (SCI), chest trauma, abdominal and pelvic trauma, and burn trauma.

A. Jain (✉) · A. Kaushal
Anesthesiology, All India Institute of Medical Sciences Bhopal,
Bhopal, Madhya Pradesh, India
e-mail: anuj.anesth@aiimsbhopal.edu.in; ashutosh.anesth@aiimsbhopal.edu.in

© The Author(s), under exclusive license to Springer Nature Singapore Pte Ltd. 2024
A. Agrawal et al. (eds.), *Special Considerations in Trauma Care*,
https://doi.org/10.1007/978-981-99-9662-9_6

Before we begin formulating a customized anesthesia plan, we need to be absolutely clear about certain basic principles for the management of any patient with major trauma.

Securing a patent airway and ensuring oxygenation should be the priority in any trauma patient.

In acute trauma, victims cannot relate their symptoms or medical history due to altered mental status (e.g., neurologic injury and/or intoxication). Every attempt should be made to identify pre-existing medical conditions by contacting the patient's primary care physician or family members. The presence of significant medical comorbidities and medical conditions requiring antiplatelet or anticoagulation should be determined.

6.2 Intoxicants and Their Interaction with Anesthetics

A significant number of RTAs happen under the effect of intoxicating substances. Intoxicating substance use may have a significant anesthetic implication. The pattern of drug abuse varies significantly across the globe, but alcohol abuse is the most prevalent among RTA victims. Various intoxicants, through their direct action on the CNS and autonomic nervous system, may make the pharmacodynamics of the anesthetic drugs unpredictable.

Ethanol Chronic alcohol usage leads to multiorgan system involvement and may cause, delayed gastric emptying and predisposition to regurgitation and aspiration, cardiomyopathy, predisposes to pneumonia and adult respiratory distress syndrome (ARDS); megaloblastic anaemia and increased fibrinolysis; electrolyte imbalances, hypokalemia and hypomagnesemia being most common; Wernicke's encephalopathy. All these physiological perturbations can have grave implications on the perioperative outcome.

Chronic alcohol abuse also causes hepatic enzyme upregulation, thereby increases the drug metabolism. Hence, chronic alcohol intake in the absence of acute intake may lead to increase requirement of anesthetic drugs [1, 2]. The duration of action of non-depolarizing muscle relaxants like vecuronium and rocuronium is likely to get enhanced in advanced alcoholic liver disease and hence should be used in conjunction with neuromuscular monitoring [3, 4]. Atracurium, cis-atracurium have organ independent metabolism [5]. Although succinylcholine is metabolized by pseudocholinesterase, even advanced liver disease is unlikely to have any clinically significant effect on its metabolism [6]. Acetaminophen should also be used with caution in these groups of patients.

Ethanol is a central nervous system depressant that acts agonistically at the *N*-methyl D-aspartate (NMDA), 5-hydroxytryptamine (5-HT3), glycine and gamma amino butyric acid (GABA) receptors [7]. Since many anesthetic agents exert their action through these receptors, the dose of general anesthetics gets reduced, but in a rather unpredictable fashion.

Cocaine Cocaine is another commonly used recreational drug. Cocaine exerts its sympathomimetic effect by preventing the reuptake of catecholamines at the adrenergic receptors [8, 9], enhances the release of catecholamines; the effect is preferentially alpha-adrenergic, leading to vasoconstriction in the peripheral and cardiac vessels, manifesting as hypertension. Approximately 5–6% of patients have cardiac ischemia at the time of presentation in emergency [10]. Three to four percent of patients also have seizures and intracranial hemorrhage [11, 12].

Euphoric symptoms of cocaine are due to enhanced levels of excitatory amino acids likely glutamate and aspartate in nucleus accumbens.

Cocaine also has sodium channels blocking action; at higher doses, the cardiac sodium channels also get affected and may manifest as bradycardia and arrhythmia [10].

Cocaine when taken along with ethanol, undergoes a transesterification reaction forming benzylmethylecgonine also called as ethyl cocaine [13]. In contrast to cocaine, which has a relatively short duration of action (30–90 min), ethyl cocaine has effects similar to cocaine, but the duration of action is approximately 12–13 h [14].

Hence, patients with cocaine intoxication may have a complex pathophysiology. The excitatory CNS effect is likely to increase the requirement of general anesthetics. The cardiovascular effects are dependent on the dose consumed and may range from hypertension to profound cardiovascular collapse.

While managing hypertension in a cocaine-positive patient, vasodilators like nitroglycerine, nitroprusside and nicardipine are agents of choice. Beta-blockers are contraindicated as they may cause unopposed adrenergic stimulation [15–17].

Among the anesthetic drugs, ketamine and succinylcholine should be avoided. Ketamine may enhance the hypertensive response of cocaine, while succinylcholine may enhance the duration of action of cocaine by sharing the pseudocholinesterase for its own metabolism.

Inhaled cocaine may cause burns in the airway mucosa and a reactive airway. Cocaine inhalers prevent exhaling the drug by applying the Valsalva maneuver and, as a result, may develop pneumothorax, pneumomediastinum and pneumopericardium [18–20].

Similarly, other psychotropic drugs like marijuana and synthetic cannabinoids may also have serious adverse implications in perioperative management, which the treating team must be aware of.

6.3 Airway Management in Trauma Patients

Trauma patients may have maxillofacial injury, blunt or penetrating neck injury, laryngeal or major bronchial disruption, cervical spine instability, etc. All these make airway management typically challenging. A pre-existing anatomical predisposition to a difficult airway may be further complicated by repeated attempts at laryngoscopy and intubation.

Since trauma patients have limited lung reserves, they are likely to develop serious hypoxemia, which can seriously jeopardize the outcome of any further management. Hence, a predefined sequential approach of airway management needs to be adopted; the American Society of Anaesthesiologists Committee on Trauma and Emergency Preparedness guidelines [21] for difficult airway management in trauma patients need to be adhered to. Some aspects of difficult airway management shall be dealt with in various sections of this chapter. While managing difficult airway in trauma, there should be a low threshold for emergency invasive airway access and surgical airway access.

Induction of anesthesia for securing a definitive airway has certain basic principles which need to be adhered to. Firstly, all the patients undergoing an emergency surgery should be considered full stomach and at risk for aspiration. Hence, rapid sequence induction should be done. For further details on rapid sequence induction, also refer to the section on management of cervical spine injury of this chapter.

Secondly, all the patients having major trauma and requiring induction of anesthesia should be considered hemodynamically unstable and to have a low intravascular volume; wide bore (16G or more) intravenous cannula, real-time invasive intraarterial blood pressure monitoring, warm intravenous fluid, vasopressor infusions and transcutaneous/defibrillation pads should be handy and applied. Hemodynamic stability is primary determinant of the anesthesia plan for induction. Since the intravascular volume is contracted, the volume of distribution for the drugs is also less; hence, less than usual doses are sufficient and administration of usual doses can lead to serious adverse effects [22, 23]. In hemodynamically stable patients, a short-acting cardioneutral hypnotic agent may be used. Etomidate, due to its least effect on hemodynamic stability, is our agent of choice, the usual dose is 0.15–0.3 mg/kg. In hemodynamically unstable patient, a dose of 0.1–0.15 mg/kg may be sufficient. Other agents like ketamine (0.5–1 mg/kg intravenously) or propofol (0.5–1.0 mg/kg) may be used. Ketamine should be used with extreme caution in patients having suspicion of amphetamine or cocaine poisoning. The epileptogenic property of ketamine makes it a less preferred agent for induction of anesthesia in trauma patient who are also likely to have head trauma.

The anaesthesiologist should have an in-depth knowledge of the salient difference between the various available In our practice, in any patient having hypotension with tachycardia, phenylephrine is vasopressor of choice; a bolus of 50–100 μg suffices, and if repeated boluses are needed, then an infusion of phenylephrine 0.1–1 μg/kg/min can be started. We use Norepinephrine infusion for patients who, in addition to vasoconstriction, also require an increase in heart rate or cardiac contractility. Vasopressin (0.01–0.04 units/min) is used for hypotension resistant to catecholamines and sympathomimetics. Vasopressin has little effect on the peripheral vascular resistance and exerts its effect mainly through splanchnic vasoconstriction. Epinephrine has a dose-dependent differential effect on the beta-adrenergic and alpha-adrenergic receptors; alpha-adrenergic receptors are stimulated at higher doses (0.1–1 μg/kg/min); at this vasopressor dose, it causes extreme tachycardia. Hence, epinephrine is usually indicated for cardiac arrest situations and anaphylactic shock.

6.4 Opioids in Trauma Patients

Although opioids are useful adjuvants to intravenous induction agents, they can worsen the hypotension during induction. Besides, opioids are comparatively slower to act and take several minutes to produce their full effect. Hence, they may not be suitable for patients with major trauma who require rapid induction and endotracheal tube insertion. Opioids are usually skipped at induction and are usually given during the maintenance phase. The most commonly used opioid is fentanyl. Hemodynamic stability is the main determinant for the dose of opioids. The usual practice is to administer fentanyl in a dose of small boluses (50 μg) every 15–20 min, and if the hemodynamics remain stable (Systolic >90 mmHg) then bigger boluses are administered. With ever-changing blood volume (due to ongoing blood loss and intravenous transfusions) the quantity of opioids administered in hemodynamically stable patients is more than usual and may vary between 10 and 30 μg/kg during the surgical procedure. Opioids have a beneficial effect on microcirculation and, hence, should be used as soon as possible [24, 25].

Since patients who are hemodynamically unstable may not tolerate an adequate dose of anesthetic agents for maintenance of anesthesia, they are at high risk for intraoperative awareness [26]. Hence, in hemodynamically labile patients, we give intermittent boluses of midazolam along with opioids [27].

6.5 Temperature Management

Trauma patients undergoing surgery are at a great risk of developing hypothermia. All efforts should be made to maintain euthermia. Active and passive warming techniques of thermoregulation should be applied wherever possible. While making efforts for maintaining euthermia, a close watch should be kept on complications of hypothermia. Even mild hypothermia (>1–2° fall in the core temperature) may predispose the patient to the development of coagulopathy [28–30], delayed metabolism of drugs [31–34], hemodynamic instability [35], infections [36], etc.

6.6 Lung Protective Ventilation

While ventilating trauma victims, the goal is to maintain a balance between oxygenation and hemodynamic stability. A tidal volume of 6–8 mL/kg is considered sufficient. A haemoglobin saturation of up to 90% or more is acceptable, hyperoxia is avoided [27, 37]. Permissive hypercapnia (etCO2 40–45 mmHg) is acceptable in the absence of brain injury. A positive end-expiratory pressure (PEEP) may lead to hemodynamic instability and hence should be used judiciously. While mechanically ventilating trauma patients, a close watch must be kept on increasing intrathoracic pressure due to worsening pneumothorax or dynamic hyperinflation of the lung (auto-PEEP). In patients with severe injury to the lung or the airway, extracorporeal membrane oxygenation (ECHMO) may be a viable option [38].

6.7 Intraoperative Fluid Management

Trauma patients may require infusion of large volume of fluids, balanced salt solution is the preferred fluid for resuscitation. Large volume of normal saline infusion may lead to hyperchloremic acidosis. In patients requiring large volume of resuscitation, a combination of crystalloid and colloids is used [39, 40]. This approach of combining crystalloids and colloids is helpful in restricting the quantity of fluid administered and is usually applicable till the blood products are being arranged. Albumin is the preferred colloid. Colloids are usually avoided in patients with traumatic brain injury. A goal-directed approach of fluid administration is considered to improve the perioperative outcome [41, 42].

Dynamic hemodynamic parameters like left ventricular volume in transoesophageal echocardiography (TEE) and respirophasic variation in the arterial pressure waveform are better than the static parameters like heart rate, blood pressure, urine output, central venous pressure and pulmonary capillary wedge pressure [43–45].

In hemorrhaging trauma patients, blood and blood products must be transfused as soon as they are available.

6.8 Anesthesia for Chest Trauma

Chest trauma may be penetrating or blunt. For emergency evaluation of a patient with chest trauma, kindly refer to the chapter on resuscitation. Initial resuscitation and management strategies are based on advanced trauma and life support (ATLS) protocols. While dealing with chest trauma, again, airway and oxygenation take precedence over breathing and circulation.

Focused assessment with sonography in trauma (FAST) is a useful systematic approach in patients with blunt trauma to the abdomen. It examines for presence of blood in the peritoneal cavity by examining the hepatorenal pouch, peri-splenic space, pericardium and pelvis. Extended FAST (e-FAST) also incorporates the sonography of anterior chest to rule out pneumothorax.

Chest trauma patients may have hemoptysis; however, life-threatening hemoptysis is uncommon [46]; expectoration of more than half a cup of blood or 100 mL in an hour is considered life-threatening [47]. Massive hemoptysis may cause airway obstruction, prevent gas exchange or may cause hemodynamic instability due to exsanguination. Patients with ongoing hemoptysis should be kept in lateral decubitus with the bleeding side down and all efforts to maintain oxygenation and hemodynamic stability need not be emphasized. Lung isolation is of paramount importance in patients with ongoing massive hemoptysis. If the bleeding side is known, then a broad cuffed endotracheal tube may be proceeded into the non-bleeding side to achieve lung isolation. Lung isolation techniques like double-lumen tubes (DLTs) or bronchial blockers may not be feasible in chest trauma-associated massive hemoptysis. DLTs become mandatory in patients who are not able to maintain adequate oxygenation with single-lumen endobronchial intubation. DLTs allow ventilation of both the lungs and prevent contamination of the other lung, but have their own set of limitations.

Non-penetrating Precordial Injury While penetrating precordial injuries are often fatal due to hemorrhage shock or cardiac tamponade. More frequently, patients making to the operating room have blunt precordial trauma. In blunt precordial trauma, there may be minimal external manifestation of an internal injury. In blunt precordial trauma, the right ventricle is most commonly injured due to its anterior location, followed by the left ventricle [46, 48]. FAST may reveal any cardiac tamponade that might have developed as a result of such injury. Cardiac tamponade should be ruled out in any hypotensive trauma patient without an obvious ongoing blood loss. The onset of hypotension is directly proportional to the rate of accumulation of blood in the pericardial cavity. If the pericardial blood is getting intermittently spilled into the pleural cavity, the symptoms may be less dramatic and may get missed on initial evaluation.

Cardiac tamponade that is making the patient hemodynamically unstable, needs to be evacuated by pericardiocentesis. However, pericardiocentesis may be challenging in case a small amount of blood is causing the tamponade physiology (cardiac tamponade in coexisting constrictive pericarditis) or if the blood in the pericardial space is clotted. While arrangements for pericardiocentesis are being made, the goal of management is to keep the heart "full, fast and strong" by administration of intravenous fluids, vasopressors, and inotropes.

Blunt trauma to the chest may cause cardiac contusion, which may manifest as minor dysrhythmias or may cause severe myocardial dysfunction. However, it rarely leads to cardiogenic shock [48, 49].

However, it is not only penetrating trauma that can causes massive intrathoracic bleed, but patients having rapid deceleration in a high-energy collision may have severe major vessel injuries, which may be an immediate threat to life. Management of severe aortic injury and penetrating cardiac injury may require thoracotomy in the emergency department and is beyond the scope of this chapter.

A penetrating injury can damage the tracheobronchial tree also, this damage may be any part of the tracheobronchial tree. Blunt trauma to the chest in high energy collision can lead to disruption of the bronchus from the trachea; a spot 2–3 cm distal to the carina on the right side being most vulnerable [50]. The presence of pneumothorax, subcutaneous emphysema, hemoptysis, and bubbling of airway from a gaping wound are signs of tracheobronchial injury. While securing the airway in patients with such injuries, the most vulnerable spot of tracheobronchial shearing should be kept in mind. Most prudent approach would be to insert an appropriately sized Double Lumen Tube. A pre-shaped styleted single lumen endotracheal tube may be easier to insert. If vision permits, a flexible fiberoptic bronchoscope may be extremely useful in the endobronchial placement of the endotracheal tube (ETT).

Pulmonary contusion is much more common injury encountered in trauma patients (65%) but has less dramatic presentation [51]. Pulmonary contusion has to be suspected in any patient having tachypnea, hypoxia, wheezing or hemoptysis.

E-FAST may give the earliest signs of pulmonary contusion; computed tomography and chest X-rays may not show any changes till several hours after the trauma. Pulmonary contusion disrupts the alveolar-capillary gas exchange interface, leading to arteriovenous shunting. Patients with pulmonary contusion may develop atelectasis and may culminate into respiratory distress syndrome. ECHMO may be necessary if the lung contusion is massive enough to cause severe impairment of gas exchange.

While dealing with any patient having blunt trauma to the chest and receiving positive pressure ventilation, a close watch should be kept on the airway pressures. An increase in driving pressures may be a harbinger of development of or worsening of pneumothorax. A small pneumothorax may convert into a tension pneumothorax.

Chest trauma may be associated with rib fractures. A rib may get fractured at more than one place and may create a flail segment. While isolated rib fractures without any underlying lung injury may be managed with multimodal analgesia techniques, a flail segment may lead to ineffective ventilation, hypoxemia, lung collapse, etc., in a spontaneously breathing patient.

6.9 Anesthesia for Orthopedic Trauma

Fractures of the long bones are very common in trauma settings and may be associated with injury to the other organs as well. While deciding the anesthesia plan for an orthopedic trauma, patient's hemodynamic status and consciousness are the two most important factors to be considered. Basic principles of advanced trauma life support are the basis for the management of orthopedic trauma.

Perioperative fat embolism needs special consideration. Subclinical fat embolism occurs in majority of patients with long bone and pelvic fractures. Fat embolism syndrome occurs in 0.5% of patients and is especially common in the patients with bilateral long bone fractures and during reaming for nailing and arthroplasties [52, 53]. Signs of fat embolism syndrome are non-specific and manifest as tachycardia, hypoxemia and altered sensorium; the management is supportive. Usually, the patients recover well but may progress to develop adult respiratory distress syndrome (ARDS) and multiorgan failure.

6.10 Anesthesia for Neurotrauma

Trauma victims are likely to have a high incidence of neurological injury. Identification and management of brain and SCI are vital in achieving a purposeful recovery in trauma patients. In a case with polytrauma, neurological injury may be difficult to rule out, and hence, anesthesia should be planned accordingly.

All the patients of trauma should be considered to have cervical spine injury unless proven otherwise; neck movement while intubation should be minimized as far as possible [54–56]. While intubating head tilt maneuvers should be avoided, the assistance of a video or a fiberoptic laryngoscope is extremely useful in minimizing neck movement in pursuit of securing the airway. Nasal route of endotracheal tube insertion should be discouraged in trauma patient due to the possibility of associated skull base fracture [57].

Induction agents like propofol, thiopentone or etomidate in titrated sleeping dose can be used to facilitate laryngoscopy and intubation. These agents cause cerebral vasoconstriction that results in decrease in cerebral blood flow (CBF), cerebral blood volume and intracranial pressure (ICP) with decrease in cerebral metabolic rate for oxygen (CMRO2) [58]. Narcotics, when used in clinical doses, cause a minimal to moderate decrease in CBF and CMRO2. Hypotension should be avoided in patients with suspected head injury as it may lead to cerebral hypoperfusion. During maintenance phase, mild hypocapnia or normocapnia (PaCO2 30–35), PaCO2 less than 30 may cause cerebral ischemia, especially in the first 24 h after neurotrauma. Inhalational agents in higher concentration (>1–1.5 MAC) are avoided as they lead to increased CBF and potential increase in ICP [58]. So, either inhalational agents up to 1 MAC or total intravenous anesthesia in the form of propofol and fentanyl/remifentanil is recommended. Normal saline is the preferred intravenous fluid of choice. Glucose-containing fluid can cause hyperglycaemia, which is an independent risk factor for poor outcomes; a blood glucose level of 80–180 mg% is desirable [59]. Hyperosmolar fluids help achieve brain relaxation; hypertonic saline is considered to have better treatment response than mannitol [60].

Extubation should be smooth with avoidance of hypertension and coughing; a concerted decision of extubation should be taken by the surgeon and the anaesthesiologist.

Traumatic brain injury may be associated with many systemic complications like diabetes insipidus, syndrome of inappropriate antidiuretic hormone secretion (SIADH) and cerebral salt wasting syndrome, which may have important perioperative implications.

Apart from traumatic brain injury, traumatic spine injury also incurs important anesthetic implications. The manifestations of SCI depend on the spinal level of trauma. While a high SCI (above C5 level) is likely to cause respiratory compromise resulting in respiratory failure, an injury at the thoracic level is likely to make the patient hemodynamically labile. Neurogenic shock that ensues almost immediately following an SCI is likely to cause hypotension, bradycardia and hypothermia and may last up to 6 weeks [61]. Although, neurogenic shock is most seen in injuries above the T5 level, it can happen even in injuries at a lower level. Almost 70% of patients in neurogenic shock have a heart rate which is less than 45/min; bradycardia is usually at its worse on Day 4 and usually recovers over 2–6 weeks after injury [62]; these patients may develop cardiac arrest during airway manipulation [63, 64].

In SCI above T5 level, as the acute phase of SCI resolves and enters into chronic phase, neurogenic shock is replaced by autonomic dysreflexia. Autonomic dysreflexia is characterized by excessive sympathetic stimulation in response to stimulus below the level of SCI. Sympathetic stimulation may follow stimulus like somatic pain, abdominal distention, faecal impaction and bladder distention.

Prolonged immobility also predisposes these patients to deep vein thrombosis.

All patients in the acute phase of SCI, should be considered at high risk of aspiration. During the spinal shock phase of SCI, gastric emptying is delayed [65]. Patients with SCI are likely to have hyponatremia due to the impairment of renal sympathetic pathway that regulates the renin-angiotensin system. Upregulation of the extra-junctional nicotinic acetylcholine receptors happens after 3 days of SCI-associated muscle denervation; succinylcholine administration in this group of patients can cause serious hyperkalaemia.

Prone surgical position for spinal surgery may significantly increase the intracranial pressure, which may be detrimental in patients also having traumatic brain injury.

During surgery for SCI, intraoperative neuromonitoring (IONM) is frequently used; inhalational agents may interfere with IONM and hence should be avoided when IONM is planned. Administration of high dose of steroid is not recommended for the purpose of spinal cord protection, although it may improve the short-term outcome if given within 8 h of the injury.

6.11 Anesthesia for Burn Trauma

Frequently, trauma victims also have burn-related injuries [64, 66]. A burn is considered severe if it is associated with major trauma or inhalational injury, burns covering more than 20% of the body surface area, high voltage electric burns or chemical burns. Burn injuries in children and elderly patients are considered severe even if covering less than 20% of BSA. Baux score (age in years + burn area in percentage) or revised Baux score (age in years + burn area in percentage + 17 * [presence of inhalational injury]) correlates with mortality [67]. Patients with more than 20% burns should be treated preferably at a dedicated burn unit. Patients with >50% burns usually do not survive [68].

Patients with severe burns require a lot of fluids for resuscitation, which may lead to ileus, abdominal compartment syndrome, pulmonary edema, ARDS, etc. [69]. Chest wall eschars may cause respiratory compromise. Limb eschars may cause vascular compromise. Burn patients may have kidney dysfunction, which may be due to dehydration, usually in adults a urine output of 0.5–1.0 mL/kg/h and in children 1.0 mL/kg/h is desirable. In patients with high-voltage electric burns double the usual target of urine output is desirable. Burn patients are at a risk of venous thromboembolism and should be prescribed thromboprophylaxis as soon as possible [69].

Although the management of cutaneous burn has improved significantly, the same cannot be said for inhalational injuries. Inhalational injuries can occur with or without cutaneous burn injuries. Wheezing, stridor, hoarseness and tachypnoea are features of significant inhalational injury. Airway edema usually worsens beyond 18 h after the initial insult; hence, airway must be secured before the airway edema sets in or worsens. An awake fiberoptic examination of the airway is indispensable tool not only for securing the airway but also for airway toileting [70, 71]. Following intubation, the head must be kept elevated to prevent positional worsening of facial and airway edema.

Usually, inhalational injuries are associated with carbon monoxide poisoning or cyanide poisoning, making pulse oximetry deceptive. The half-life of carbon monoxide is 4–6 h, but administration of normobaric 100% oxygen reduces it to 45–60 min.

Especial ventilation modes like airway pressure release ventilation (APRV) and volumetric diffusive ventilatory (VDR) mode are considered superior to the conventional modes in the management of inhalational injury patients [72].

Adjuvant treatments like bronchodilators, inhaled *N*-acetylcysteine, inhaled heparin, nitric oxide, and corticosteroids have been found to be of limited utility in preventing progression of the lung injury following inhalational trauma [73–76].

6.12 Anesthesia for Pregnancy Trauma Victims

Pregnant females are more prone for trauma. For physical and physiological reasons, certain basic principles need to be taken care of while managing such patients. Every female in the childbearing age must be considered pregnant unless proven otherwise. Pregnant females must be considered full stomach and hence are prone for aspiration. Females with uterus above the umbilicus are prone for supine hypotension syndrome and, hence, must be placed either in a left lateral position or with a wedge under the right buttock. While managing hypotension, fluid and blood product administration must be given preference over vasopressors. During early pregnancy exposure to anesthetic agents may lead to miscarriage, hence appropriate consent is a must. Repeated or prolonged exposure to anesthetic agents increases the risk of developmental abnormalities. Although most of the anesthetics have been shown to be teratogenic in animal models, they have not been replicated in human-based studies, when administered on a discrete basis [77–86].

Sugammadex is a new reversal agent to reverse the action of steroidal neuromuscular blockers. Sugammadex chelates progesterone and hence may lead to shedding of uterine endometrium if administered early in the pregnancy or an irritable myometrium if administered in later part of the pregnancy [87]. Neuromuscular agents do not cross the placenta and, hence, do not have any significant effect on the newborn. Opioids can cross the placental barrier and may make the newborn dull, mandating care in a neonatal ICU.

Conclusion Road traffic accidents (RTAs) may cause serious and life-threatening multisystem involvement, which may require the highest level of care. Airway compromise, and hemorrhage are the most common acute cause of death. Hypothermia, massive blood transfusion and infections are the most common complications in the intermediate time frame. Neurotrauma has special anesthesia considerations, and these implications may remain relevant several weeks after the initial trauma.

References

1. Chapman R, Plaat F. Alcohol and anaesthesia. Continu Educ Anaesth Crit Care Pain. 2009;9(1):10–3.
2. Spies CD, Rommelspacher H. Alcohol withdrawal in the surgical patient: prevention and treatment. Anesth Analg. 1999;88(4):946–54.
3. Hunter JM, Parker CJ, Bell CF, Jones RS, Utting JE. The use of different doses of vecuronium in patients with liver dysfunction. Br J Anaesth. 1985;57(8):758–64.
4. van Miert MM, Eastwood NB, Boyd AH, Parker CJ, Hunter JM. The pharmacokinetics and pharmacodynamics of rocuronium in patients with hepatic cirrhosis. Br J Clin Pharmacol. 1997;44(2):139–44.
5. De Wolf AM, Freeman JA, Scott VL, et al. Pharmacokinetics and pharmacodynamics of cisatracurium in patients with end-stage liver disease undergoing liver transplantation. Br J Anaesth. 1996;76(5):624–8.
6. Thomas SD, Boyd AH. Prolonged neuromuscular block associated with acute fatty liver of pregnancy and reduced plasma cholinesterase. Eur J Anaesthesiol. 1994;11(3):245–9.
7. Aguayo LG, Peoples RW, Yeh HH, Yevenes GE. GABA(A) receptors as molecular sites of ethanol action. Direct or indirect actions? Curr Top Med Chem. 2002;2(8):869–85.
8. Tella SR, Schindler CW, Goldberg SR. Cardiovascular effects of cocaine in conscious rats: relative significance of central sympathetic stimulation and peripheral neuronal monoamine uptake and release mechanisms. J Pharmacol Exp Ther. 1992;262(2):602–10.
9. Tella SR, Schindler CW, Goldberg SR. Cocaine: cardiovascular effects in relation to inhibition of peripheral neuronal monoamine uptake and central stimulation of the sympathoadrenal system. J Pharmacol Exp Ther. 1993;267(1):153–62.
10. Hollander JE, Hoffman RS, Gennis P, et al. Prospective multicenter evaluation of cocaine-associated chest pain. Cocaine Associated Chest Pain (COCHPA) Study Group. Acad Emerg Med. 1994;1(4):330–9.
11. Koppel BS, Samkoff L, Daras M. Relation of cocaine use to seizures and epilepsy. Epilepsia. 1996;37(9):875–8.
12. Brody SL, Slovis CM, Wrenn KD. Cocaine-related medical problems: consecutive series of 233 patients. Am J Med. 1990;88(4):325–31.
13. Bourland JA, Martin DK, Mayersohn M. In vitro transesterification of cocaethylene (ethylcocaine) in the presence of ethanol. Esterase-mediated ethyl ester exchange esterase-mediated ethyl ester exchange. Drug Metab Dispos. 1998;26(3):203–6.
14. Herbst ED, Harris DS, Everhart ET, Mendelson J, Jacob P, Jones RT. Cocaethylene formation following ethanol and cocaine administration by different routes. Exp Clin Psychopharmacol. 2011;19(2):95–104.
15. Richards JR, Lange RA, Arnold TC, Horowitz BZ. Dual cocaine and methamphetamine cardiovascular toxicity: rapid resolution with labetalol. Am J Emerg Med. 2017;35(3):519.e511–4.
16. Öcal L, Çakir H, Tellice M, İzci S, Alizade E, Esen AM. Successful treatment of cocaine-induced cardiotoxicity with carvedilol therapy. Herz. 2015;40(1):159–61.
17. Lo KB, Virk HUH, Lakhter V, et al. Clinical outcomes after treatment of cocaine-induced chest pain with beta-blockers: a systematic review and meta-analysis. Am J Med. 2019;132(4):505–9.
18. Maeder M, Ullmer E. Pneumomediastinum and bilateral pneumothorax as a complication of cocaine smoking. Respiration. 2003;70(4):407.
19. Savader SJ, Omori M, Martinez CR. Pneumothorax, pneumomediastinum, and pneumopericardium: complications of cocaine smoking. J Fla Med Assoc. 1988;75(3):151–2.
20. Uva JL. Spontaneous pneumothoraces, pneumomediastinum, and pneumoperitoneum: consequences of smoking crack cocaine. Pediatr Emerg Care. 1997;13(1):24–6.
21. Hagberg CA, Kaslow O. Difficult airway management algorithm in trauma updated by COTEP. ASA Newsl. 2014;78:56.
22. Sikorski RA, Koerner AK, Fouchè-Weber LY, Galvagno SM. Choice of general anesthetics for trauma patients. Curr Anesthesiol Rep. 2014;4:225–32.

23. Egan ED, Johnson KB. The influence of hemorrhagic shock on the disposition and effects of intravenous anesthetics: a narrative review. Anesth Analg. 2020;130(5):1320–30.
24. Dutton RP. Resuscitative strategies to maintain homeostasis during damage control surgery. Br J Surg. 2012;99(Suppl 1):21–8.
25. Lin JY, Hung LM, Lai LY, Wei FC. Kappa-opioid receptor agonist protects the microcirculation of skeletal muscle from ischemia reperfusion injury. Ann Plast Surg. 2008;61(3):330–6.
26. Schneider G. [Intraoperative awareness]. Anasthesiol Intensivmed Notfallmed Schmerzther. 2003;38(2):75–84.
27. Messina AG, Wang M, Ward MJ, et al. Anaesthetic interventions for prevention of awareness during surgery. Cochrane Database Syst Rev. 2016;10(10):CD007272.
28. Valeri CR, Khabbaz K, Khuri SF, et al. Effect of skin temperature on platelet function in patients undergoing extracorporeal bypass. J Thorac Cardiovasc Surg. 1992;104(1):108–16.
29. Wolberg AS, Meng ZH, Monroe DM III, Hoffman M. A systematic evaluation of the effect of temperature on coagulation enzyme activity and platelet function. J Trauma. 2004;56(6):1221–8.
30. Rajagopalan S, Mascha E, Na J, Sessler DI. The effects of mild perioperative hypothermia on blood loss and transfusion requirement. Anesthesiology. 2008;108(1):71–7.
31. Heier T, Caldwell JE. Impact of hypothermia on the response to neuromuscular blocking drugs. Anesthesiology. 2006;104(5):1070–80.
32. Caldwell JE, Heier T, Wright PM, et al. Temperature-dependent pharmacokinetics and pharmacodynamics of vecuronium. Anesthesiology. 2000;92(1):84–93.
33. Heier T, Caldwell JE, Sessler DI, Miller RD. Mild intraoperative hypothermia increases duration of action and spontaneous recovery of vecuronium blockade during nitrous oxide-isoflurane anesthesia in humans. Anesthesiology. 1991;74(5):815–9.
34. Leslie K, Sessler DI, Bjorksten AR, Moayeri A. Mild hypothermia alters propofol pharmacokinetics and increases the duration of action of atracurium. Anesth Analg. 1995;80(5):1007–14.
35. Frank SM, Higgins MS, Breslow MJ, et al. The catecholamine, cortisol, and hemodynamic responses to mild perioperative hypothermia. A randomized clinical trial. Anesthesiology. 1995;82(1):83–93.
36. Kurz A, Sessler DI, Lenhardt R. Perioperative normothermia to reduce the incidence of surgical-wound infection and shorten hospitalization. Study of Wound Infection and Temperature Group. N Engl J Med. 1996;334(19):1209–15.
37. Baekgaard JS, Isbye D, Ottosen CI, et al. Restrictive vs liberal oxygen for trauma patients—the TRAUMOX1 pilot randomised clinical trial. Acta Anaesthesiol Scand. 2019;63(7):947–55.
38. Della Torre V, Robba C, Pelosi P, Bilotta F. Extra corporeal membrane oxygenation in the critical trauma patient. Curr Opin Anaesthesiol. 2019;32(2):234–41.
39. Myburgh JA, Finfer S, Bellomo R, et al. Hydroxyethyl starch or saline for fluid resuscitation in intensive care. N Engl J Med. 2012;367(20):1901–11.
40. Annane D, Siami S, Jaber S, et al. Effects of fluid resuscitation with colloids vs crystalloids on mortality in critically ill patients presenting with hypovolemic shock: the CRISTAL randomized trial. JAMA. 2013;310(17):1809–17.
41. Benes J, Giglio M, Brienza N, Michard F. The effects of goal-directed fluid therapy based on dynamic parameters on post-surgical outcome: a meta-analysis of randomized controlled trials. Crit Care. 2014;18(5):584.
42. Gan TJ, Soppitt A, Maroof M, et al. Goal-directed intraoperative fluid administration reduces length of hospital stay after major surgery. Anesthesiology. 2002;97(4):820–6.
43. Ansari BM, Zochios V, Falter F, Klein AA. Physiological controversies and methods used to determine fluid responsiveness: a qualitative systematic review. Anaesthesia. 2016;71(1):94–105.
44. Funk DJ, Kumar A. If the central venous pressure is [x], call me … maybe. Crit Care Med. 2013;41(7):1823–4.
45. Marik PE, Cavallazzi R. Does the central venous pressure predict fluid responsiveness? An updated meta-analysis and a plea for some common sense. Crit Care Med. 2013;41(7):1774–81.

46. Mondoni M, Carlucci P, Job S, et al. Observational, multicentre study on the epidemiology of haemoptysis. Eur Respir J. 2018;51(1):1701813.
47. Ibrahim WH. Massive haemoptysis: the definition should be revised. Eur Respir J. 2008;32(4):1131–2.
48. Orliaguet G, Ferjani M, Riou B. The heart in blunt trauma. Anesthesiology. 2001;95(2):544–8.
49. Maron BJ, Estes NA III. Commotio cordis. N Engl J Med. 2010;362(10):917–27.
50. Rossbach MM, Johnson SB, Gomez MA, Sako EY, Miller OL, Calhoon JH. Management of major tracheobronchial injuries: a 28-year experience. Ann Thorac Surg. 1998;65(1):182–6.
51. Devitt JH, McLean RF, Koch JP. Anaesthetic management of acute blunt thoracic trauma. Can J Anaesth. 1991;38(4 Pt 1):506–10.
52. Mellor A, Soni N. Fat embolism. Anaesthesia. 2001;56(2):145–54.
53. Giannoudis PV, Tzioupis C, Pape HC. Fat embolism: the reaming controversy. Injury. 2006;37(Suppl 4):S50–8.
54. Crosby ET. Airway management in adults after cervical spine trauma. Anesthesiology. 2006;104(6):1293–318.
55. Hauswald M, Sklar DP, Tandberg D, Garcia JF. Cervical spine movement during airway management: cinefluoroscopic appraisal in human cadavers. Am J Emerg Med. 1991;9(6):535–8.
56. Keller C, Brimacombe J, Keller K. Pressures exerted against the cervical vertebrae by the standard and intubating laryngeal mask airways: a randomized, controlled, cross-over study in fresh cadavers. Anesth Analg. 1999;89(5):1296–300.
57. Jung JY. Airway management of patients with traumatic brain injury/C-spine injury. Korean J Anesthesiol. 2015;68(3):213–9.
58. Cole CD, Gottfried ON, Gupta DK, Couldwell WT. Total intravenous anesthesia: advantages for intracranial surgery. Neurosurgery. 2007;61(5 Suppl 2):369–77; discussion 368–377.
59. Fogelholm R, Murros K, Rissanen A, Avikainen S. Admission blood glucose and short term survival in primary intracerebral haemorrhage: a population based study. J Neurol Neurosurg Psychiatry. 2005;76(3):349–53.
60. Han C, Yang F, Guo S, Zhang J. Hypertonic saline compared to mannitol for the management of elevated intracranial pressure in traumatic brain injury: a meta-analysis. Front Surg. 2022;8:765784.
61. Ditunno JF, Little JW, Tessler A, Burns AS. Spinal shock revisited: a four-phase model. Spinal Cord. 2004;42(7):383–95.
62. Lehmann KG, Lane JG, Piepmeier JM, Batsford WP. Cardiovascular abnormalities accompanying acute spinal cord injury in humans: incidence, time course and severity. J Am Coll Cardiol. 1987;10(1):46–52.
63. Raw DA, Beattie JK, Hunter JM. Anaesthesia for spinal surgery in adults. Br J Anaesth. 2003;91(6):886–904.
64. Yoo KY, Jeong CW, Kim SJ, Jeong ST, Shin MH, Lee J. Cardiovascular and arousal responses to laryngoscopy and tracheal intubation in patients with complete spinal cord injury. Br J Anaesth. 2009;102(1):69–75.
65. Kao CH, Ho YJ, Changlai SP, Ding HJ. Gastric emptying in spinal cord injury patients. Dig Dis Sci. 1999;44(8):1512–5.
66. Santaniello JM, Luchette FA, Esposito TJ, et al. Ten year experience of burn, trauma, and combined burn/trauma injuries comparing outcomes. J Trauma. 2004;57(4):696–700; discussion 691–700.
67. Osler T, Glance LG, Hosmer DW. Simplified estimates of the probability of death after burn injuries: extending and updating the baux score. J Trauma. 2010;68(3):690–7.
68. ABA Board of Trustees, Committee on Organization and Delivery of Burn Care. Disaster management and the ABA Plan. J Burn Care Rehabil. 2005;26(2):102–6.
69. Wise R, Jacobs J, Pilate S, et al. Incidence and prognosis of intra-abdominal hypertension and abdominal compartment syndrome in severely burned patients: pilot study and review of the literature. Anaesthesiol Intensive Ther. 2016;48(2):95–109.
70. Latenser BA. Critical care of the burn patient: the first 48 hours. Crit Care Med. 2009;37(10):2819–26.

71. Kasten KR, Makley AT, Kagan RJ. Update on the critical care management of severe burns. J Intensive Care Med. 2011;26(4):223–36.
72. Faucher LD, Conlon KM. Practice guidelines for deep venous thrombosis prophylaxis in burns. J Burn Care Res. 2007;28(5):661–3.
73. Sheridan RL, Hess D. Inhaled nitric oxide in inhalation injury. J Burn Care Res. 2009;30(1):162–4.
74. Enkhbaatar P, Murakami K, Cox R, et al. Aerosolized tissue plasminogen inhibitor improves pulmonary function in sheep with burn and smoke inhalation. Shock. 2004;22(1):70–5.
75. Adhikari N, Burns KE, Meade MO. Pharmacologic treatments for acute respiratory distress syndrome and acute lung injury: systematic review and meta-analysis. Treat Respir Med. 2004;3(5):307–28.
76. Palmieri TL. Use of beta-agonists in inhalation injury. J Burn Care Res. 2009;30(1):156–9.
77. Cohen-Kerem R, Railton C, Oren D, Lishner M, Koren G. Pregnancy outcome following non-obstetric surgical intervention. Am J Surg. 2005;190(3):467–73.
78. Czeizel AE, Pataki T, Rockenbauer M. Reproductive outcome after exposure to surgery under anesthesia during pregnancy. Arch Gynecol Obstet. 1998;261(4):193–9.
79. Dolovich LR, Addis A, Vaillancourt JM, Power JD, Koren G, Einarson TR. Benzodiazepine use in pregnancy and major malformations or oral cleft: meta-analysis of cohort and case-control studies. BMJ. 1998;317(7162):839–43.
80. Duncan PG, Pope WD, Cohen MM, Greer N. Fetal risk of anesthesia and surgery during pregnancy. Anesthesiology. 1986;64(6):790–4.
81. Fisher SC, Siag K, Howley MM, Van Zutphen AR, Reefhuis J, Browne ML. Maternal surgery and anesthesia during pregnancy and risk of birth defects in the National Birth Defects Prevention Study, 1997-2011. Birth Defects Res. 2020;112(2):162–74.
82. Friedman JM. Teratogen update: anesthetic agents. Teratology. 1988;37(1):69–77.
83. Kort B, Katz VL, Watson WJ. The effect of nonobstetric operation during pregnancy. Surg Gynecol Obstet. 1993;177(4):371–6.
84. Lind JN, Interrante JD, Ailes EC, et al. Maternal use of opioids during pregnancy and congenital malformations: a systematic review. Pediatrics. 2017;139(6):e20164131.
85. Mazze RI, Källén B. Reproductive outcome after anesthesia and operation during pregnancy: a registry study of 5405 cases. Am J Obstet Gynecol. 1989;161(5):1178–85.
86. Visser BC, Glasgow RE, Mulvihill KK, Mulvihill SJ. Safety and timing of nonobstetric abdominal surgery in pregnancy. Dig Surg. 2001;18(5):409–17.
87. Et T, Topal A, Erol A, Tavlan A, Kılıçaslan A, Uzun ST. The effects of Sugammadex on progesterone levels in pregnant rats. Balkan Med J. 2015;32(2):203–7.

Craniocerebral Trauma

7

Chirag Solanki

7.1 Introduction

Craniocerebral trauma (CCT) consists of a wide spectrum of mechanisms, pathology, severity, physiology and sequela. It is the most common cause of morbidity and mortality globally. Being the major cause of disability in young adults, predominantly males, it leads to loss of many valuable work-related life years. The incidence of CCT is increasing, due to industrialization and an increase in vehicular population, but unfortunately, the outcome has not improved significantly over the years, especially in developing countries, despite the progression of the medical field. The size of this preventable problem takes a toll on the economy of a nation due to psychosocial and financial burden caused.

Craniocerebral injury can be divided into two main components: cranial vault injuries and traumatic brain injuries (TBI). The management of craniocerebral injuries has evolved over the years. It is imperative for every neurosurgeon to be well-versed with the management, contemporary treatment options and guidelines for this most common injury. The knowledge about this silent epidemic, its epidemiology, severity and outcome would help us to structure health care services as well as rehabilitation programs.

7.2 Epidemiology

CCT is one of the major public health problems. In a recent review the incidence of CCT varies from 47 to 849 per 100,000 population per year. It has been estimated that annually, 64–74 million cases are present to healthcare facilities worldwide [1, 2]. The global incidence, according to the 2010 GBD project report, was around 200

C. Solanki (✉)
Consultant Neurosurgeon, Marengo CIMS Hospital, Ahmedabad, Gujarat, India

© The Author(s), under exclusive license to Springer Nature Singapore Pte Ltd. 2024

A. Agrawal et al. (eds.), *Special Considerations in Trauma Care*,
https://doi.org/10.1007/978-981-99-9662-9_7

cases per 100,000 per year, which translates to around 15 million cases per year [2]. On the other hand, analysis of the 2016 GBD study showed global incidence of 369 cases per 100,000 people, which showed a significant increase in incidence [3]. In the same study, the incidence in India was reported to be 455 cases per 100,000 population. This was believed to be underestimated due to non-documentation of mile cases, which do not report to emergency department or even the hospital. In a recent report, the global incidence is estimated at 939 cases per 100,000 people. The annual incidence as proportion of population was found to be highest (1.6%) in SEAR countries [2]. The exact incidence of CCT in India remains clouded due to lack of quality national registry as well as large-scale epidemiological studies. According to a report published in 1991, at that time, in India, there were 1% of total vehicles of the world, but India contributed to 6% of total road traffic accidents (RTA) in the world [4]. Considering the steep rise in the number of vehicles in India, there would be a proportional increase in the number of RTAs in India.

CCT is more frequently, around 60–70%, found to affect young adults 20–40 years of age. The most common cause of head injury is RTA followed by falls and assaults. The proportion of mild CCT is around 80% and of severe CCT around 8% [2].

CCT is the leading cause of death worldwide, more than one-third of all injury-related deaths [5–7]. A recent national review reported one-third of all deaths in hospitals are due to injuries and more than half of them have CCT [8, 9]. Almost all patients with severe CCT, 50% of patients with moderate and around 20% of those with mild CCT suffer from physical or psychosocial disabilities, who require further measures for rehabilitation [10].

7.3 Biomechanics and Pathophysiology of CCT

Craniocerebral injury is transient or persistent brain dysfunction with or without involvement of the cranial vault due to suprathreshold loading as a result of head movement and/or collision between the head and an object or a surface. This is actually a continuum of events rather than a one-time occurrence (Fig. 7.1).

The mechanical load is the initiator of craniocerebral injury cascade. It leads to dynamic changes in head motion, which in turn is transduced to brain leading to various types of injuries (Fig. 7.2).

There are different types of loads that lead to different types of injuries due to different loading conditions, i.e. rate, force and impact area. Based on the same the mechanical loading can be classified as shown in Fig. 7.3. The endpoint of this mechanical load is primary injury, which in turn initiates the process of secondary injury.

The components of secondary injury are summarized in Table 7.1.

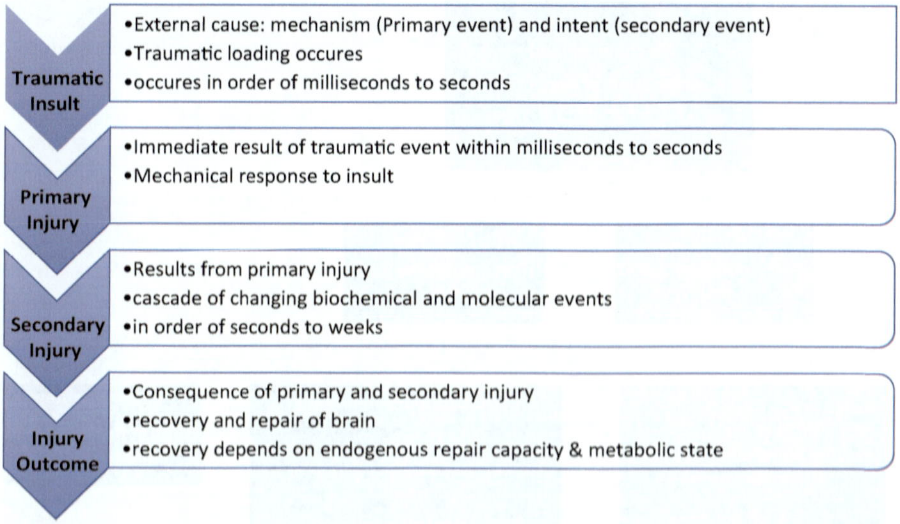

Fig. 7.1 Craniocerebral injury continuum

Fig. 7.2 Event biomechanics of primary injury

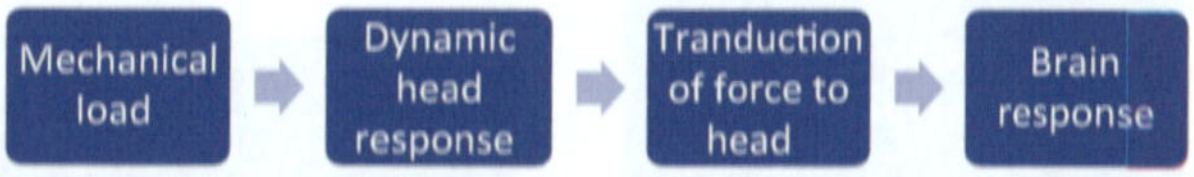

7.4 Classifications of CCT

1. **Classification by mechanism**
   (a) Closed/blunt injury:
   - It is caused by direct force to head along with acceleration, deceleration, or rotational forces.
   - Common causes are road traffic accidents, falls, and assaults.

   (b) Blast injury:
   - It is caused by high-pressure waves generated by explosives. A significant amount of mechanical, thermal, and electromagnetic energy is transferred to cranium.
   - It causes damage to blood vessels, blood-brain barrier and gray white matter junction.

   (c) Penetrating injury:
   - Common causes are gunshot wounds, shrapnel, and knife injuries.
   - It is a direct injury due to penetration along with force applied to the small area of vault.
2. **Clinical classification based on Glasgow Coma Scale (GCS):**

Severity of injury	GCS
Mild	13–15

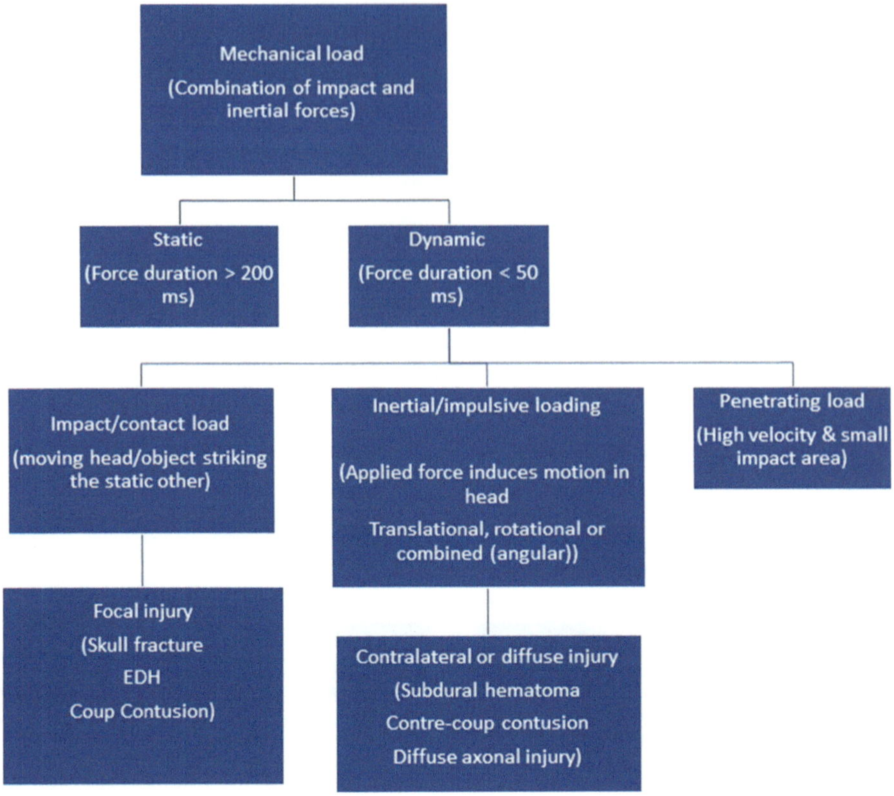

Fig. 7.3 Types of mechanical loading

Severity of injury	GCS
Moderate	9–12
Severe	3–8

3. **Classification based on location of structural damage or hemorrhage:**
   ***Cranial Vault Injuries*:**
   (a) **Subgaleal Hematoma:**
   - It is the bleeding into the subgaleal space and appears as a boggy swelling over the scalp.
   - In most the instances, it does not require any treatment.

   (b) **Skull Fractures:**
   - It can be caused by both blunt and penetrating injuries.
   - It is classified into closed and open/compound fracture based on the integrity of overlying scalp skin.
   - The skull base fractures and those involving inner table of frontal sinuses are a risk factors for cerebrospinal fluid leak.

Table 7.1 Components of secondary insult following craniocerebral trauma

Components	Pathological process
Chemical imbalance	– Abnormal ion homeostasis: mitochondrial damage and aberrant cell signaling – ↑ Excitatory neurotransmitters: excitotoxicity and network disturbances
Impaired metabolism	– Hypoxia and impaired perfusion – Fluctuation in glucose metabolism and metabolic demand
Molecular degradation	– Enzyme activation: cellular damage, membrane damage and impaired signaling – Free radicals: degradative process
Diffuse axonal injury and axonal damage	– Impaired axolemmal permeability – Cytoskeletal damage: impaired axonal transport and axonal swelling – Oligodendrocyte damage: myelin degradation, white matter changes and impaired network function
Vascular dysfunction	– Blood-brain barrier disruption – Vascular leakage and micro-bleeding: toxicity, hypoxia and hematoma – Uncoupling of CBF and metabolism: hyperemia, ↓ CPP, edema, raised ICP
Inflammation	– Microglia activation, pro- and anti-inflammatory processes
Cerebral edema	– Osmolality changes, high hydrostatic pressure and cellular swelling
Cell death and cytotoxicity	– Apoptosis and autophagy – Necrosis

***Traumatic Brain Injuries (TBI)*:**

(c) **Extradural Hematoma (EDH):**
- It is a collection of blood in epidural space.
- Usually, it is of arterial origin with middle meningeal artery being the most common source.
- It does not cross suture lines and typically it appears biconvex on imaging.
- It has got relatively better postsurgical outcome.

(d) **Subdural Hematoma (SDH):**
- It is a collection of blood in subdural space. It may be acute or chronic.
- It is caused mainly by tears in the bridging veins.
- It extends over the entire hemisphere and is of concavo-convex shape.
- It has got relatively poor outcome as compared to EDH.

(e) **Diffuse Axonal Injury (DAI):**
- It is the microscopic injury to axons at gray-white matter junction due to the inertial loading, mainly in acceleration–deceleration forces.
- On presentation, it may appear as a severe type of injury but overall long-term prognosis is better than that of acute SDH.

(f) **Traumatic Subarachnoid Hemorrhage (tSAH):**
- It is collection of blood in subarachnoid space.
- It is considered a poor prognostic factor in severe TBI.

(g) **Intraventricular Hemorrhage (IVH)**
- Post-traumatic intraventricular hemorrhage can cause acute or delayed hydrocephalus.
- It also is considered a poor prognostic factor in severe TBI.

(h) **Contusions:**
- It is the parenchymal hemorrhage, coup or contrecoup, typically located in frontal and temporal lobes.
- When the hematoma is extending to the surface and is associated with acute subdural hematoma, it is termed as "burst lobe".
- It should be differentiated from the post-traumatic hemorrhagic venous infarct, which is of mixed density type and located in the territory of major cortical veins like vein of Labbe.

7.5 Management of Craniocerebral Injuries

Craniocerebral injuries have the best prognosis when managed timely. These timely interventions are pivotal in preventing the secondary brain insult caused by various factors, as discussed above. There are several guidelines published for the management of these injuries. The brain trauma foundation guideline (fourth edition) is widely followed around the world. But, in the case of developing countries like India, there might be feasibility issues in widely implementing these guidelines. In response to that, a multiorganizational committee, of the members from the American Association of South Asian Neurosurgeons and American Association of Physicians of Indian Origin, formed consensus recommendations for the Indian subcontinent. Very recently, the Neurotrauma Society of India in collaboration with Neurological Society of India, has published "National Guidelines for the Management of Traumatic Brain Injury".

In these guidelines, authors have laid down specific recommendations for prehospital management as well as for in-hospital care at various levels of hospital setups. We have summarized the recommendations as detailed recommendations are out of scope of this chapter. So, readers are requested to refer to this publication for detailes of these recommendations.

7.5.1 Prehospital Management Guidelines

Prehospital emergency care is a crucial link in the chain of CCT care. The initial 60 min, i.e. "the golden hour", are of immense importance by which the patient should be transported to the nearby trauma care facility. It is important to educate and train the personnel involved in prehospital care to improve the outcomes.

The principal tasks to be accomplished by the prehospital management team are as follows:

- Reduced time to give prehospital care.

- Perform full spinal immobilization.
- Securing and maintaining the airway and providing high flow of oxygen.
- Maintain systolic blood pressure >90 mmHg by stopping external bleeding, splinting long bone fractures and higher rate of infusion of isotonic fluids.
- Recognition of severe injuries and injuries with potential to cause rapid decompensation.
- Efficient triage of multiple victims.
- Early stabilization and swift transport to a trauma care facility.

7.5.2 In-Hospital Management Guidelines

The first line of management on arrival to hospital would be to follow standard "ABC"—"airway, breathing, circulation" protocol. The details regarding the same can be found in these guidelines as well as in other resources.

As mentioned earlier, the primary goal of management of CCT would be to limit the secondary brain injury. To achieve that goal, optimization of oxygenation and maintaining blood pressure and intracranial pressure to achieve adequate cerebral perfusion pressure is of paramount importance. Also, maintaining temperature and glucose levels as well as treatment of seizures and other potential causes of secondary brain insult are of great importance.

Once the patient is stabilized, the next step is to evaluate the presence or absence and determine the severity of craniocerebral injuries. The computerized tomographic scan (CT) is the investigation of choice in an emergency setting due to adequacy of information provided as well as the rapidity by which the CT scan can be performed. The indications for performing the CT scan, National Guidelines for the Management of Traumatic Brain Injury, Neurotrauma Society of India, 2022, are as follows.

- GCS score less than 13 on the initial assessment.
- GCS score less than 15 at 2 h after the injury.
- Amnesia for the event.
- Suspected penetrating or depressed fracture.
- Suspected base of skull fracture (hemotympanum, "panda" eyes, cerebrospinal fluid leakage from the ear or nose, Battle sign).
- Post-traumatic seizure.
- Focal neurological deficit.
- Two or more episodes of vomiting.
- Patient on antiplatelet drugs or anticoagulants.
- History of coagulopathy.
- Persistent headache, nausea, giddiness, and restlessness.
- Before clearance for anesthesia for other injuries (do not delay emergency surgery to control hemorrhagic shock).
- Tense anterior fontanelle (in infants).

In case of worsening of GCS or development of fresh neurological deficit, bradycardia or hypertension, persistent headache, vomiting or restlessness, or initial abnormal CT scan may warrant for a repeat CT scan at 24-h intervals or earlier. Based on CT scan findings, the severity of CCT can be determined. Based on clinical and radiological severity of injury, the decision regarding necessity of surgical intervention is made. Although there are several recommendations regarding surgical intervention in literature like volume of EDH of more than 30 cm^3, width of SDH of more than 10 mm or midline shift of more than 5 mm etc., are in place, the final decision-making does not depend on these absolute numbers. It is the overall clinical judgement of a neurosurgeon, based on clinical status as well as radiological findings, which determines the surgical decision. The details regarding surgical interventions are out of the scope of this chapter. Once the patient is admitted, regardless of surgical intervention, it is important to monitor the patient closely and manage fluid and electrolyte balance, ventilation, anticonvulsants and other drugs and raised ICP.

The management of raised ICP is of pivotal importance to maintain CPP and prevent secondary brain injury. The general principles of management of raised ICP are as follows:

- Elevation of head above heart level to facilitate venous return.
- Maintenance of neck in a neutral position.
- Adequate control of temperature, BP and maintaining smooth airway and breathing.
- Prevention of post-traumatic seizures.
- Maintaining proper fluid and electrolyte balance with special consideration to maintain normal sodium levels.

In case of clinical or radiological evidence of raised ICP mannitol or hypertonic saline or both in combination may be used. Mannitol is considered to be more effective in intermittent doses, not more than 6 h apart, with a total dose of 1–2 g/kg per day. This is because the effect of mannitol starts within 5–10 min with peak effect at around half an hour and lasts for 6 h. It is considered that Hypertonic saline, on the other hand, can be administered either continuously or as bolus dose with the target serum sodium level upto 150 mEq/L. In many studies and reviews, hypertonic saline is found to be superior in reduction of ICP. It also has got the advantage in patients with hypovolemia, renal diseases, pediatric patients, and prolonged treatment, as compared to mannitol.

There are specific situations where it is recommended to monitor ICP. The preferred method of monitoring of ICP is via externalized intraventricular catheter. It also has got the advantage of drainage of CSF, which may help to reduce the ICP when required. The following are the indications for ICP monitoring as per national guidelines.

- All salvageable patients with GCS of 3–8 and abnormal CT.

- In patients with GCS of 3–8 with normal CT if two or more of the following are present:
  - Age >40 years.
  - Unilateral or bilateral motor posturing.
  - SBP <90 mmHg.

The use of anticonvulsants as a prophylactic measure is recommended only for a week. This is because they are found to be effective only to prevent early post-traumatic seizures. The routine use of prophylactic antibiotics is not advisable. In the setting of agitation, for smooth ventilation or for procedures like intubation, splinting etc., sedation might be considered. It is advisable to use short-acting sedatives and, preferably, in an emergency room or ICU setting, as close monitoring of patients is must when sedatives are used.

7.6 Assessment of Severity of Injury

Once the patient is stabilized, the detailed documentation of severity of injury has to be done. Although there is no universally accepted system of documentation for all stages of TBI, Glassgow Coma Scale (GCS) is the most widely accepted system for documentation of severity. But, it also has got limitations. In case of neuromuscular blockade, state of intubation or sedation the assessment of the total score or component score (i.e. verbal score) would not be possible. It is observer-dependent score and more than 30% of inter-observer inaccuracies have been documented [11]. Apart from GCS, there are many other systems for characterization of injury.

- FOUR scores (Full Outline of Unresponsiveness): It includes eye response, motor response, brainstem reflexes and respiration.
- ACDU scale (Alert, confused, drowsy, unresponsive).
- AVPU scale (Alert, response to voice, response to pain, unresponsive).
- LCFS (Levels of cognitive functioning scale); it is also known as Rancho Los Amigos levels of cognitive functioning.
- MPAI-4 (Mayo Portland adaptability inventory): It is mainly designed for follow-up assessment. It measures three subsets—ability (sensory, motor, cognitive abilities), adjustment (mood, interpersonal interactions) and participation (social contacts, initiation, money management).
- Coma/Near-coma scale: There are eight parameters based on stimuli of sound, light, smell and nasal swab.
- DOCS (Disorders of consciousness scale): There are eight subscales based on stimuli responses).

7.7 Assessment of Outcome

The assessment of outcome is equally important and it helps in formulating a suitable and individualized rehabilitation program for patients. The most commonly used outcome assessment scores are GOS (Glasgow Outcome Scale), GOSE (Glasgow Outcome Scale Extended), DRS (Disability Rating Scale) and KPS (Karnofsky Performance Scale). The GOSE is an extension of GOS, in which the moderate and severe disabilities and also good recovery are each subdivided into two scores.

Apart from these, CRS-R (Coma Recovery Scale-Revised), also known as JFK Coma Recovery Scale, FIM (Functional Independence Measure), FAM (Functional Assessment Measure), Galveston Orientation and Amnesia Test and O-Log (Orientation Log) are other available systems for assessment of outcome. The details regarding all the mentioned scales and scores can be found in literature and are out of scope of this chapter.

7.8 Neurorehabilitation After CCT

Neurorehabilitation is an important aspect of continuum of care of patients with CCT. It should be an integral part of in-patient services provided to head injury patients. The ideal setup of neurorehabilitation requires a team of various specialists to provide complete care to a patient. The complete rehabilitation team consists of neurosurgeon, neurologist, orthopedic surgeon, chest physician, urologist, gastroenterologist, psychiatrist, physiatrist, neuropsychologist, speech therapist, physical therapist, pain physician, occupational therapist, orthotist, rehabilitation nurse, and a social worker.

The role of neurorehabilitation therapy is important deciding factor in moderate and severe brain injuries for better functional outcomes. The following are the important rehabilitation measures for better mobility and function:

- The muscle strengthening program is important for functional mobility skills.
- Balance training with or without virtual reality helps improve sitting, maintaining balance of head and dynamic standing balance.
- The vestibular rehabilitation using gaze and habituation exercises, compensatory training and correcting benign paroxysmal positional vertigo gradually corrects balance impairment as well as symptoms of vertigo.
- The body weight-supported treadmill training is considered highly effective in recovery of ambulation.
- The use of orthoses and specialized positioning may be used to prevent contractures and bed sores, help in mobility and maintain patient safety.
- The role of neuropsychologist and psychiatrist is important in mitigating behavioral impairments as well as psychiatric disturbances like depression and psychosis, related to post-traumatic stress and disabilities.

- The role of a neurosurgeon is indispensable in managing cranioplasty, post-cranioplasty complications, post-traumatic hydrocephalus or chronic subdural hematoma, refractory spasticity requiring surgical intervention, and other possible long-term surgical issues.
- Post-traumatic headaches not responding to traditional treatment, refractory seizures, involuntary movements, autonomic disturbances, and other issues need a neurologist's assistance.
- Issues like myositis ossificans, fixed contractures, and deformities require orthopedic intervention.
- The issues related to chronic bedridden states like bed sores, pneumonia, deep vein thrombosis and venous thromboembolism, recurrent urinary tract infection, neurogenic bladder, bladder, and bowel incontinence, etc., require specialty support from pulmonologist, urologist, and plastic surgeon.
- If there is likely to be prolonged dependency on tube feeding, then the gastroenterologist's help is required for placement of percutaneous endoscopic gastrostomy (PEG) or feeding jejunostomy (FJ).

7.9 Conclusion

In nutshell, the craniocerebral trauma is a global issue of concern. With provision of improved emergency care and improvements in protocol-based treatment have improved outcomes in craniocerebral injuries, at least in western world. In developing nations, it needs a robust system of prehospital management, hospital treatment protocol, and post-hospitalization rehabilitation to reduce mortality and morbidity, and to have a good overall functional outcome. Equal importance has to be given for prevention of these grave injuries by improving vehicle safety rules, improving road safety, and by using technology and artificial intelligence.

Acknowledgement and Suggested Readings Brain Trauma Foundation (BTF) guidelines for severe traumatic brain injury, fourth edition, 2016.

- National Guidelines for the Management of Traumatic Brain Injury, Neurotrauma Society of India (An NTSI-NSI Initiative), 2022.

References

1. Iaccarino C, Gerosa A, Viaroli E. Epidemiology of traumatic brain injury. Traumatic brain injury. 2021 [cited 2022 Jul 12]. p. 3–11. https://link.springer.com/chapter/10.1007/978-3-030-78075-3_1.
2. Dewan MC, Rattani A, Gupta S, Baticulon RE, Hung YC, Punchak M, et al. Estimating the global incidence of traumatic brain injury. J Neurosurg. 2019;130(4):1080–97.
3. James SL, Bannick MS, Montjoy-Venning WC, Lucchesi LR, Dandona L, Dandona R, et al. Global, regional, and national burden of traumatic brain injury and spinal cord injury,

1990-2016: a systematic analysis for the global burden of disease study 2016. Lancet Neurol. 2019;18(1):56–87. http://www.thelancet.com/article/S1474442218304150/fulltext.

4. Head injuries: a neglected field in India. Natl Med J India. 1999;4(2):53–4. https://pubmed.ncbi.nlm.nih.gov/29751451/.
5. Traumatic brain injury in the United States: emergency department visits, hospitalizations, and deaths, 2002-2006. [cited 2022 Jul 11]. https://stacks.cdc.gov/view/cdc/5571.
6. Parikh S, Koch M, Narayan RK. Traumatic brain injury. Int Anesthesiol Clin. 2007;45(3):119–35. https://pubmed.ncbi.nlm.nih.gov/17622833/.
7. Report to congress: traumatic brain injury in the United States | Concussion | Traumatic brain injury | CDC Injury Center. [cited 2022 Jul 12]. https://www.cdc.gov/traumaticbraininjury/pubs/tbi_report_to_congress.html.
8. Gururaj G. Epidemiology of injuries—a population based survey in Bangalore. In: Proceedings of the 6th world conference on injury prevention and control montreal, 2002.
9. World Health Organization. Injury prevention and control. An epidemiological survey of injuries in area of Municipal Corporation of Delhi, New Delhi. SEA injuries-5, 2003.
10. Gururaj G. An epidemiological approach to prevention: pre-hospital care and rehabilitation in neurotrauma. Neurol India. 1995;43(3):95–105.
11. Zuercher M, Ummenhofer W, Baltussen A, Walder B. The use of Glasgow Coma Scale in injury assessment: a critical review. Brain Inj. 2009;23(5):371–84. https://pubmed.ncbi.nlm.nih.gov/19408162/.

Trauma to the Skull Base

8

Abhinav Srivastava

Over the last few decades, there has been an increase in the incidence of the head injury due to faster means of transportation and also occupational accidents. Skull base injuries are invariably associated with the head injury caused by force of severe magnitude. Skull base injuries are frequently associated with blunt type of trauma in 90% of the cases in comparison to penetrating type of injuries such as caused by gunshot [1].

The injury varies from small linear fracture in cases associated with force of lesser magnitude, to very complex craniofacial damage with associated brain contusions, intracranial hematomas, dural tear, and vascular injury in injuries associated with force of considerable high force. The clinically inaccessible location of the skull base has caused challenges in the diagnosis and further treatment. Improvements in the diagnostic tool such as CT scan have increased the diagnostic accuracy of the skull base trauma, which was missed in earlier years.

The management of the skull base trauma requires coordinated move among different departments, namely, neurosurgeon, ENT surgeon, neuroradiologists, and maxillofacial surgeons.

The parts that are commonly involved with skull base trauma are orbit and paranasal sinus in anterior skull base, cavernous sinus, and intracavernous segment of carotid artery in middle part of the skull base sometimes even leading to carotid-cavernous fistula. Injury to the posterior aspect of the base of the skull involves laceration of the adjoining venous sinuses and may also cause instability of the craniocervical junction. The petrous bone is generally involved by trauma of high magnitude with involvement of both the middle and posterior part of the skull base. A detailed cranial nerve examination is of paramount importance in every case of skull base trauma and should be performed in conscious and cooperative patients.

A. Srivastava (✉)
Department of ENT, Rohilkhand Medical College and Hospital, Bareilly, UP, India

© The Author(s), under exclusive license to Springer Nature Singapore Pte Ltd. 2024
A. Agrawal et al. (eds.), *Special Considerations in Trauma Care*, https://doi.org/10.1007/978-981-99-9662-9_8

8.1 Anterior Skull Base Fracture

The most common mode of injury is direct frontal trauma causing fractures of the forehead and orbital roof with likely involvement of the cribriform plate.

It has two components (Fig. 8.1):

(a) Frontal component: The fractures in the region are confined to the upper third of the facial bone along with the superior orbital rim.
(b) Basal component: The fracture involves the cribriform plate along with ethmoidal roof and planum sphenoidale.

8.2 Classification of Frontobasal Fractures [2]

Type I: It is a linear fracture that is basically parallel to the cribriform plate, then it may extend further in posterior direction along the Sella and the petrous ridge there by separating the anterior and middle cranial fossa from that of the posterior cranial fossa. It can usually be caused with injury of a relatively lower magnitude. This is generally located more medially, and injury being confined to the medial third of the supra-orbital rim. It carries very less chances of associated complications like CSF rhinorrhea and associated intracranial injury.

Type II: They are located further laterally and are linear and vertical in orientation, involving frontal aspect of the calvarium and also anterior part of the skull base. It may further extend to involve the lateral two-thirds of the supra-orbital rim, the squamous portion of the temporal bone, the orbital roof, and the lateral orbital

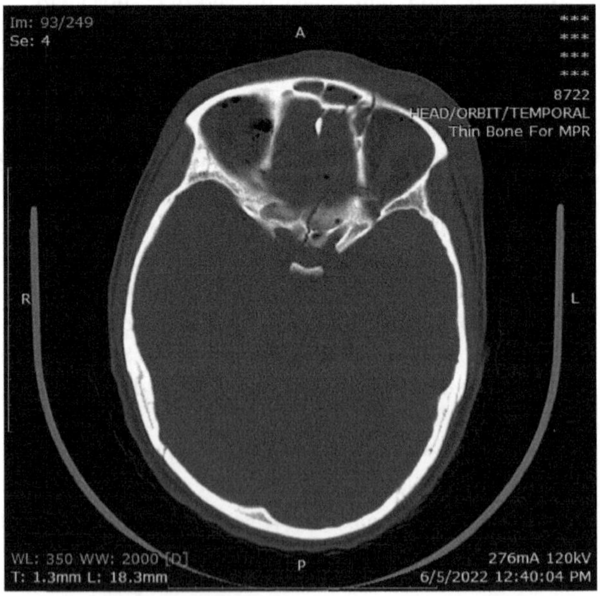

Fig. 8.1 Axial CT scan showing fracture of the anterior skull base

wall and may also involve the orbital apex. CSF leak is frequently associated with this type of fracture and may also be associated with certain intracranial injuries.

Type III: This type involves both the central as well as the lateral frontobasillar fractures and often in comminution with the entire frontal bone, orbital roof, and lateral cranial vault. This type of fracture is usually associated with impact of higher magnitude and carries the highest chance of CSF leak and associated intracranial injury.

Periorbital ecchymosis is one of the findings suggesting the trauma of the skull base and is also known as blepherohematoma. Depending on the impact and extent of the injury, it may also involve both sides. Anosmia is usually remain not detected initially due to the grave nature of the injury, and it is put to notice by the patient as the recovery progresses and sometimes after the complete recovery and the reason for this anosmia is attributed to the damage caused to the olfactory nerve following trauma. Associated CSF leakage occurs as a result of concomitant injuries of the bone and the adjoining duramater leading to the egress of the CSF. The site is variable and can be in the paranasal sinus in frontobasal fractures, middle ear, and mastoid in temporal bone fractures. Episodes of meningitis may follow in cases of persistent CSF leakage.

Impression It is clear from the above classification system that as the type progresses from I to III, more structures are involved both laterally and posteriorly. As a result, one will witness midface injuries more often with II and III type of fractures and are a result of impact of higher velocity trauma with vector from the lateral direction or with inferior frontal or supraorbital vector. So, the classification of the fracture is a very useful tool to interpret that type III fractures are associated with injury of relatively greater magnitude and carries a high chance of association with complications like intracranial hematoma and CSF leak.

8.3 Middle (Central) Skull Base Fractures

Types:

(a) Sagittal or oblique fracture
(b) Transverse fracture

Mechanism It is the extension of the frontobasal fractures as a result of the frontal impact along the sagittal or oblique vector passing through the central part of the skull base with involvement of the Sella and sphenoid sinus and may also involve the temporal bone.

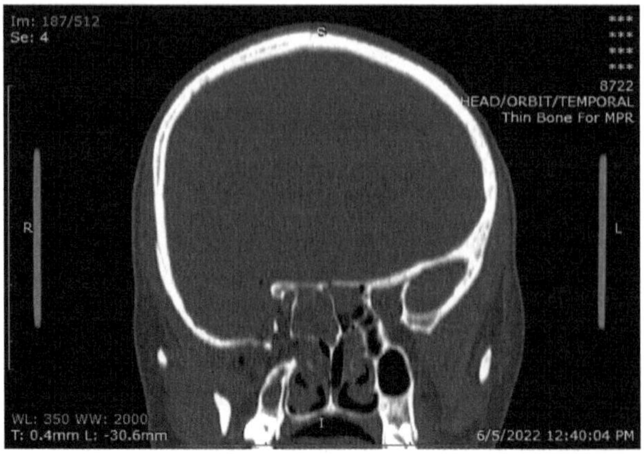

Fig. 8.2 Fracture of central skull base involving sphenoid sinus

It is caused as a result of the high-velocity impact in lateral direction to the lateral part of frontal bone, zygoma, temporal, or parietal bone, this may result in transverse fracture in coronal plane, which may further extend to the sphenoid sinus. It may further extend laterally if the impact is of even higher magnitude thereby involving the greater wing of the sphenoid bone, and squamosal part of temporal bone (Fig. 8.2).

If the transverse fracture is more toward in the anterior direction, then it may involve the posterior aspect of the anterior cranial fossa, with extension to the clinoid processes, and may involve orbital apex and the superior orbital fissure of both sides. This may also be associated with injuries involving cranial nerves and or vessels.

On the contrary, if the position of the fracture is more in the posterior direction, then it may cause involvement of the bilateral temporal bones which may further extend to involve sphenopetrosal synchondrosis, posterior portion of the sphenoid sinus, and/or the clivus. Injury of the mastoid process may lead to ecchymosis over the mastoid process known as Battle's sign.

Oblique type of central skull base fractures is mostly associated with fractures of the facial bones with type II and III frontobasal fractures and may be associated with CSF leak.

- Transverse type of fractures is more commonly associated with injury to vascular structures and damage to cranial nerves of varying degrees.

It is rare to see fracture of the clivus in cases involving central and posterior part of skull base fractures and it accounts in about 2% of all cranial fractures. A point of concern is the high mortality in up to 8% of cases and this is attributed to close proximity to the brainstem. High incidence of neurological manifestation with/without vascular injuries is also associated with it [3].

8.4 Clival Injury

There are two characteristic patterns of fracture [4]:

(a) Transverse or oblique fracture: These are caused as a result of lateral force of considerable magnitude which might result in crushing type of injury, and such types of injuries are commonly associated with injuries involving cranial nerves and may also cause injury of the internal carotid artery.
(b) Longitudinal fracture: These are seen in association with injuries at the cranio-cervical junction, and retro clival hematoma.
    - A hallmark of the clival fracture is the sixth cranial nerve palsy which is located in Dorello canal within the clivus. It may also be associated with other cranial nerve injuries.
    - There is less association of CSF leaks by extension of the fracture line to the sphenoid sinus.

As a result of the high-velocity impact, these are generally associated with intra-cranial injuries which may include associated multi-compartmental hemorrhage, contusion of the temporal lobe parenchyma, and even diffuse axonal injuries. All of these associated findings with complications should be managed accordingly.

Anterior middle cranial fossa epidural hematoma also known as benign Venom epidural hematoma occurs in concurrence with the injury of the greater wing of the sphenoid bone.

8.5 Posterior Skull Base Fractures

Mechanism There is a lateral and/or the posterior blow to the occipital region, and this may involve the occipital bone with possible extension to the petrous part of the temporal bone.

There occurs a wide variety of injuries due to presence of both vascular and neural structures. It includes the formation of hematoma in the extra and subdural region as well as in the cerebellar parenchyma. Hematoma in the epidural area of the posterior fossa is often venous which is mostly a result of the injury to the adjoining venous sinuses (transverse or sigmoid venous sinuses) or the jugular bulb.

It further predisposes to the formation of the thrombosis in the dural venous sinus. It may also be associated with long-term complications of formation of dural arteriovenous fistula and it can present with progressive worsening intracranial hypertension, venous infarction, or hemorrhage. There may also occur injuries of the lower cranial nerves.

8.5.1 Evaluation

The evaluation follows the standard protocol of trauma evaluation and this includes assessment first, a primary survey and as soon as the patient is stabilized secondary survey is undertaken which lays stress on the complete physical and neurological examination. A meticulous cranial nerve examination should be performed in all conscious and cooperative patients. Cranial nerve (CN) II, i.e., optic nerve can be assessed by visual acuity. Presence of extraocular movement of each eye confirms the integrity of CN III, IV, and VI as well as absence of damage to the extraocular muscles following trauma. Presence of hypoesthesia usually on one side of the face suggests damage to CN V of that side. Weakness of the muscles of the facial expression may be caused by facial nerve injury of that side as well as by injury of the muscles and must be distinguished by topo-diagnostic test of facial nerve function.

Assessment of the cranial nerve function in comatose patients is challenging and relies on testing the brain stem reflexes. The integrity of the optic and oculomotor nerves can be evaluated by the "**swinging flashlight test,**" which tests the intactness of the afferent pathway of CN II and efferent parasympathetic pathway of CN III. A case of damage of the unilateral afferent pathway of CN II is revealed by bilateral, and equal pupillary constriction in response to light given to the eye with intact vision. However, on providing the light toward the affected eye with diminished vision, pupils of both the eye will dilate. This phenomenon is well known as Marcus Gunn pupil.

The extraocular movements in a comatose patients can be tested with the help of oculocephalic (or "doll's-eye") reflex. The corneal reflex is tested by touching the cornea with a wisp of cotton; the afferent fibers of trigeminal nerve (CN V) send the signals to the brain and facial nerve (CN VII) responds to it by blinking. Cranial nerve VIII (vestibulocochlear nerve) is tested by performing cold-water caloric test, CN IX and CN X are tested by gag reflex.

The extent of skull base injuries can be tentatively assessed by quick surveillance of the face and skull along with the palpation of the calvarium and all the bony landmarks. The presence of ecchymosis over the mastoid process and/or periorbital area suggests the presence of the skull base fracture and may even be present with good score on Glasgow Coma Scale (GCS). The presence of cerebrospinal fluid (CSF) leak is also an indication suggestive of skull base fracture with associated dural tear, the condition usually presents with rhinorrhea in anterior skull base fracture, and/or otorrhea and paradoxical rhinorrhea (CSF leak as a result of temporal bone fracture seeps through Eustachian tube and presents as rhinorrhea) with middle skull base fracture. The leakage is usually around the time of injury but the presentation may be delayed which may range from days to months. Post-trauma meningitis which may also be recurrent also indicates presence of CSF leakage. CSF admixed with blood presents a diagnostic challenge and can be seen as a ringed pattern on a clean gauze also known as **halo sign**. This is as a result of easy spread of lighter CSF from heavier blood products. Though the test is nonspecific but is a confirmatory and instantaneous for the presence of CSF leak. One can also send the CSF for beta-2-transferrin protein, the test is time taking and relatively costly.

Deficits in olfaction are one of the occult injuries following anterior skull base injury and are recognized much later after injury. On the contrary, paresthesia and sensory deficits may be more commonly recognized in relatively early period following trauma. Central skull base fractures as discussed usually involve the superior orbital fissure, supraorbital foramen, with extension to Sella, or clivus, and manifest with paresis or paralysis of nerves supplying the orbital structures and thus manifesting ocular findings. Other findings may include hypesthesia in the sensory distribution of ophthalmic (V1) and maxillary (V2) component of the trigeminal nerve, cranial nerve paresthesia, and even Horner's syndrome. Multiple cranial neuropathies are mostly seen in cases involving fractures of the central and posterior region of the skull base.

Facial nerve injuries are usually associated with the fracture of the temporal bone, the fracture can be both longitudinal and transverse thereby injuring the nerve at internal auditory canal or labyrinthine segment and geniculate ganglion, respectively. Other cranial nerves like glossopharyngeal, vagal, spinal accessory, and hypoglossal nerve injuries are associated with fractures that traverse the jugular or hypoglossal foramina [5] (Fig. 8.3).

So, a through systematic approach should be followed for diagnosing skull base injury. This approach is not only confined in the emergency room but also in the intensive care unit (ICU), high dependency unit (HDU), and in the follow-up period as some of the complications like CSF leaks may manifest even months later.

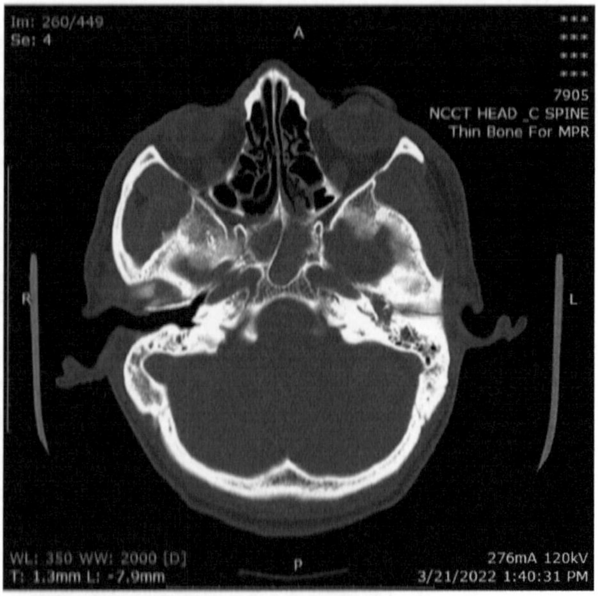

Fig. 8.3 Axial CT scan showing transverse fracture of temporal bone

8.5.2 Imaging Modalities for the Assessment of Skull Base Injuries

In the emergency set-up, for evaluating the skull base injuries, thin slice high-resolution CT scan (HRCT) is the gold standard with its added advantage of evaluating intracranial injuries. HRCT helps in assessing the integrity of the neurovascular foramina and evaluating the likely source of CSF leakage (*ethmoidal fovea is one of the weakest sites for CSF leak in anterior skull base*).

Magnetic resonance imaging (MRI) is reserved for assessing the integrity of the cranial nerves, and inner ear.

8.6 Management

Surgical intervention is not always indicated in cases with injury to the skull base and many times it is an incidental finding requiring no active intervention. The timing of the surgery depends on many factors such as the general condition of the patient, presence of other associated life-threatening injuries including intracranial hematomas, type of injury, i.e., open or closed, signs of orbital injury, and presence of CSF rhinorrhea.

Based on the radiological assessment, definite management (Conservative or surgical) is planned. If the surgical intervention is to be planned, then also pre-op radiological assessment is essential for planning the approach of the surgery.

In cases of **anterior skull base injury**, the approach must try to fulfill the following criteria:

(a) Wide exposure of the dural defect.
(b) Feasibilty to address associated intracranial injury through same approach.
(c) Preservation of the olfactory sense.

As per the case, the following approaches can be used:

(a) Transfrontal extradural approach.
(b) Transfrontal intradural approach.
(c) Transfacial approach.
(d) Endoscopic approach for orbital injury, and repair of CSF leak.

In case of **central skull base trauma**, immediate or early surgical treatment is indicated for open depressed fracture with or without dural injury as well as for expanding intracranial hematoma. CSF which may be observed as otorrhea and/or paradoxical rhinorrhea due to dural injury to the middle ear can be planned for surgery after evaluating HRCT and the approach to the middle fossa can be:

(a) Transcranial.
(b) Subtemporal approach to the middle fossa.

(c) Trans-mastoid.
(d) Combination of all.

Other **associated** complaints which need to be addressed are:

(a) **Hearing loss**: The hearing loss can be conductive due to rupture of the tympanic membrane, and/or discontinuity of the ossicular chain. Sensorineural hearing loss results from injury to the cochlea and/or internal auditory canal.
(b) **Vascular injury**: Internal carotid artery is likely to be injured in the carotid canal which may range from arterial wall dissection and may also result in formation of carotid cavernous fistula. This may require intervention by interventional radiologist.
(c) **Facial nerve injury**: They are mostly associated with transverse type of temporal bone fracture. Management depends on the general condition of the patient and degree of facial nerve palsy. Mild nonprogressive paresis can be managed conservatively but complete paralysis not improving conservatively and clear evidence of temporal bone fracture indicates the need for facial nerve exploration and repair.

Injury involving the **posterior skull base** may involve fractures of the petrous bone (mainly the transverse fracture) and may also extend to the occipital bone thereby affecting the posterior fossa and this increases the chances of injury of major venous sinus such as the sigmoid sinus and also jugular bulb. This may result in epidural hematoma which may manifest late and is evident on repeat CT scans. This is of paramount importance in comatose patients where a repeat CT scan is justified if one finds a fracture of the posterior skull base. In case of epidural hematoma, surgical intervention with the repair of the dural venous sinus should be taken early. Injury involving the jugular foramen may lead to multiple cranial nerve deficits and may result in dysphagia, unilateral or bilateral abductor vocal cord paralysis leading to even airway compromise, and may require dependency on tracheostomy for a longer period of time. These cases also require rehabilitation of swallowing function.

Trauma to the **craniocervical junction** may accompany skull base fracture and should be kept in mind. Associated injury of the cervical spine complex may involve bone, joints, ligaments, and vascular structures. Clinical examination along with radiological investigation helps in diagnosing the injury and an expert in spine surgery should be consulted.

Fracture of the maxilla, zygoma, and mandible should be managed accordingly by the concerned specialty.

References

1. Blevins NH, Jackler RK. Facial, auditory, and vestibular nerve injuries associated with basilar skull fractures. In: Youmans RJ, editor. Neurological surgery. 4th ed. Philadelphia: Saunders; 1996. p. 1865–78.
2. Manson PN, Stanwix MG, Yaremchuk MJ, et al. Frontobasal fractures: anatomical classification and clinical significance. Plast Reconstr Surg. 2009;124:2096–106.
3. Ochalski PG, Spiro RM, Fabio A, et al. Fractures of the clivus: a contemporary series in the computed tomography era. Neurosurgery. 2009;65(6):1063–9.
4. Menku A, Koc RK, Tucer B, et al. Clivus fractures: clinical presentations and courses. Neurosurg Rev. 2004;27(3):194–8.
5. Lehn AC, Lettieri J, Grimley R. A case of bilateral lower cranial nerve palsies after base of skull trauma with complex management issues: case report and review of literature. Neurologist. 2012;18(3):152–4.

Temporal Bone Fractures

9

Vishudh Mohan, Vidhu Sharma, and Amit Goyal

9.1 Introduction

The human skull is one of the most complicated structures in the human body. It has functions of protection, support, and motion. It encases a plethora of major structures of the head and neck. An adult human skull comprises approximately 22 bones but also 6 associated bones which are 3 ossicles of each ear. Some authors considered the hyoid bone as part of the associated bones of the skull. The temporal bone (two in number) is the part of neurocranium made up of eight bones. The temporal bone consists of five parts—the petrous, mastoid, tympanic, squamous parts, and styloid process.

The petrous bone is one of the hardest bones in the human body, which contains many vital structures such as the cochleovestibular system and facial nerve, carotid artery, and in close relation with multiple venous sinuses and veins. Temporal bone (Fig. 9.1) trauma is a common manifestation of head and neck trauma. More than 90% of temporal bone fractures are associated with head and neck injuries. Among head injuries involving the cranial base, 18–40% showed temporal bone involvement [1]. Due to this most of the time, the initial screening and management part will be taken under neurosurgery, emergency medicine, maxillofacial, or orthopedics departments. We recommend a thorough evaluation by a specialist ENT surgeon to rule out initial signs of temporal bone fracture. Clinical manifestations of temporal bone fracture will vary from asymptomatic presentation to a daring emergency like a carotid injury. Jugular vein injury is one of the emergencies which should be diagnosed promptly to prevent progression and long-term sequelae such as aseptic thrombus formation and shock.

V. Mohan · V. Sharma · A. Goyal (✉)
Department of Otorhinolaryngology, All India Institute of Medical Sciences Jodhpur, Jodhpur, Rajasthan, India

© The Author(s), under exclusive license to Springer Nature Singapore Pte Ltd. 2024
A. Agrawal et al. (eds.), *Special Considerations in Trauma Care*,
https://doi.org/10.1007/978-981-99-9662-9_9

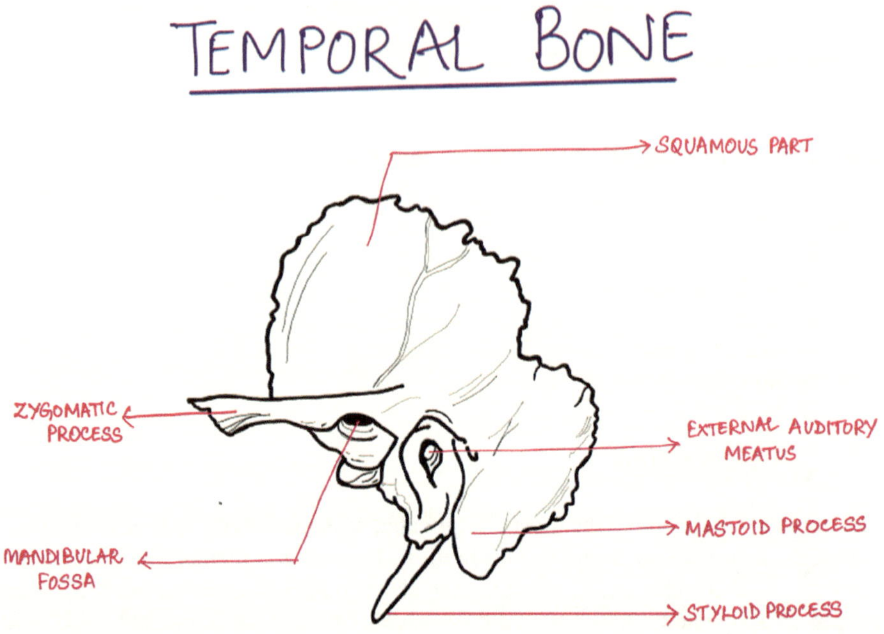

Fig. 9.1 Diagrammatic representation of parts of temporal bone

Hearing loss [2] is only one of the complications, lifelong morbidity to mortality has been seen among patients who have suffered from temporal bone trauma. Hence early triage and thorough clinical and radiological correlation are essential for the management of the spectrum of injuries associated with a temporal bone fracture.

9.2 Classification

Previously temporal bone fractures were classified based on the relation of the fracture line with the plane of the long axis of the petrous bone. This classification was given by Ulrich. According to his cadaveric dissections and other observations given by anatomists, more than 80% of the fractures are longitudinal, the rest being transverse [3].

In transverse fractures, the fracture line is at right angles to the long axis of the petrous bone, and the direction of force is from anterior to posterior direction. The common mechanism is an occipital or frontal blow injury.

The common mechanism for longitudinal fractures (Fig. 9.2) is a lateral blow to the head and the line of the fracture is parallel to the petrous ridge [4].

In children, there is a relative increase [5] in transverse fractures; around 40% are transverse fractures (Fig. 9.3).

However, with the invention of sophisticated radiology imaging systems, various studies found that most of these injuries are mixed or oblique types and can not be

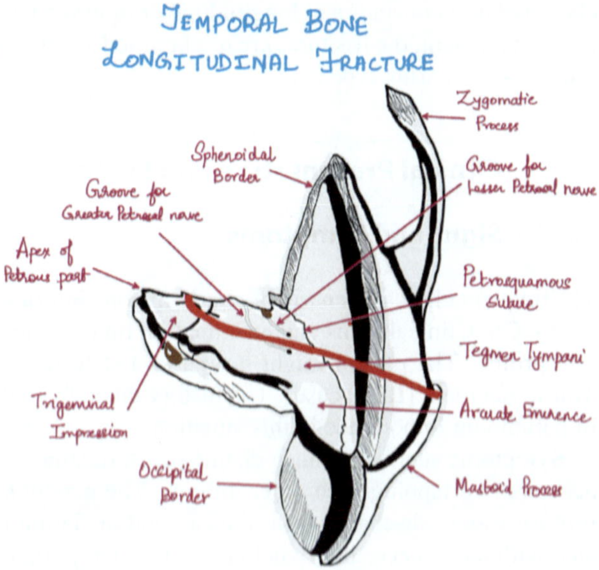

Fig. 9.2 Diagrammatic representation of temporal bone fracture showing longitudinal fracture—red line indicates fracture line

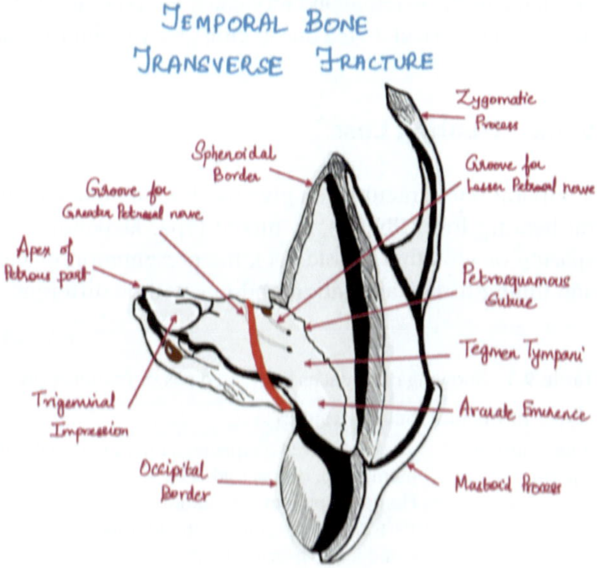

Fig. 9.3 Diagrammatic representation of temporal bone fracture showing transverse fracture—red line indicates fracture line

classified into conventional longitudinal or transverse types. Hence, to decide about the management, the fractures are re-classified as otic capsule involving/violating or otic capsule sparing type [6].

9.3 Clinical Presentation and Evaluation

9.3.1 Signs and Symptoms

The frequent clinical scenario of temporal bone injuries is a case of polytrauma with poor GCS. Clinical signs and examination findings are more important than symptom profile. The patient might not be in a state to give a proper history in Road Traffic Accident (RTA) cases. The history taken from the attendees of the patient is of paramount importance in this situation.

Symptoms such as balance disturbances, dizziness, tinnitus, headache, and earache are overlapping with other injuries. The patient's complaints of hearing loss, profuse watery discharge from the ear, and deviation of face or symptoms associated with facial nerve injury help to suspect temporal bone trauma.

Irrespective of the mode of injury, haemotympanum, haemotorrhoea, and laceration or edema to the external auditory canal are common [7]. Another sign is discoloration over the postauricular area due to emissary vein injury, known as Battle's sign [8].

9.3.2 Hearing Loss

Temporal bone fracture can give rise to conductive hearing loss (CHL), sensorineural hearing loss (SNHL), or mixed type. Depending on whether it is otic capsule sparing or violating (Table 9.1), the presentation of hearing loss and the otoscopic and tuning fork examination findings will be different.

Table 9.1 Showing differences between types of fractures (newer classification system)

Types of fracture	Salient features
Otic capsule sparing	Areas involved—squamosal part, external auditory canal, tympanic membrane, or mastoid cells Hemotympanum is common Perforation of tympanic membrane Conductive hearing loss Nystagmus—rare and less intense
Otic capsule violating	External auditory canal is usually unaffected. Jugular foramen or foramen magnum involvement is more common Sensorineural hearing loss Facial nerve injury is more common CSF otorrhoea is more common Nystagmus—common and intense (third degree) Perilymph fistula Temporal lobe contusion/middle cranial fossa injuries

Otic capsule violating type usually presents as sensorineural hearing loss (moderate to severe) or mixed hearing loss if it is associated with edema or haematoma of the middle ear or the canal wall. Injury to the cochlear artery or direct insult to the cochleovestibular nerve complex or labyrinthine fistula can also be the cause of SNHL. Studies are showing a small percentage of people later in life present with SNHL in the contralateral ear, the most common cause for the same is the activation of inner ear antigens resulting in an autoimmune response [9].

Conductive hearing loss is possibly due to haematoma, edema, or effusion inside the middle ear which usually gets absorbed as the days progress, and hearing improves, but ossicular disruption causes permanent conductive hearing loss. Among ossicular chain injuries, incudostapedial joint dislocation is the most common pathology in cases of temporal bone trauma [10].

Bedside tuning fork tests help in the diagnosis of hearing loss including type and severity [10]. It is always advisable to get pure tone audiometry once the patient is stable, for documentation purposes and diagnosis of higher frequency hearing loss which may be missed during routine tuning fork tests.

Once the patient's airway, spine, and haemodynamics are stabilized, clinical examination including detailed otological examination can be performed.

One should look for ear discharge—type of discharge whether bloody or watery; profuse or continuous watery or blood-tinged can be CSF. In suspected cases ear packing should not be attempted, the patient should be kept in a lateral position with the injured ear facing up. If it is frank blood, the ear should be mopped and a thorough examination of the external auditory canal for any laceration, edema, or EAC wall fracture should be performed. One should look for the morphology of the tympanic membrane. A swollen out, lusterless, reddish violaceous tympanic membrane is usually an indicator of haematoma in the middle ear cavity due to temporal bone fracture. At times TM would be ruptured which can be seen as perforation, an experienced otologist can differentiate it from an existing old perforation by examination of the margins as epithelialized margins are suggestive of chronic otitis media.

9.3.3 CSF Fistula

The site of the CSF fistula [11] will be different based on the type of injury. In otic capsule-sparing fractures, the site will be from the middle ear cleft, fracture of the epitympanum, or tegmen tympani often resulting in CSF otorrhoea [12]. If associated tympanic membrane perforation is present, CSF otorrhoea will be the major presentation.

Examination will not be complete without examining the nose and paranasal sinuses. With an intact tympanic membrane, CSF rhinorrhoea will be the main presentation, otoscopic findings in such cases will be a bulge in the tympanic membrane with or without fluid level.

9.3.4 Facial Nerve Palsy

Facial nerve palsy or paresis is a common reason for an ENT referral other than bleeding or cerebrospinal fluid (CSF) leak from ear. As patients are commonly admitted under trauma or neurosurgery departments, a prompt reference to ENT is often delayed if symptoms of facial nerve palsy or significant otorrhoea are not present.

Seven percent of temporal bone fractures result in facial paralysis [4]. In most of the cases, facial paralysis is of an incomplete type as seen in almost one-third of all the cases. The incidence is almost similar among all the age groups [1].

At the first contact with the doctor, one-third of the patients will show facial paralysis, and rest show deterioration as the days progress. Perigeniculate region is most commonly involved, irrespective of the mode of injury, followed by tympanic segment and second genu, respectively [13]. The intracranial part of facial nerve is covered by the bony fallopian canal; hence edema of the facial nerve results in compression and causes paresis.

Topodiagnostic Tests

Used to determine the anatomical level of peripheral nerve injury involvement, the principle of the topodiagnostic tests [14] is that any injury distal to the site of origin of a branch of the facial nerve will spare the function of that branch (Fig. 9.4).

Schirmer tear test will test the lacrimation (by measuring meniscus volume and residual tear volume), which is by the greater superficial petrosal nerve, which arises just after the labyrinthine segment of the facial nerve and before tympanic segment, all other branches of the facial nerve arise distal to this. Hence any injury at this position will result in dysfunction of chorda tympani and nerve to stapedius causing loss of taste sensation in anterior two-thirds of the tongue, decreased submandibular gland salivary flow rate and hyperacusis. The most common traumatic injury is seen proximal to the geniculate ganglion followed by proximal tympanic and labyrinthine segments, therefore most of the patients have mixed symptoms.

Stapedial reflex is otherwise known as an acoustic reflex which checks for the amplitude of the reflex and tests some functions of the facial nerve and cochlear nerve complex. Presence of reflex below 60 dB often indicates recruitment due to cochlear pathology but the absence of ipsilateral reflex usually indicates facial nerve injury or cochlear nerve injury or dissection. Ipsilateral signals with absent contralateral signals often indicate brainstem lesions.

Taste test—Absence of taste in the anterior two-thirds of the tongue indicates chorda tympani injury.

Hearing and balance—Internal acoustic meatus injury will be associated with combined injury to the vestibulocochlear complex resulting in SNHL and vertigo [2].

Sub-mandibular salivary flow rate assessment is usually not performed on a bedside basis. It is usually invasive, requiring cannulation of the salivary duct.

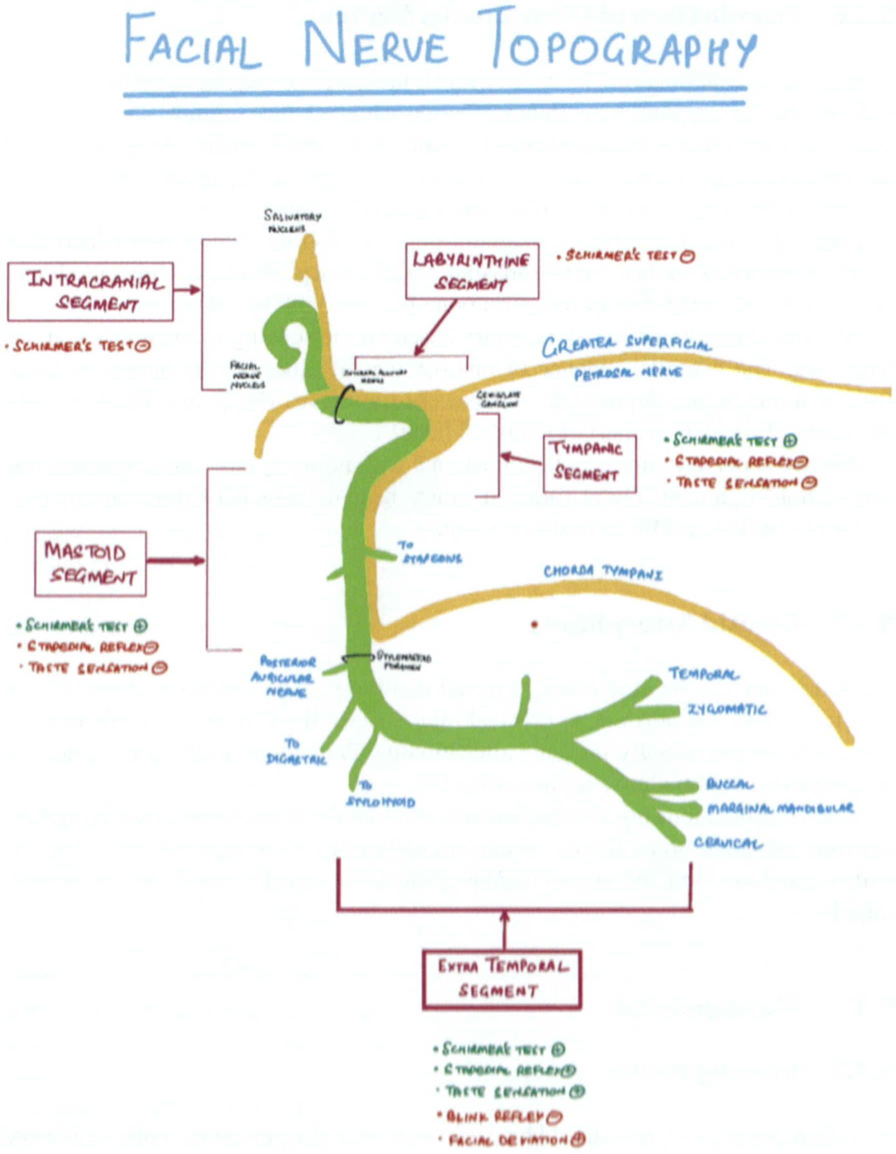

Fig. 9.4 Showing facial nerve topography and topodiagnostic tests inferences at different levels of injury

9.3.5 Vertigo

The most common type of vertigo is post-traumatic BPPV (positional type) [15] intractable or progressive vertigo with intense nystagmus indicates labyrinthine fistula or severe damage to vestibule.

9.3.6 Examination of Other Cranial Nerves

Cranial nerve examination [16] is very much important in any head and neck injury in RTA case. In temporal bone trauma, there is a high chance of injury to the petrous apex, and internal acoustic canal which results in the involvement of trigeminal and vestibulocochlear complex. Involvement of CP angle and jugular foramen also results in other cranial nerve involvement especially abducens and other lower cranial nerve palsies. The foramen magnum injury is also not uncommon which may result in transient or late vertebrobasilar insufficiency. Hence a clinician should approach a suspected case of temporal bone fracture with broad vision.

All cranial nerves are at risk of injury based on the severity of the injury that has happened. The overall incidence of involvement of other cranial nerves is 7.8%. Jugular foramen area injury causes palsies of the nerves IX, X, and XI along with a fracture of the petrous part of temporal bone.

Abducens nerve injury is noted in patients with injury at Dorello's canal near the petroclinoid ligament. Dural foramen injury near the Meckel's cave and petrous pyramid results in a fifth cranial nerve injury.

9.3.7 Carotid Artery Injury

Carotid injury can be suspected on initial neurological examination suggestive of deficits, Horner's syndrome, or cervical injury. Carotid—Cavernous fistula is a late complication that usually presents after months. Patients present with pulsatile or nonpulsatile exophthalmos or chemosis [17].

Late complications are also not uncommon like the formation of endolymphatic hydrops, otogenic brain abscess, recurrent meningitis of otogenic origin, otogenic hydrocephalous, and meningocoele/encephalocoele usually involving the temporal lobe.

9.4 Management

9.4.1 Investigations

A bedside tuning fork test should be performed once the patient is vitally stable and conscious. Documentation of hearing at the first contact is of paramount importance not only for diagnosis and prognosis but also due to the legal implications.

High-resolution computerized tomography of temporal bone with 0.5 mm thick slices [18] will provide an anatomy of all important structures and should be done in all head and neck trauma cases with a suspected temporal bone fracture in conjunction with NCCT brain [19].

MRI is not performed routinely in Indian scenarios [20] where resources are limited and all patients might not afford it. Also, there is no direct indication for

MRI in a case of temporal bone trauma. In a suspected case of temporal lobe contusion or multiple cranial nerve palsies, MRI is helpful for surgical planning.

In penetrating injuries like gunshot wounds, a CT angiography should be considered as the major arteries maybe involved.

A neurologic injury should be addressed first, especially in patients with intracranial injury, poor GCS, and polytrauma. Common intracranial injuries include subdural haematoma, subarachnoid haemorrhage, pneumocephalus, and brain contusions.

Airway, breathing, and circulation should be stabilized in any case of trauma.

9.4.2 Facial Nerve Injury

Conservative or surgical management depends on the clinical, topodiagnostic, and electrodiagnostic tests [21]. Nowadays radiological investigations have no direct role in determining surgical decompression. Most of the time tissue edema and collection of haematoma cause transient compression of the facial nerve which results in the decreased firing of nerve axons. This usually improves over a period of time with conservative management. Despite a complete degree of facial nerve palsy, better outcomes have been shown with conservative management, especially if palsy was immediate in onset. Irrespective of the level of facial nerve palsy a full course of corticosteroids on tapering dose and physiotherapy are beneficial. Supportive therapy for the prevention of exposure keratitis should be considered [1]. The decision to surgically explore the facial nerve is by grading the injury as to whether it is reversible or irreversible. House Brackman grading system gives the clinical status of the facial nerve, and the same scale is used for the prognosis also. A neuropraxia often improves very fast; however, axonotmesis may not warrant a complete recovery but gradual improvement is seen.

Neurotmesis, otherwise Sunderland V degree injury, complete transection of the nerve may show an absence of electric activity, even though the different grades of the partial transection cannot be diagnosed by an electrodiagnostic test.

The surgical decision is usually taken on the basis of ENOG, which is to be done after 3 days, before that often, Wallerian degeneration can take place. A reduction of more than 90% compared with opposite facial nerve amplitude along with House Brackman grading 6 or worsening facial nerve status of a patient with ongoing conservative treatment can be a consideration for surgical decompression [13]. Different schools of thought are present regarding when to do decompression surgery, many institutions follow their guidelines, but all guidelines are based on clinical-electrodiagnostic tests [22].

The most common approach is the transmastoid approach, especially for otic capsule-sparing fractures with ossicular involvement.

9.4.2.1 Transmastoid Approach

The transmastoid approach involves tympanomastoid exploration with delineation of the facial nerve. The fallopian canal course should be identified by doing a canal wall down mastoidectomy. The fallopian canal should be opened for at least 180° of its circumference to release edema. The facial canal course should be examined for any breach in the endoneurium or epineurium. The major landmarks for this approach are the horizontal semicircular canal, digastric ridge, fossa incudes, and short process of the incus. Both tympanic and mastoid segments including geniculate ganglion can be assessed by this approach.

9.4.2.2 Middle Cranial Fossa Approach

It can be used as a combined approach with transmastoid and is usually beneficial in a situation where the lesion is present at the level of internal acoustic meatus, meatal, or labyrinthine segment. The greater superficial petrosal nerve, anterior semicircular canal, and Bills bar are the major landmarks.

Translabyrinthine approach—Rarely used, this approach is only performed when the entire cochlea vestibular nerve has been damaged by the trauma and to visualize the entire course of the facial nerve.

Tension-free repair of the facial nerve segment is the best and most accepted method, intraoperatively nerve can be mobilized and one should use a nerve monitor if available. If repair is planned, early repair is always advisable. Complete transection of the nerve often shows poor results with primary repair.

In case tension-free repair is not possible, cable grafting using greater auricular or sural or antebrachial cutaneous nerves can be tried.

In cases of the long-standing condition of facial nerve palsy cross-face nerve grafting, nerve transfers using hypoglossal or spinal accessory nerve, regional muscle transfer or free muscle transfer can be tried [23]. Temporalis and masseter can be used as regional muscles whereas gracillis, and latissimus dorsi can be used for free muscle transfer. Facial reanimation can be tried at any duration of facial paralysis.

9.4.3 Hearing Loss

Surgical exploration is indicated when the patient is symptomatic with 30 dB hearing loss and above persistently. For better results, ossiculoplasty can be done with or without a prosthesis. The air-bone gap is better improved with traumatic ossicular damage compared to chronic otitis media. The type of ossiculoplasty to be done is based on the site and the amount of injury to the ossicles.

Rehabilitation with a cochlear implant has a very favorable response among many patients with SNHL.

9.4.4 Vertigo

The most common cause of vertigo is due to concussion cerebralis. Temporary vascular flow alteration in the vestibular and basilar artery is associated with transient vestibuloneuropathy. Another common cause is BPPV, which can be classically diagnosed with DIX-Hallpike maneuver.

Patients need bed rest and advised to avoid vigorous body movements in the acute phase with supportive care.

Pharmacotherapy is broadly classified into vertigo suppression drugs [24] (antihistamines, sympathomimetics, antiemetics, psychotherapeutic drugs, etc.) and drug-modifying underlying pathology (cerebroactive drugs, vasodilators, diuretics, etc.).

Betahistine, cinnarizine, and prochlorperazine are the most commonly used drugs based on severity. A corrective positional maneuver like Epley's maneuver should be performed after ruling out cervical injuries and vertebral-basilar insufficiency. Later patients are advised for Cow Thorne-Cooksey exercises which improve the overall balance system.

Otic capsule involving injuries usually result in vertigo which is not relieved spontaneously, usually it needs definitive surgery in later stages.

9.4.5 CSF Fistula

In otic capsule disrupting fractures CSF fistula usually connects with the posterior cranial fossa and conservative management fails in most circumstances.

In unnoticed cases, the patient might present with features of meningitis, in such cases prompt treatment with broad-spectrum antibiotics followed by CSF fistula repair should be done.

In traumatic cases, 2–3 weeks of conservative observation can be tried as traumatic CSF fistula heals more commonly within this period. If it persists or the patient is symptomatic, one should consider definitive surgical treatment.

The clear watery discharge should be collected under sterile precautions and should be sent for culture, Beta-2-transferrin, and glucose oxidase tests. The most common organism in secondary bacterial meningitis is pneumococcus.

An HRCT temporal bone with CSF cisternogram is considered preoperatively for localization of the defect [12]. MRI and MR Cisternogram (which is a non-invasive modality) are also useful in few cases. The radiological investigation allows the surgeon to rule out meningocoele, meningoencephalocoele, and status of the middle ear. In most of the cases, a retrotympanic approach suffices for the repair, the defect must be repaired with temporalis fascia graft and should be obliterated with fat and tissue glue. In the case of brain herniation middle cranial fossa approach or inferior retrotympanic or combined approaches can be considered. And based on the bony defect size, the repair strategy is different. In larger bony defects, cartilage graft or bone cement is used. In the case of labyrinthine fistula, based on the size, the defect should be repaired promptly by different techniques like recapping, and resurfacing.

Auditory canal stenosis and cholesteatoma formation may be seen years after the trauma. The hypothesis behind the formation of cholesteatoma is traumatic implantation of squamous layer of tympanic membrane into the middle ear or entanglement of epithelial tissues along the fracture line. The cholesteatoma formation is extensive in traumatic cases compared to COM.

9.4.6 Vascular Injury

Sigmoid sinus and jugular vein injuries are seen as direct injury resulting in rupture of the venous sinus valve and thrombosed vessels. Carotid-cavernous fistula is rare, though carotid injury is most commonly noticed in fractures of the petrous segment [25].

In suspected cases of carotid artery injury anticoagulant agents should be started before development of ischemia. This will prevent major thromboembolic phenomena and reduce the chances of hemiplegia/hemiparesis. Antithrombotic agents are considered if carotid artery injury is diagnosed radiologically.

9.5 Summary

Temporal bone trauma is one of the major emergencies. Prompt assessment and early diagnosis can prevent further complications. As the most common causes are road traffic accidents, a multidisciplinary approach is necessary.

References

1. Gordin E, Lee TS, Ducic Y, Arnaoutakis D. Facial nerve trauma: evaluation and considerations in management. Craniomaxillofac Trauma Reconstr. 2015;8(1):1–13.
2. Djalilian HR. Symptoms: hearing loss and vertigo after trauma. Hear J. 2015;68(10):10.
3. Ishman SL, Friedland DR. Temporal bone fractures: traditional classification and clinical relevance. Laryngoscope. 2004;114(10):1734–41.
4. Diaz R, Cervenka B, Brodie H. Treatment of temporal bone fractures. J Neurol Surg Part B Skull Base. 2016;77(5):419–29.
5. Shapiro RS. Temporal bone fractures in children. Otolaryngol Neck Surg. 1979;87(3):323–9.
6. Nosan D, Beneckejr J, Murr R. Current perspective on temporal bone trauma. Otolaryngol Head Neck Surg. 1997;117(1):67–71.
7. Backous DD, Minor LB, Niparko JK. Trauma to the external auditory canal and temporal bone. Otolaryngol Clin N Am. 1996;29(5):853–66.
8. Tubbs RS, Shoja MM, Loukas M, Oakes WJ, Cohen-Gadol A. William Henry Battle and Battle's sign: mastoid ecchymosis as an indicator of basilar skull fracture: historical vignette. J Neurosurg. 2010;112(1):186–8.
9. Lazarini PR, Camargo ACK. Idiopathic sudden sensorineural hearing loss: etiopathogenic aspects. Braz J Otorhinolaryngol. 2006;72(4):554–61.
10. Patel A, Groppo E. Management of temporal bone trauma. Craniomaxillofac Trauma Reconstr. 2010;3(2):105–13.
11. Wood CP, Hunt CH, Bergen DC, Carlson ML, Diehn FE, Schwartz KM, et al. Tympanic plate fractures in temporal bone trauma: prevalence and associated injuries. Am J Neuroradiol. 2014;35(1):186–90.
12. Hicks GW, Wright JW, Wright JW. Cerebrospinal fluid otorrhea. Laryngoscope. 1980;90(S25):1–25.
13. Quaranta A, Campobasso G, Piazza F, Quaranta N, Salonna I. Facial nerve paralysis in temporal bone fractures: outcomes after late decompression surgery. Acta Otolaryngol (Stockh). 2001;121(5):652–5.

14. Bento RE, Vellutini EAS, Pahl FH, Tedesco-Marchese AJ, Formigoni GS, Navarro HC, et al. Topodiagnóstico na paralisia facial periférica. Arq Neuropsiquiatr. 1985;43(3):275–80.
15. Di Cesare T, Tricarico L, Passali GC, Sergi B, Paludetti G, Galli J, et al. Traumatic benign paroxysmal positional vertigo: personal experience and comparison with idiopathic BPPV. Int J Audiol. 2021;60(5):393–7.
16. Damodaran O, Rizk E, Rodriguez J, Lee G. Cranial nerve assessment: a concise guide to clinical examination. Clin Anat. 2014;27(1):25–30.
17. Li C, Green L, Wang J, Tully D, Woliansky J, Gumm K, et al. Factors associated with blunt internal carotid artery injury in petrous temporal bone fractures. Injury. 2022;53(6):2023–7.
18. Bešenski N. Traumatic injuries: imaging of head injuries. Eur Radiol. 2002;12(6):1237–52.
19. Little SC, Kesser BW. Radiographic classification of temporal bone fractures: clinical predictability using a new system. Arch Otolaryngol Neck Surg. 2006;132(12):1300.
20. Davey S, Maheshwari C, Raghav S, Singh N, Muzammil K, Pandey P. Impact of Indian public health standards for rural health care facilities on national programme for control of deafness in India: the results of a cohort study. J Fam Med Prim Care. 2018;7(4):780.
21. Coker NJ. Facial electroneurography: analysis of techniques and correlation with degenerating motoneurons. Laryngoscope. 1992;102(7):747–59.
22. Vajpayee D, Mallick A, Mishra AK. Post temporal bone fracture facial paralysis: strategies in decision making and analysis of efficacy of surgical treatment. Indian J Otolaryngol Head Neck Surg. 2018;70(4):566–71.
23. Volk GF, Pantel M, Guntinas-Lichius O. Modern concepts in facial nerve reconstruction. Head Face Med. 2010;6(1):25.
24. Strupp M, Brandt T. Diagnosis and treatment of vertigo and dizziness. Dtsch Ärztebl Int. 2008;105(10):173–80. https://www.aerzteblatt.de/10.3238/arztebl.2008.0173.
25. Lazaridou M, Bourlidou E, Kontos K, Mangoudi D. Carotid-cavernous fistula as a complication of facial trauma: a case report. Craniomaxillofac Trauma Reconstr. 2015;8(3):239–45.

Facial Trauma

10

Kuldeep Vishwakarma, Ravi Sankar Manogaran, Govind Bhuskute, Saurabh Kumar Rawat, and Abhishek Dubey

10.1 Soft Tissue Trauma

Soft tissue injuries of facial structures in facial trauma often occur in the setting of more severe trauma, and there is always a chance to miss these injuries. Cases of maxillofacial trauma that are not associated with airway obstruction or significant bleeding should be addressed only after life-threatening injuries have been managed. The treating physician must examine facial structures such as facial nerve injury (Fig. 10.1a), parotid duct transection (Fig. 10.1b), eyelid laceration, canalicular injuries, ocular injuries, and intra-oral examination with assessment of dental occlusion. The eyes should be examined for visual acuity, pupillary size, hemorrhage of the conjunctiva and fundus, penetrating injury, contact lenses (remove before edema occurs), dislocation of the lens, ocular movements, foreign bodies, and muscle entrapment (Fig. 10.2). The degree and manner of force delivered by the impact on the skeletal tissue play a role in the severity or complexity of the resultant injury. The entire scalp and head should be examined for lacerations, contusions, and evidence of fractures.

The microvascular replantation of well-preserved tissues of avulsions and amputations of the ear, nose, lips, and scalps are viable options for these structures. Salivary fistulas and sialoceles resulting from salivary gland parenchymal injuries often respond to conservative management. Parotid duct injuries without loss of its segments need primary approximation, while in cases of loss of segment in the proximal portion need, complete ligation of the duct. If the distal portion is lost, the

K. Vishwakarma · S. K. Rawat
Department of Oral and Maxillofacial Surgery, Apex Trauma Centre, Sanjay Gandhi Postgraduate Institute of Medical Sciences, Lucknow, UP, India

R. S. Manogaran (✉) · G. Bhuskute · A. Dubey
Neuro Otology Unit, Department of Neurosurgery, Sanjay Gandhi Postgraduate Institute of Medical Sciences, Lucknow, UP, India

© The Author(s), under exclusive license to Springer Nature Singapore Pte Ltd. 2024
A. Agrawal et al. (eds.), *Special Considerations in Trauma Care*,
https://doi.org/10.1007/978-981-99-9662-9_10

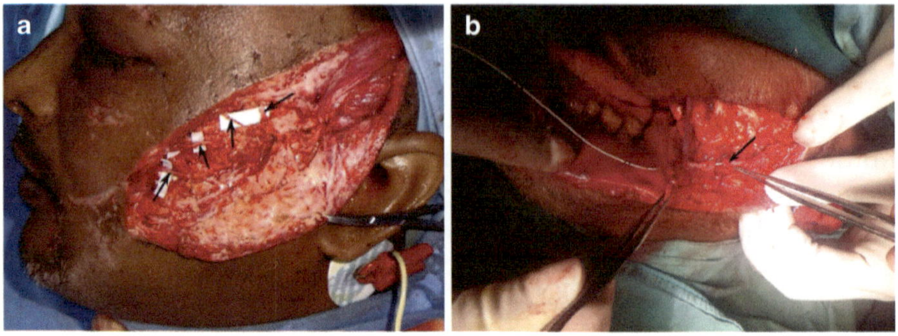

Fig. 10.1 (**a**) Laceration through cheek showing repaired branches of the facial nerve (arrows). (**b**) Cheek laceration showing severed parotid duct (arrow)

Fig. 10.2 A 4-year-old kid with right orbital floor fracture and entrapment of inferior rectus muscle resulting in reduced movement of the right eye in upward gaze

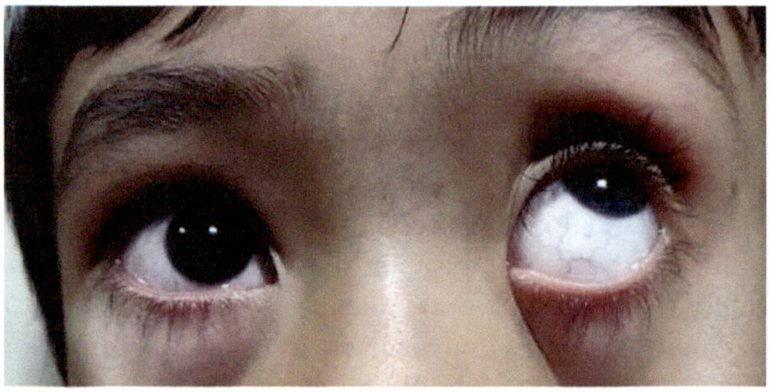

duct can be replanted in the oral cavity. In the penetrating injuries of facial nerves, if the gap is less than 1 cm can be repaired primarily as soon as the patient is stable with fine monofilament sutures. In greater than 1 cm gap, a nerve graft (cable graft) to span defect is needed. The aim of treating soft tissue injuries should be a cosmetically acceptable repair to both patients and the physician with the possible pre-injury appearance and function.

10.2 Nasal Trauma

The nasal bone is one of the most common facial bones to get fractured in the event of facial trauma. Midline position and outward projection of the nose make it vulnerable to blunt and penetrating trauma. Anatomically nasal architecture is made up of cartilaginous as well as bony parts. It is divided into three parts—the upper one-third formed by the nasal bones attached to the frontal bone superiorly and the perpendicular plate of ethmoid in the midline. The middle 1/3rd is made by the upper lateral cartilage and in the midline by attachment of septal cartilage with the upper lateral cartilage. The lower 1/3rd comprises the lower lateral cartilage forming the columella and nasal tip. This division of external nasal anatomy helps identify the subset involved and directs the management plan accordingly.

10.2.1 Pathophysiology

Nasal fractures can be classified based on the direction of the force of trauma into lateral and frontal injury. For example, a blow to the nose from a lateral aspect is more likely to cause nasal fracture than a frontal blow as the cartilages dissipate the oncoming force.

There are multiple systems of classification of nasal bone fractures described in the literature. The extent of lateral deviation of nasal dorsum fracture can be described using the following grading system:

1. Grade 0: bones perfectly straight
2. Grade 1: bones deviated less than half of the width of the bridge of the nose
3. Grade 2: bones deviated half to one full width of the bridge of the nose
4. Grade 3: bones deviated greater than one full width of the bridge of the nose
5. Grade 4: bones almost touching the cheek

The greater the grade of lateral deviation, the more it is unlikely to be managed using closed fracture reduction.

In his study of nasal bone fractures done on cadavers, Murray described seven grades of fracture patterns.

Class 1—Simple nasal depression. The fracture lines parallel the dorsum and naso-maxillary suture without septal fracture. This type of injury usually does not require any reduction and can be managed conservatively.

Class 2—involves a fracture of both nasal bones with a fracture line running across the bones and an additional line parallel to the nasal dorsum. The septal fracture may be encountered in the upper 3 cm of the perpendicular plate of the ethmoid. This fracture pattern may be associated with CSF leak following relatively trivial nasal trauma.

Class 3—involves a comminuted fracture of nasal bones with the extension of fracture line onto the bony and cartilaginous septum in a C-shaped fashion extending from a perpendicular plate of the ethmoid, vomer extending anteriorly to the cartilaginous septum. It may be associated with lateral deviation of the nasal dorsum to a distance greater than one-half width of the bridge of the nose (Grade 2 as described above).

Class 4—is similar to class 3 fracture; however, the extent of nasal bone fracture is less. There is also overriding of the bony-cartilaginous portion of the nasal dorsum with lateral deviation. The closed reduction does not always give adequate cosmetic results in this fracture type.

Class 5—the frontal force of trauma causing nasal bone fracture pushing the midline portion of nasal bones inwards with splaying of nasal bones at nasomaxillary suture line.

Class 6—cartilaginous fracture caused by frontal fracture involving the upper and lower lateral cartilage and the quadrilateral cartilage of the septum. The fracture line of the septal cartilage extends posteriorly toward the vomer parallel to the maxillary crest.

Class 7—cartilaginous fracture with septal cartilage fracture extending toward the perpendicular plate of the ethmoid.

10.2.2 Clinical Assessment

History of trauma with exact information of how and when it occurred is mandatory for documentation in medicolegal cases and determining the optimal time for reducing fractures. Patients should also be asked about nasal complaints like persistent pain with the nasal blockade, suggestive of a septal hematoma. Displaced nasal fractures can be associated with nasal obstruction. It is also vital to ask the patient about unilateral or bilateral clear or blood-tinged nasal discharge to rule out traumatic CSF rhinorrhea. Knowledge about prior nasal trauma and nasal surgeries should also be noted. Anosmia, hyposmia, visual deterioration, or orbital displacement must be investigated to complete the assessment.

The nose and paranasal sinuses should be thoroughly done, starting with an external nasal examination. The external nasal framework should be examined and recorded in four views—frontal, right lateral, left lateral, and basal. The deviation of the nasal dorsum has to be recorded by describing in which a third of the deviation exists. Following this, performing anterior rhinoscopy and ruling out septal hematoma is mandatory. Palpation of nasal bone and septum should be done to feel the crepitus and cartilage overriding. This helps in knowing the class of fracture and formulating management protocol. CSF rhinorrhea has to be ruled out in all cases.

Isolated nasal bone fractures do not require any imaging for their confirmation if a thorough clinical assessment is made. However, one must consider a CT scan if there is suspicion of skull base fracture or depressed skull fracture and if the patient has a focal neurological deficit. For example, in a grossly comminuted nasal fracture with associated facial trauma, CT nose and paranasal sinus with the 3D reconstruction of the face helps plan surgery to achieve maximum functional and cosmetic results.

10.2.3 Management

Management of nasal fracture can be divided into—a conservative approach, closed reduction, or septorhinoplasty. Timing of nasal bone fracture, type, the extent of the fracture, displacement of the nasal dorsum, symptoms at presentation, and soft tissue edema dictates the approach used.

As a consensus, if the patient presents within a few hours of trauma, soft tissue edema makes the accurate assessment of nasal deformity difficult. Hence after ruling out septal hematoma and CSF rhinorrhea, the patient is reassessed after 5–7 days once the edema subsides. In patients with pre-existing nasal deformity, a formal septorhinoplasty can be planned on a routine basis. However, in patients pursuing professions with a risk of nasal trauma, it is advised to correct the nasal deformity once there is no other obvious risk of repeat trauma.

In patients presenting after 6–8 weeks of trauma when the nasal bones ossify, it is impossible to achieve an optimal fracture reduction using closed reduction and requires septorhinoplasty (Chart 10.1).

Fracture reduction can be achieved under local and general anesthesia depending on the patient and surgeon factors. Infiltration of the local anesthetic agent can distort nasal deformity leading to inaccurate correction. However, there is no significant difference in the results achieved using local or general anesthesia.

The indications for the closed reduction in adult patients are:

1. Unilateral or bilateral nasal bone fracture.
2. Fracture of the nasal-septal complex with nasal deviation less than half the width of the nasal bridge.

The indications for open reduction are:

1. Extensive fracture-dislocation of the nasal bones and septum.
2. Nasal pyramid deviation exceeding one-half the width of the nasal bridge.
3. Fracture and dislocation of the caudal septum.
4. Open septal fracture.
5. Persistent deformity after closed reduction.

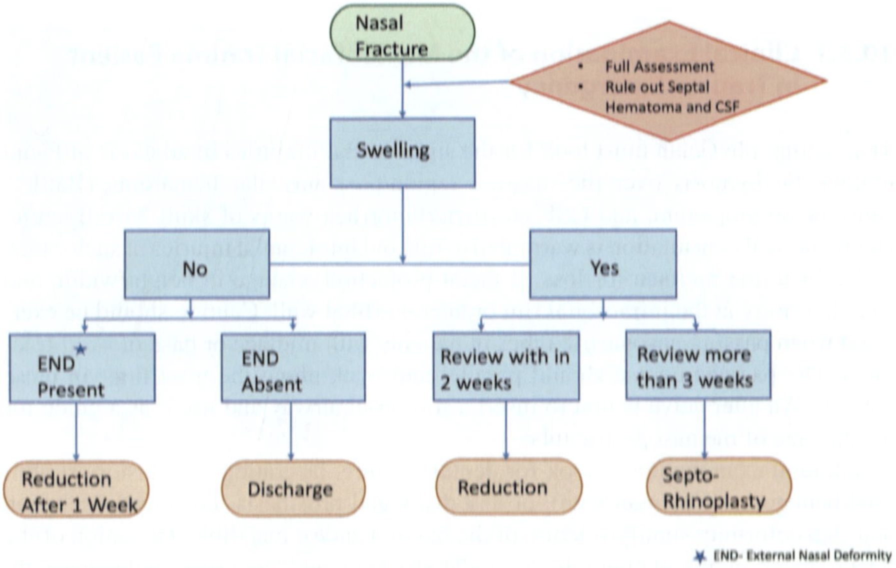

Chart 10.1 Flowchart for nasal fracture management

The closed reduction follows the principle of distraction, realignment, and distal fracture segment reduction. Nasal bones can be realigned by giving firm finger pressure or using forceps. Walsham forceps are designed to deal with impacted nasal bones, whereas the Asch forceps are suitable for reducing the nasal septum. However, they are also helpful in restoring the alignment of impacted nasal bones.

Open reduction techniques include septoplasty, septorhinoplasty with osteotomy, and postoperative stabilization of fractures using splints and nasal packs.

10.3 Maxillofacial Trauma

Maxillofacial trauma can be defined as any external injury to the face. It may occur in isolation but frequently involves other adjacent anatomical areas like the cranium, orbital contents, ears, and neck. Due to the differences in social, cultural, environmental, and risk factors, the trauma's incidence and etiology vary from one country to another. The incidence of motor vehicle accidents (MVA) is higher in developing countries, whereas in the western world, interpersonal violence is the leading cause of maxillofacial injuries [1, 2], and sports-related injuries are more commonly seen in teenage boys or young [3].

Guglielmo Salicetti and Gilmer are thought to be the first to use intermaxillary wires to treat mandible fractures. The advent of rigid bone plates has dramatically changed how mandibular and other facial fractures are treated [4]. The technique of rigid internal fixation was advanced and popularized by the AO/ASIF (Arbeitsgemeinschaft fur Osteosynthesefragen/Association of the Study of Internal Fixation) in Europe in 1970.

10.3.1 Clinical Examination of the Maxillofacial Trauma Patient in Trauma Emergency

The treating physician must look for the signs of skull injuries in all cases of facial trauma. Ecchymosis over the mastoid region/post auricular hematoma (Battle's sign), hemotympanum, and CSF otorrhea/rhinorrhea warns of skull base fracture. Neurosurgical consultation is warranted to rule out intracranial injuries in such cases.

Evaluate the midface for loss of facial projection, change in height/width, and step deformity at the infraorbital rim or lateral orbital wall. Caution should be exercised when passing nasogastric tubes in patients with midface or base of skull fractures. The passage course should parallel and track along the nose floor in these patients. An alternative is first to insert a soft nasal airway and use it as a guide for the passage of the nasogastric tube.

Intraoral examination to look for dental fracture, lacerations, occlusion, sublingual hematoma (Coleman sign), or any dislodged prosthesis. Deranged occlusion and step deformity signify fracture of the maxilla and/or mandible. Deviation of the lower jaw on mouth opening, preauricular swelling, and tenderness indicates mandibular condyle fracture (Fig. 10.3).

10.3.2 Radiographic Examination

Maxillofacial trauma can be complex and proper treatment requires accurate evaluation and assessment of the patient. Plain radiographs have a minimal value in facial trauma patients, particularly for evaluating the mid-face and orbital fractures because of the superimposition of other anatomical structures. Orthopantomogram (OPG) can be used in cases of isolated mandible fracture (Fig. 10.4).

However, if available, multidetector computed tomography is the most accurate imaging technique and is considered the standard for identification of facial fractures, as well as associated injuries. Three-dimensional reformatting allows for better conceptualization, pre-surgical planning, patient education, and postoperative assessment (Fig. 10.5).

Plain radiographs (PA skull, lateral skull, OMV, SMV, Towney's projection) are of limited value in the assessment and treatment planning of complex facial trauma. However, they can be considered if the facility of CT is not available.

10.3.3 Management

The protocol proposed by Advanced Trauma Life Support (ATLS) is the gold standard for the initial assessment and management of polytrauma patients (Table 10.1). Although the priority of maxillofacial injuries is usually subordinated to more critical, life-threatening injuries, the role of the maxillofacial surgeon in the primary and secondary survey of patients with maxillofacial injuries should be emphasized [5]. Joshi et al. [6] studied the association between head injury and facial trauma and found a significant increase in the risk of head injury with an increase in the number of maxillofacial fractures. Post-traumatic brain and C-spine injuries should always be suspected and managed accordingly with the concerned specialty before managing maxillofacial injuries.

This section aims to highlight the role of the maxillofacial surgeon in the ABCDEs.

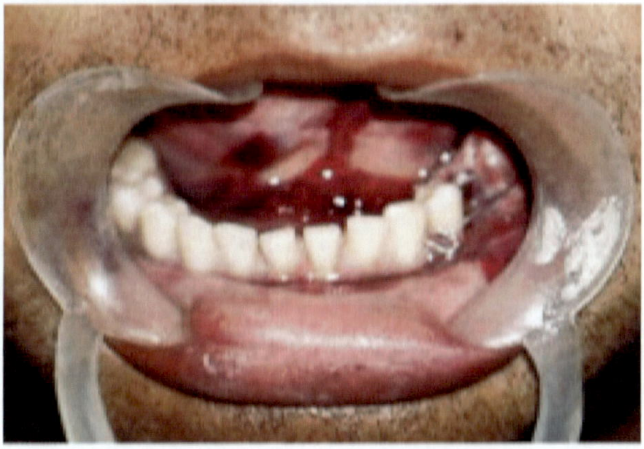

Fig. 10.3 Intraoral photograph of a patient with mandible parasymphysis fracture showing Coleman's sign (sublingual hematoma) and deranged occlusion

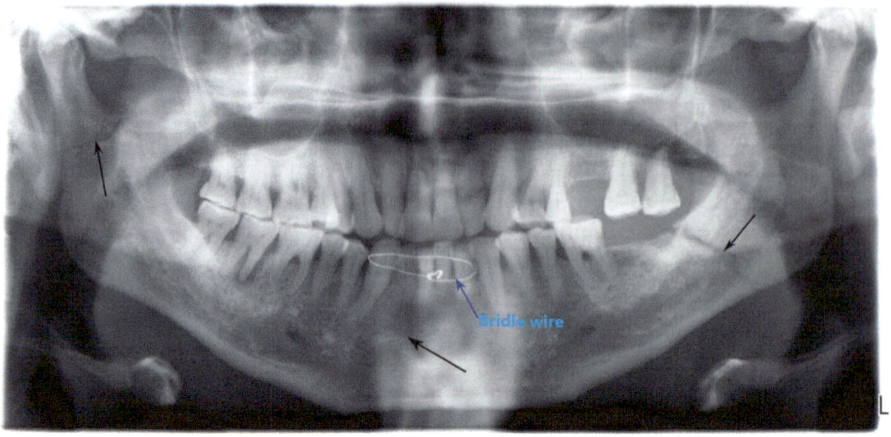

Fig. 10.4 Orthopantomogram showing fracture symphysis, left angle, and right sub-condyle of the mandible

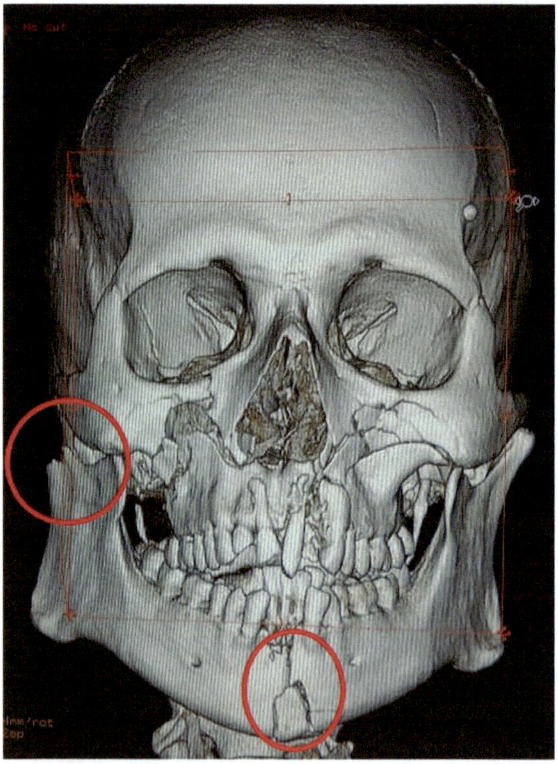

Fig. 10.5 3D reformatted image depicting pan facial fracture (bilateral Le Fort 1, symphysis and right subcondyle of mandible) with flaring of mandible resulting in increased lower facial width

Table 10.1 Trauma initial assessment and management checklist

A = Airway with restriction of cervical spine motion
B = Breathing and ventilation
C = Circulation with hemorrhage control
D = Disability
E = Exposure with environmental control

10.3.4 Inadequate Airway

Obstruction of the airway can be attributed to the avulsed tooth, dislodged or fractured prosthesis, blood clot, bone fragments, vomit, and foreign bodies. The oral cavity and upper airway should be appropriately evaluated after suctioning out saliva and blood clots. In addition, a chest X-ray should rule out tooth/foreign body/ or prosthesis aspiration. "Tongue fall" in cases of bilateral fracture of parasymphysis or body of the mandible and impacted/"Floating maxilla" due to LE FORT fractures causing displacement in the posterior region, eventually can contribute to decreased or occluded airway. Primary stabilization of displaced bony fracture ends with wires/arch bars helps relieve the obstructed airway.

10.3.5 Hemorrhage Control

In the immediate period following trauma, control of any facial hemorrhage and nasal bleeding are the primary concern related to the maxillofacial surgeon. Any facial wound must be inspected, and control of bleeding must be achieved with the help of pressure dressing and stay sutures. Sutures, staples, or Raney clips may help control bleeding from large scalp flaps.

Nasal bleeds may require anterior nasal packing and sometimes posterior nasal packing (Fig. 10.6a, b). If these measures fail to control hemorrhage, consider the patient for selective embolization. The packing should be removed in 3 days to avoid the risk of toxic shock syndrome secondary to *Staphylococcus aureus* infection. To prevent septal necrosis and subsequent saddle nose deformity, septal hematoma must be treated immediately by drainage and intranasal packing.

Bridle wiring around the tooth adjacent to the fractured jaw bone will temporarily stabilize and control the bleeding from the exposed medulla of fractured ends (Fig. 10.7).

10.3.6 Closed Reduction Techniques

Immobilization of fractured bone ends is achieved with the help of adjacent stable structures without direct surgical access to the fracture site. Various techniques of closed reduction are as follows:

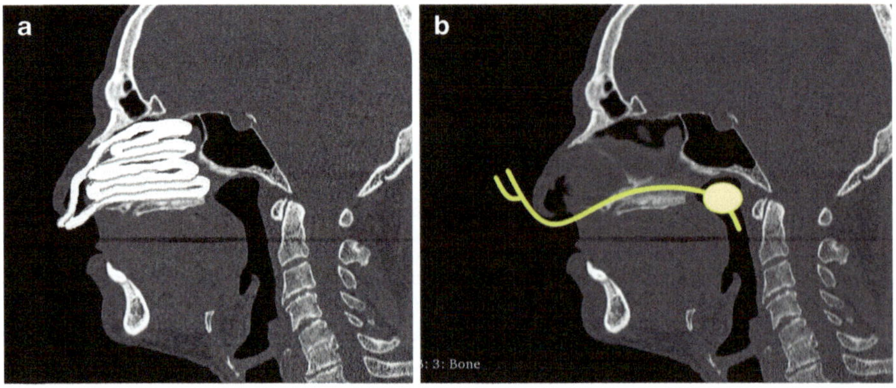

Fig. 10.6 (**a**) Anterior nasal packing (ribbon gauze impregnated with an antibiotic ointment or a lubricant can be used. Usually removed after 24–48 hours). (**b**) Posterior nasal packing (Foleys catheter can be used along with anterior nasal packing)

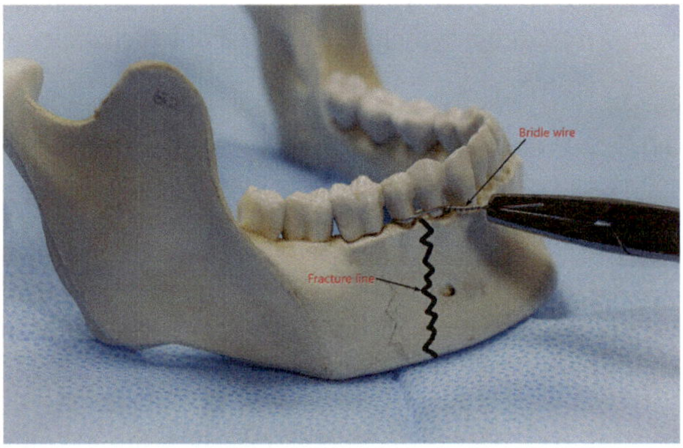

Fig. 10.7 Bridle wiring around the teeth to temporally stabilize the fracture

1. Suspension wiring—Pyriform aperture suspension wiring, infraorbital rim suspension wiring, frontal suspension wiring, circumzygomatic wiring
2. Intermaxillary fixation: Erich arch bar, Risdon wiring, Ivy loop wiring
3. Cap splint
4. Gunning splint and circum-mandibular wiring for edentulous mandible fracture
5. External pin fixation—used in comminuted mandibular fractures, infected mandibular fractures, gunshot wounds with associated comminuted mandibular fractures, and tissue loss. However, these devices have a minimal role because of the development of rigid and load-bearing osteosynthesis systems and microvascular reconstruction techniques.

Maxillomandibular Fixation (MMF) or Intermaxillary Fixation (IMF): It is the most commonly used technique for closed reduction. It utilizes the patient's occlusion as a guide for dental reduction, and immobilization is achieved with the help of arch bars, IMF screws, or eyelet wiring (Fig. 10.8). It can be employed either as an aid in reducing fractures or as a definitive treatment for mandibular fractures in instances where operative treatment is not feasible. The duration of IMF depends upon the morphology of the fracture and the patient's age.

10.3.7 Limitations and Contraindications of IMF

- Inability to tolerate intermaxillary fixation.
- Obtund patients, developmentally delayed patients, and chronic alcoholics.
- Patients are prone to nausea and vomiting and are at risk for aspiration.

10.3.8 Open Reduction and Internal Fixation (ORIF)

Traditionally maxillofacial fractures were managed nonoperatively by immobilization of the jaws which results in secondary bone healing through callus formation. This treatment modality hinders normal jaw function and as there happens to be constant micromovement between the fractured bone ends thereby may be associated with complications of infection and nonunion. ORIF is indicated in unfavorable and grossly displaced fractures or patients with contraindicated intermaxillary fixation. Advantages like primary bone healing, faster recovery, and early return to function favor ORIF over closed reduction techniques. Here the fractured bones are surgically exposed utilizing extraoral or intraoral incisions. The bones are then anatomically reduced, and fixation hardware is used to stabilize the fracture long enough to allow healing or "union."

Ideal fixation hardware should be biocompatible, autoclavable, rigid, radiopaque, and should be compatible with future magnetic resonance imaging (MRI). The most commonly used material for fixation hardware is medical-grade titanium alloy.

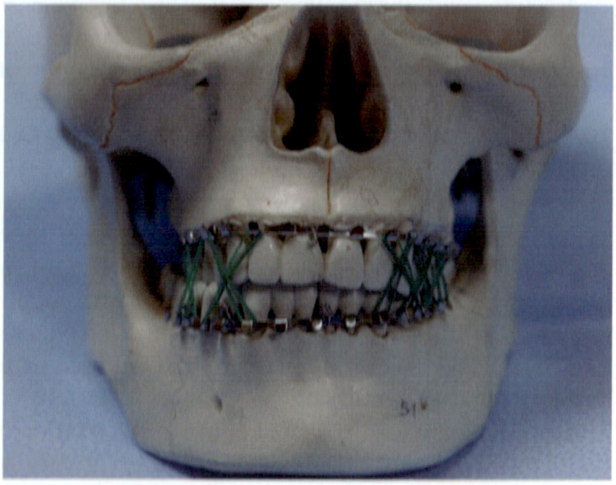

Fig. 10.8 Intermaxillary fixation (IMF) utilizing Erich arch bar and elastic

Bioresorbable fixation implants such as (polylactic acid) are also available and can be used in pediatric patients and in cases of less biomechanical requirements. But these implants are bulkier and more costly as compared with titanium implants.

10.3.9 Principles of ORIF

To understand the principles of ORIF, it is essential to get familiar with the buttress system of the maxillofacial skeleton. These buttresses can be grouped as vertical, horizontal, and transverse (Fig. 10.9). These are the pillars through which the forces of the mastication are transmitted to the cranium. Surgical treatment of maxillofacial fractures aims to restore these buttress systems.

Maxime Champy 1976 described the ideal lines of osteosynthesis for mandible and monocortical fixation devices. The placement of fixation hardware along these lines balances the tension and compression forces and offers the best biomechanical advantage (Fig. 10.10).

10.3.10 Fixation Schemes for Maxillofacial Fractures

10.3.10.1 Nonrigid Fixation

Nonrigid fixation "stabilizes the fracture fragments during function but may allow some inter-fragmentary motion." Miniplates and microplates, when used with monocortical screws, are an example of nonrigid fixation. The midface skeleton does not have any significant destabilizing muscular forces compared to the mandible; hence most of the fixation scheme used in mid-face is functionally stable fixation.

10.3.10.2 Rigid Fixation

A form of fixation that is strong enough to prevent interfragmentary motion between the fractured ends during function. It is also known as mechanically stable fixation. Example—Two miniplates at angle and body region of the mandible, lag screw fixation, and fixation utilizing high profile reconstruction plate.

10.3.10.3 Load Bearing Versus Load Sharing Osteosynthesis

Load-bearing fixation uses high-strength, rigid plates and screws that are strong enough to bear an entire load of masticatory function without any reliance on load sharing between bone fragments themselves; in other words, no buttressing is required for load-bearing constructs. It is indicated in the instances of mandible fracture with continuity defect, comminuted fracture, and atrophic mandible fracture. High-profile (2.5 or 2.8 mm) reconstruction plates with at least three bi-cortical screws on either side of the fracture line are used as fixation hardware to achieve load-bearing osteosynthesis.

The functional load is shared between the fixation device and the bone in load-sharing osteosynthesis. The bone must be solid with good buttressing to share the

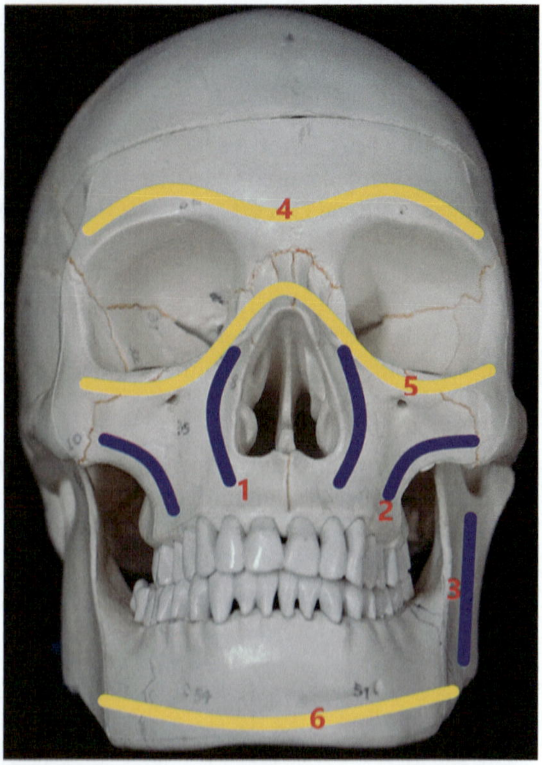

Fig. 10.9 Buttress system of the facial skeleton; vertical buttress, in blue (1—nasomaxillary, 2—zygomaticomaxillary, 3—vertical ramus of mandible) and horizontal buttress, in yellow (4—frontal, 5—infraorbital rim and zygomatic arch, 6—lower border of mandible)

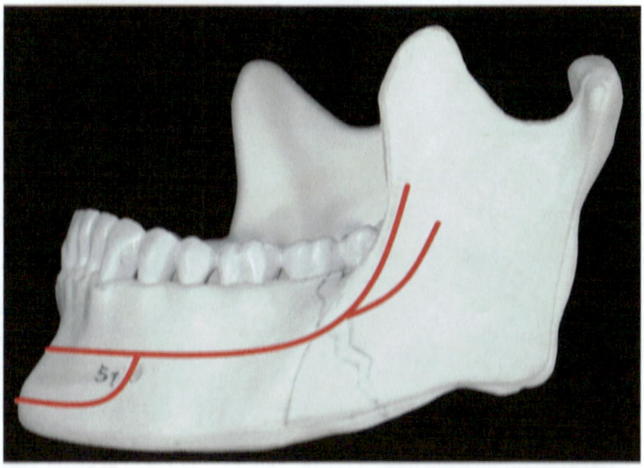

Fig. 10.10 Champy's ideal lines of osteosynthesis

loads. It is indicated in the case of a simple linear fracture of the mandible. For example, 1.5 and 2 mm miniplates and lag screws are used in load-sharing osteosynthesis.

10.3.10.4 Le Fort Fracture

The most commonly used classification for midface fracture is based upon the experiments of Rene Le Fort (1869–1951, France) where cadavers were exposed to frontal impact (Table 10.2) The fracture lines follow a definite pattern and are classified as Le Fort 1, 2 and 3 (Fig. 10.11a, b).

Le Fort 1 Fracture: The fracture line runs transversely through the maxilla commencing from the lateral margin of the pyriform aperture, above the roots of the teeth, below the zygomatic buttresses, and separating the pterygoid plates at the lower third.

10.3.10.5 Signs and Symptoms of Lefort I fracture

- Edema of upper lip and midface
- Epistaxis
- Ecchymosis of upper vestibule
- En bloc mobility of maxillary dentoalveolar segment

Table 10.2 The Le Fort classification

Le Fort 1 fracture (horizontal/low-level fracture)
Le Fort 2 (pyramidal fracture/mid-level fracture)
Le Fort 3 (craniofacial disjunction/high-level fracture)

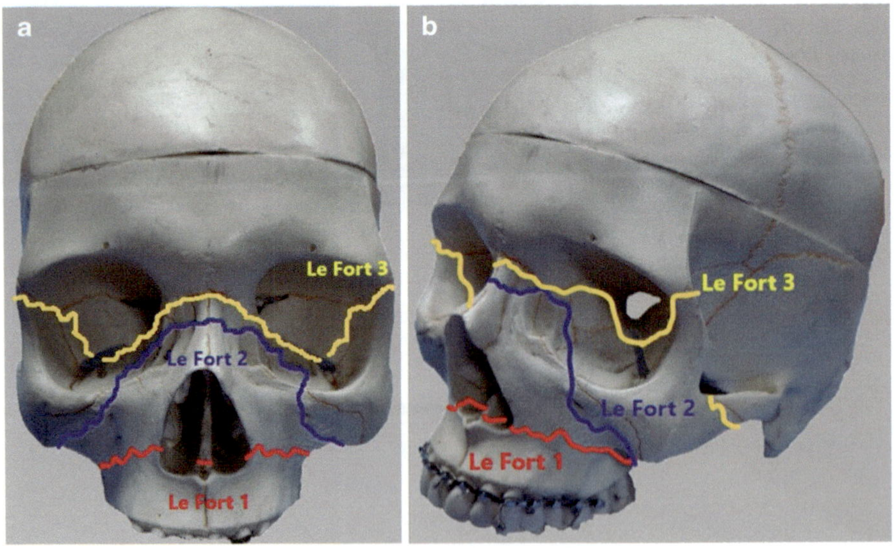

Fig. 10.11 (**a**, **b**) Le Fort fracture pattern along three-level (Le Fort 1; red, Le Fort 2; blue, Le Fort 3; yellow)

- Oronasal communication in case of an accompanied palatal split
- Step deformity and tenderness at zygomatic buttress intraorally
- Deranged occlusion
- Anterior Open bite in case of the impacted maxilla

Le Fort 2 Fracture: The fracture line begins at the thin middle area of the nasal bridge and involves the lacrimal bone crossing the infraorbital rim medial to or through the infraorbital foramen runs below the zygomatic buttress and fractures the pterygoid plates in the middle.

10.3.10.6 Signs and Symptoms of Lefort II fracture

- Edema of the midface.
- B/L circumorbital edema and ecchymosis—Raccoon eyes
- Epistaxis, septal hematoma
- Step deformity and tenderness at the infraorbital rim and zygomatic buttress intraorally
- En bloc mobility of midface with mobility of segments felt at nasal bridge and infraorbital rim
- Oronasal communication is associated with a palatal split
- Deranged occlusion
- Anterior open bite in case of the impacted maxilla
- Possible CSF rhinorrhea

Le Fort 3 Fracture: The fracture line commences at the bridge of the nose and runs into the orbit along the medial wall, floor, and then through the lateral wall and the frontozygomatic suture, and the zygomatic arches. It also fractures the pterygoid plates at the base, separating the entire midfacial skeleton from the cranial base (craniofacial disjunction).

10.3.10.7 Signs and Symptoms of Lefort III fracture

- Gross edema of the face
- B/L circumorbital edema and ecchymosis—Raccoon eyes
- Epistaxis, septal hematoma
- Step deformity and tenderness at the nasal bridge, frontozygomatic suture
- En bloc mobility of midface with mobility of segments felt at the frontonasal and frontozygomatic suture
- Oronasal communication if associated with a palatal split
- Deranged occlusion
- Anterior open bite in case of the impacted maxilla
- Elongation and flattening of the face
- Enophthalmos and diplopia
- Possible CSF rhinorrhea

10.3.11 Principles of Le Fort Fracture Management

10.3.11.1 Observation

Nonmobile or minimally mobile Le Fort fractures with unaffected occlusion in compliant patients with good dentition. These patients have been advised a liquid and non-chewable diet for 3–4 weeks.

Closed Treatment/IMF Minimally displaced fractures in a compliant patient amenable to IMF.

10.3.11.2 Open Reduction and Internal Fixation (ORIF)

Practically the ideal Le fort fracture lines are a rare phenomenon because most of the trauma nowadays is high-energy trauma that results in comminution and a variety of permutations and combinations of fracture patterns are seen. ORIF is indicated in instances of mobile maxilla resulting in deranged occlusion. The goal of treatment is to restore the buttress system of the midface in an anatomically correct position. The height, width, and projection of the face must be re-established. In the midface, 1.5 mm miniplates with monocortical screws are used for fixation along the vertical pillars (nasomaxillary buttress, zygomaticomaxillary buttress, and frontozygomatic buttress) (Fig. 10.12).

10.3.11.3 Mandible Fracture

The mandible is the second most common bone to fracture in the facial skeleton after the nasal bones. Mandible fracture can be classified on the basis of anatomic region or degree of comminution and displacement.

10.3.11.4 Anatomic Classification

Based upon the anatomic region of the mandible involved it can be classified as symphysis, parasymphysis, body, angle, ramus, condylar process, coronoid process, and dentoalveolar fracture (Fig. 10.13).

10.3.11.5 Signs and Symptoms

The etiology/mechanism of injury is important as it may indicate the location and severity of the mandible fracture. Various clinical signs also dictate the possibility of a fracture.

1. Step deformity over the lower border of mandible with tenderness and swelling.
2. Mobility across the tooth-bearing regions indicates a fracture.
3. **Deranged occlusion:**
   (a) Anterior open bite—could be the result of bilateral condyle or bilateral angle fractures.
   (b) Unilateral open bite—may be because of contralateral angle, condyle fracture, or because of ipsilateral hemarthrosis of the temporomandibular joint.
   (c) Posterior crossbite—symphysis fracture and bilateral condyle fractures with splaying of the posterior segments.

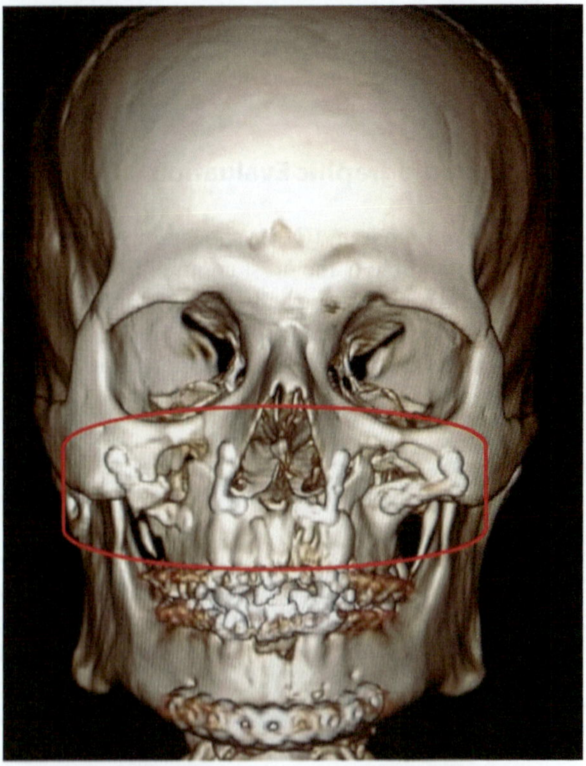

Fig. 10.12 Fixation at Le Fort 1 level, bilateral nasomaxillary, and zygomaticomaxillary buttress restoration

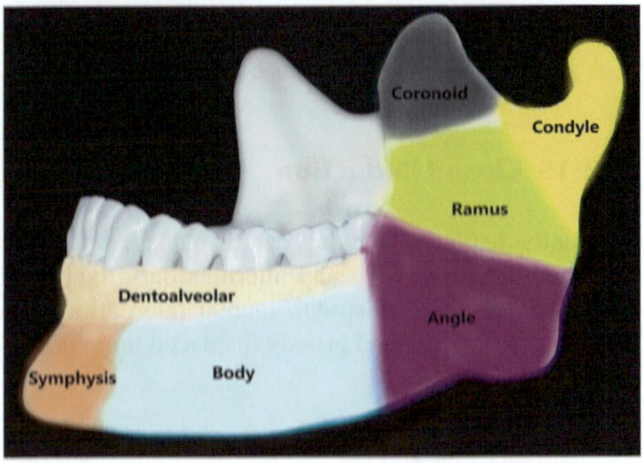

Fig. 10.13 Classification of the mandible fracture according to anatomic region (Symphysis: bounded by vertical lines distal to canines, body, angle, ramus, condyle, coronoid, dentoalveolar fracture)

4. Range of motion on mouth opening
   (a) Decreased because of pain and protective muscle spasm.
   (b) Deviation on mouth opening to the ipsilateral side of the condyle fracture.
5. **Sublingual hematoma** may be present in case of a symphysis or body fracture.
6. Anesthesia, paresthesia, or dysesthesia over the lower lip and mental region.

7. Loss of teeth because of avulsion or fracture of the crown of teeth.
8. Pain and tenderness in the temporomandibular joint region may indicate a condylar process fracture or intra-articular hematoma.

10.3.12 Radiographic Evaluation

The orthopantomogram (OPG) showing the entire dentition along with the maxilla and entire mandible is the most commonly used in the diagnosis of mandible fracture. Towne's view is especially recommended for sub-condylar fractures. CT face with 3D reconstruction depicts the fracture in different planes and is a good tool for detecting medial or lateral overlap or anteromedial displacement of proximal condylar fragment.

10.3.13 Management of Mandible Fracture

The decision-making in the management of mandible fracture must consider various factors like location of the fracture, degree of displacement of fractured fragments, quality of the bone, and general condition of the patient. The ultimate goal is to restore the anatomic form in terms of lower facial height, width, and projection and to restore the function of mastication by achieving good premorbid occlusion.

10.3.14 Observation

Greenstick/incomplete fractures with stable occlusion.

A soft (non-chewable) diet is advised for 4–6 weeks.

10.3.15 Closed Reduction

Minimally displaced fractures can be managed non-operatively by closed reduction with the help of arch bar and intermaxillary fixation (IMF). Contraindications for IMF include seizure disorder, mental retardation, chronic alcoholics, respiratory diseases like COPD, and grossly displaced unfavorable fractures.

10.3.16 Techniques for Closed Reduction

- Risdon wiring
- Ivy loop wiring
- Erich arch bars
- IMF screws

Duration of IMF depends upon the number of fractures, age of the patient, and type of fracture. Usually, for adult patients and single fractures, IMF of a 3–4-week duration is sufficient. For another accompanying fracture, an additional week must be added. In elderly patients, IMF for 6–8 weeks might be required.

Particular caution must be exercised in the case of pediatric patients with mandibular fracture and accompanying condylar fracture. In such cases, IMF is contraindicated; instead, an active mobilization of the mandible is advised to prevent TMJ ankylosis.

10.3.17 Open Reduction and Internal Fixation (ORIF)

It is indicated in cases of grossly displaced and/or comminuted mandible fracture or in cases where closed reduction utilizing IMF is contraindicated. It allows the patient to return early to function.

10.3.17.1 Surgical Access

- Symphysis and body and angle region—intraoral vestibular incision. In grossly displaced and multiple fractures, an extraoral submandibular incision can be utilized.
- Sub condylar fracture—retromandibular transparotid, preauricular, anterior parotid approach.

During the extraoral approach to the body or condylar region of the mandible, particular caution should be exercised to preserve the facial nerve branches.

10.3.18 Fixation Methods

- Body fracture: 2 mm miniplates in the juxtaalveolar region with at least two screws on either side of the fracture.
- Symphysis, parasymphysis fracture: two miniplates should be placed to counter torsion forces (Fig. 10.14e).
- Angle fracture: 2 mm miniplate at external oblique ridge via intraoral incision (Fig. 10.14c).
- Condylar fracture: two plates in nonparallel fashion, one along the posterior border and another along with the sigmoid notch. Other specialized fixation plates available for fixation of sub condylar fracture are trapezoidal plates, delta plates, lambda plates, Strut plates, etc. (Fig. 10.14d).

In the case of bilateral fractures, one fracture should be treated using rigid fixation, whereas the other can be fixed utilizing a nonrigid fixation scheme. Comminuted fracture, bone of poor quality, seizure patients with heavy muscle forces must be treated utilizing load-bearing hardware (Fig. 10.14a, b).

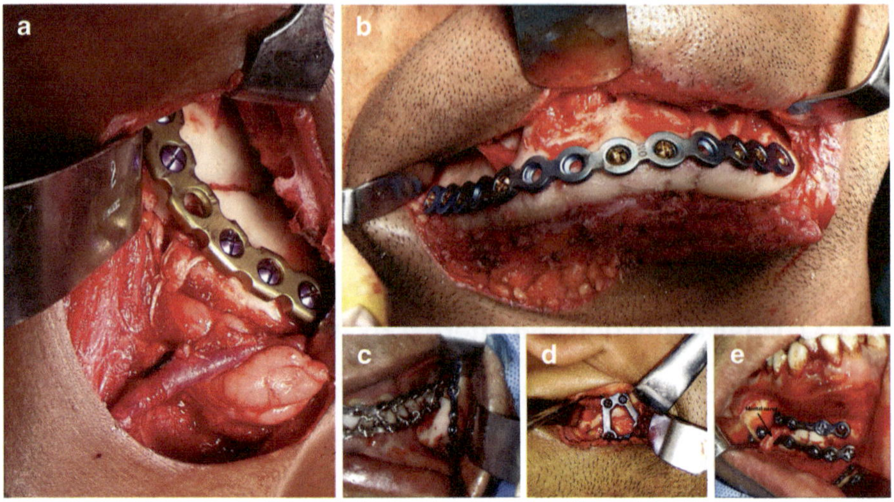

Fig. 10.14 Various fixation schemes of the mandible fracture; (**a**) extraoral fixation of angle fracture utilizing 2.4 mm reconstruction plate, (**b**) extraoral fixation of bilateral parasymphysis fracture using single 2.5 mm reconstruction plate, (**c**) intraoral fixation of angle fracture with single miniplate along the external oblique ridge, (**d**) fixation of subcondylar fracture of mandible utilizing trapezoidal condylar plate through retromandibular transparotid approach, (**e**) intraoral fixation of parasymphysis fracture using two miniplates

10.3.19 Special Considerations

10.3.19.1 Atrophic Mandibular Fracture

After the teeth are lost, the alveolar bone gets resorbed, and only the basal bone remains. However, there are many anatomical and biomechanical differences in the atrophic mandible compared with the adult mandible.

- Increased wishbone effect (flexion during function) in the atrophic mandible.
- Decreased vascularity (predominant blood supply is the periosteal one, whereas, in the adult mandible, the main blood supply comes from an inferior alveolar artery (endosteal)).

The patients with atrophic mandible are usually elderly and may not be fit for general anesthesia. External fixators can be used to temporarily stabilize the fracture till the patient is optimized for definitive surgery. As the bones are of poor quality and lack buttressing, the ORIF with load-bearing osteosynthesis utilizing high-profile locking reconstruction plates offers a distinct advantage in this patient group [7, 8]. The management strategy to be followed is to:

- Minimize periosteal stripping.
- Utilize more rigid and load-bearing osteosynthesis material (2.4 mm locking reconstruction plate).

- Screws are fixed away from the fracture, usually in the angle and symphysis region where a good stock of bone is present.
- Consider bone grafting in a severely atrophic mandible.

10.3.20 Pediatric Maxillofacial Fracture

The bone in this age group is more elastic and tends to bend (green stick fracture) rather than fracture. However, high-energy trauma may result in fracture with displaced fragments. The principles for the management of maxillofacial fractures in this age group are the same but require special attention because of the presence of developing/unerupted tooth buds in the jaw bones and growth. Most of the incomplete and simple fractures in this age group can be managed conservatively with observation and closed reduction techniques (IMF with arch bars or Risdon wiring, cap splints). However, severely displaced fractures need to be addressed operatively. The treatment duration in pediatric patients is less than in the adult population due to rapid healing and robust periosteum. If IMF is used, it can be removed in 2–3 weeks.

Intracapsular condylar fracture is more common in children. In such a case, IMF must be avoided; instead, an active mobilization of the jaw should be advised to prevent the occurrence of TMJ ankylosis. If a condylar fracture is accompanied by another body or symphysis fracture, then ORIF with fixation at the lower border of the mandible away from the tooth buds is desirable to enable active mouth-opening exercises.

In orbital floor fracture, muscle entrapment is more common in children because of the elastic nature of the bone. In such cases, emergency surgical exploration with the release of the muscle must be performed within 24–48 h.

References

1. Montovani JC, de Campos LM, Gomes MA, de Moraes VR, Ferreira FD, Nogueira EA. Etiology and incidence facial fractures in children and adults. Braz J Otorhinolaryngol. 2006;72(2):235–41.
2. Motamedi MH. An assessment of maxillofacial fractures: a 5-year study of 237 patients. J Oral Maxillofac Surg. 2003;61(1):61–4.
3. Elhammali N, Bremerich A, Rustemeyer J. Demographical and clinical aspects of sports-related maxillofacial and skull base fractures in hospitalized patients. Int J Oral Maxillofac Surg. 2010;39(9):857–62.
4. Winstanley RP. The management of fractures of the mandible. Br J Oral Maxillofac Surg. 1984;22:170.
5. Perry MT, Moutray T. Advanced Trauma Life Support (ATLS) and facial trauma: can one size fit all? Part 4: "Can the patient see?" Timely diagnosis, dilemmas, and pitfalls in the multiply injured, poorly responsive/unresponsive patient. Int J Oral Maxillofac Surg. 2008;37:505–14.
6. Joshi UM, Ramdurg S, Saikar S, et al. Brain injuries, and facial fractures: a prospective study of incidence of head injury associated with maxillofacial trauma. J Maxillofac Oral Surg. 2018;17:531–7. https://doi.org/10.1007/s12663-017-1078-8.

7. Salem JE, et al. Analysis of 523 mandibular fractures. Oral Surg Oral Med Oral Pathol. 1968;26:390.
8. Ellis E III, Price C. Treatment protocol for fractures of the atrophic edentulous mandible. J Oral Maxillofac Surg. 2008;66:421–35.

Trauma to Neck

11

Abhinav Srivastava

11.1 Why Study Neck Trauma?

The last few decades have witnessed an increase in the incidence of road traffic accidents (RTAs), thereby resulting in an increase in the incidence of neck trauma. There are other causes of neck injury also, such as sports injury, homicidal and suicidal hanging, and interpersonal violence involving the use of sharp and blunt weapons.

Anatomically, the neck extends from the skull base to the clavicle and is constituted by the aerodigestive tract along with neurological and vascular structures anteriorly and laterally and cervical vertebrae with spinal cord posteriorly. The platysma is a thin layer of skeletal muscle enveloping the neck and extends from the inferior border of the mandible to the subcutaneous tissues overlying the superior part of the pectoralis major muscle.

The strategic location of the neck makes it more susceptible to injury. It is a narrow conduit for the major blood vessels supplying the head and neck region, and the aerodigestive tract and various neurological structures also pass down from the head. The presence of these structures of vital importance makes the neck a very important aspect in a trauma. Being a narrow region, the injuries can be very difficult to manage, particularly the airway which requires immediate action to save a life.

Neck trauma poses a challenge in the emergency room because of the presence of so many above mentioned vital structures in a very confined and closed space such that the escape of all the structures from trauma is much less. Apart from these, spinal injuries are also frequently associated with patients presenting with polytrauma.

Handling patients with neck trauma is very critical and requires some special precautions, especially in view of suspected spinal injuries which are reasonably

A. Srivastava (✉)
Department of ENT, Rohilkhand Medical College and Hospital, Bareilly, UP, India

© The Author(s), under exclusive license to Springer Nature Singapore Pte Ltd. 2024

A. Agrawal et al. (eds.), *Special Considerations in Trauma Care*,
https://doi.org/10.1007/978-981-99-9662-9_11

associated in such cases of multiple injuries. In cases of associated spinal injury, excessive manipulation of the neck along with its inadequate immobilization during shifting may lead to the causation of additional neurological damage and may lead to a worsening of the patient's condition even converting an incomplete to a complete spinal transaction. Therefore, optimal management at such a critical time setting is of paramount importance for a favorable clinical outcome.

Neck trauma can be broadly classified into hanging, blunt, and penetrating trauma. Though they have different pathophysiology with a little but important difference in the line of management, the initial focus rests on the early protection of the compromised airway. Blunt trauma is found to be more common than penetrating trauma. The incidence of penetrating neck injury is estimated to be 5–10% of all the trauma cases in the emergency department and carries a mortality rate as high as 10% [1, 2].

There are always standardized guidelines for the management of the airway, but in practice, this may vary from place to place because of the difference in available resources and also the extent of training of the healthcare workers.

11.2 Mode of Injury

As mentioned, there are three modes of neck trauma:

(a) **Blunt trauma:** It is mainly caused because of RTAs and sports. As there is no obvious breach in the skin, the presentation related to laryngeal, vascular, and digestive tract injury is often delayed. A matter of most concern in these types of blunt neck trauma is associated with occult cervical spinal injury. In cases of motor vehicle accidents, the seatbelt may also be responsible for causing shearing trauma to the neck. A relatively high magnitude of energy is involved in the causation of this type of injury.

(b) **Penetrating trauma:** It is mainly caused by gunshot and stab wounds, and it invariably implies that there is a breach in platysma. The trauma is associated with even low energy penetration and has the potential to injure the vital structures present in the neck. Monson and colleagues divided the neck into three zones, which are discussed further in this chapter [3].

(c) **Near-hanging or strangulation:** The mechanism of this type of injury involves suffocation, and choking along with excessive manipulation of the cervical spine in a distracted manner which causes an increase in the jugular venous pressure thereby preventing the venous return from the brain this all results in loss of consciousness. A force of considerable amount during hanging is the cause of spinal cord injury.

Note: One important thing to be kept while managing a case of penetrating injury of the neck is patient will never die of asphyxia as during tracheal injury, the airway is always patent. Instead, the patient succumbs to either hemorrhagic shock or aspiration of blood. Therefore, a major concern in such cases should be centered on the prevention of blood seepage into the trachea, and this can be best done immediately by doing an emergency tracheostomy along with clamping of major damaged blood vessels to prevent hypovolemic shock.

11.3 Anatomical Zones in Cases of Penetrating Neck Injury

Division of neck in different anatomical zones for cases of penetrating neck trauma was first described by "Monson and Colleagues" in 1969 [3]. The classification deals with the injury in the anterior triangle of the neck of both sides, that is, from one anterior border of sternocleidomastoid to the other side including the anterior midline, mandible above, and clavicle with upper border of sternum below.

In penetrating trauma, this zone distinction has anatomic, diagnostic, and management implications. This system of dividing the neck into different zones is of great value in deciding the treatment plan for cases presenting with penetrating neck trauma.

The neck can be divided into three zones (Fig. 11.1):

Zone 1: This is one of the most critical zones and carries a greater threat to life because of a lot many structures of vital importance are present between the

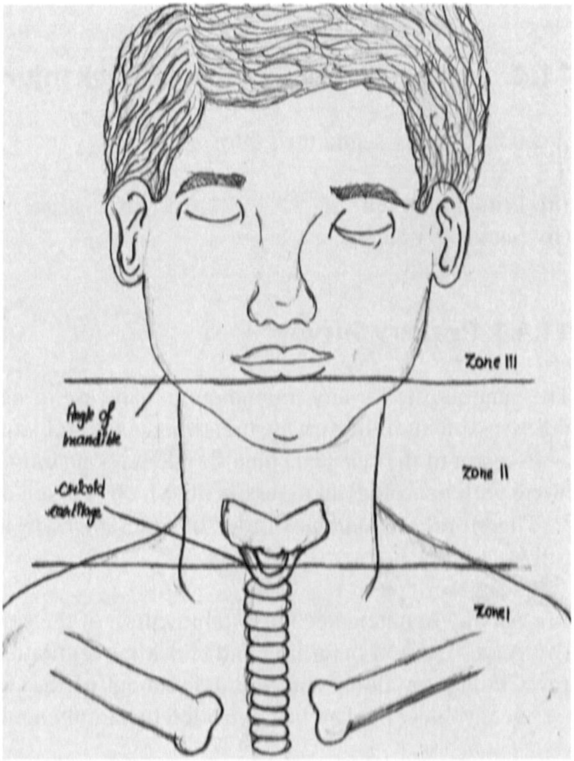

Fig. 11.1 Division of neck in three zones in penetrating injury

clavicle and cricoid cartilage. The strategic location of the clavicle guarding the thoracic inlet makes surgical access to this site a major challenge. The zone has the origin of the common carotid artery, vertebral, subclavian, and innominate vessels, brachial plexus, the trachea, esophagus, thoracic duct, and the apex of the lung.

Zone 2: The zone is the largest of all three and is found to be the most commonly injured region of the neck. This area lies between the cricoid cartilage below and the angle of the mandible above. Fortunately, the zone has relatively easy access for clinical assessment and also for surgical exploration. This region has carotid and vertebral arteries, internal jugular veins, the trachea, and the esophagus. As per some recent studies, this zone is the most commonly injured and is seen in 38–67% [4].

Zone 3: The area is confined between the angle of the mandible and the skull base and contains the distal part of the carotid and vertebral arteries and also the nasopharyngeal part of the pharynx. As the area is in close proximity to the skull base, it is very difficult to physically examine and is a very challenging issue for surgical exploration.

A point to remember: It is not necessary that the zone of the external wound correlate with the injury of the internal structures. This depends on and is governed by the point of entry and the vector of injury [5].

11.4 Assessment of a Case of Neck Injury

It can be broadly segmented into:

(a) Primary survey
(b) Secondary survey

11.4.1 Primary Survey

The general rule for any trauma applies in case of neck trauma also. It begins with the assessment of the airway, breathing, and circulation in a sequential manner. The assessment of the cervical spine should be done immediately along with “A” airway along with neurological assessment, which is again assessed in a secondary survey.

Therefore, the standard order of assessment in any case of neck trauma is as follows:

(a) Airway maintenance with stabilization of the cervical spine
(b) Assessment of breathing and checking ventilation
(c) Circulation along with the assessment of the hemorrhage/shock. In an emergency, bleeding can be controlled by simply applying manual pressure over the

wound rather than wasting time in finding bleeder in vain and blindly clamping vessels which may result in more injury

(d) Disability; neurological status
(e) Exposure/environmental control

A senior anesthetist along with a head and neck surgeon should intervene in such cases as early as possible. The priorities of the primary survey aim at the identification of any threatened or obstructed airway and its appropriate management with preferably a tracheostomy with a cuffed tracheostomy tube or, in case of its non-availability, an endotracheal tube can also be used with a caution that the tip of the tube to be adjusted just above the level of carina and equal ventilation of both lungs to be assured and this should be replaced with cuffed tracheostomy tube as soon as possible because, with endotracheal tube, there is increase chances of slipping in one of the lung resulting in one lung ventilation. The site of tracheostomy should be just distal to the site of neck injury or tracheal injury.

One should be very particular in assessing the red flag signs and symptoms which include:

Symptoms

- Stridor
- Dysphagia
- Dyspnea
- Dysphagia
- Odynophagia

Signs

- Respiratory distress
- Ecchymosis of neck
- Surgical emphysema of the neck and thorax
- Deviation of trachea to either side
- Hemoptysis of any amount
- Rapidly expanding neck hematoma
- Loss of laryngeal prominence

The presence of any of the clinical features may sequentially lead to the appearance of other new signs and symptoms. Therefore, a complete examination should be sought in both the primary and secondary surveys.

Following blunt injury, there may be variable presentation ranging from mild pain in the neck to severe respiratory obstruction presenting in the emergency department as stridor. Signs may also vary from normal or near normal to rapidly expanding neck swelling in the form of hematoma or surgical emphysema.

Sometimes patients initially present with dysphonia which may later progress to dyspnea and stridor due to progressive edema of the laryngeal mucosa. Hemoptysis following blunt trauma is a sign of injury of the laryngeal mucosa and is a point of concern for possible impending respiratory obstruction.

Blunt injury to the laryngotracheal framework frequently presents with swelling in the neck with loss of laryngeal prominence, which may be associated with subcutaneous emphysema due to a breach in the airway. Bleeding from the damaged vessels is another cause of progressive edema in the neck.

Tracheal deviation is generally rare to see but is a very serious finding and is mostly due to associated pneumothorax which sometimes goes unnoticed and is discovered when saturation does not become normal and or patient's complaints of breathlessness even after tracheostomy.

Laryngotracheal separation is one of the grave findings, and sometimes there is only a partial continuity of the laryngotracheal unit. In these cases, blind intubation should always be avoided as it may convert partial airway breach into complete dislodgement and result in false passage resulting in one-way entry of air outside the airway and inadvertently causing pressure over the airway thereby further deteriorating the airway. Applying cricoid pressure while doing laryngoscopy for intubation may displace the laryngotracheal fractures into complete separation, which makes airway stabilization even more challenging.

Providing positive pressure ventilation with the help of a face mask or by supraglottic airway devices in an emergency poses a significant risk of creating a leakage of air in the vicinity thereby further compromising the airway.

Flattening of the laryngeal prominence is one of the definite signs of laryngeal injury often associated with pain in the neck with associated dysphonia. Arytenoid dislocation following blunt trauma of the neck can also occur, and it carries the best prognosis if diagnosed within 24 hours, and management includes the relocation of the joint under vision. If addressed after 72 h, then as fibrosis has set in, it might require the use of a laser to release the bands.

11.5 Investigation and Management

Once the patient is stabilized, then the case should be evaluated with pan endoscopy under general anesthesia and all injuries should be documented. The extent of involvement of injury could involve the larynx, trachea, bronchus, and esophagus. Once all the injury is assessed and documented along with radiology, then a comprehensive approach is made to explore and repair the neck.

Injuries involving zones I and III should be evaluated and taken up more selectively due to difficulty in its anatomic accessibility. The evaluation of such cases includes angiography, bronchoscopy, and/or esophagoscopy and contributions from different specialties.

Injuries involving zone II are constituted in the majority of cases who present with penetrating neck injuries. All cases of such types should always undergo mandatory surgical exploration.

Neck injury can also be approached by a "**no zone**" approach. This approach provides superior outcomes in patients presenting with penetrating neck injury. This may be because this approach entails the clinicians to assess the entire neck region right from the skull base to the clavicle on both sides as a single entity. This is further followed by its management in a priority-wise approach. This type of management of penetrating neck injuries is a selective approach, and due consideration is given to the clinical findings along with the physiological status of the patient.

Small mucosal injuries and/or un-displaced laryngeal fractures are to be managed conservatively.

On surgical exploration, if an injury is identified with no soft tissue loss, then it needs to be repaired primarily with simple absorbable sutures. Laryngeal tissue should be repaired with a non-absorbable suture-like proline of finer size 4-0 or less.

If there is a severely displaced fracture involving laryngeal cartilages, then the laryngeal lumen should be maintained and supported with a stent of appropriate size. If the stent is not available, then a small segment of a smaller endotracheal tube can also be used as a stent and left for few days. Placing the stent also provides some added benefits such as bolstering the soft tissues and arytenoids and preventing the formation of hematomas, web, and synechia.

Fortunately, injuries involving cervical esophageal are less common, and this is attributed to its central location which protects it. These injuries present with minimal to no symptoms and often go unnoticed. The high degree of suspicion in neck trauma and proper follow-up of systematic management prevent its complications. All such patients with suspected esophageal injuries must refrain from oral diet for at least 72 h along with broad-spectrum intravenous antibiotics.

If, during the course of treatment, patients develop signs and symptoms suggestive of esophageal perforation and/or demonstrated by radiology, then immediate repair must be planned. If the cervical esophagus is only involved, then it can easily be accessed through the neck. If the injury is further down, then the help of a cardiothoracic surgeon should be taken immediately. If the esophageal leak is not diagnosed or treated promptly, then it may lead to mediastinitis. The formation of abscesses or empyema may also occur as a result of leakage of the gastric contents through the perforated esophagus.

Answer to the timing of the repair of these esophageal injuries mainly depends on the time since injury. Patients who are diagnosed with esophageal injury within 12 h of injury may be managed by primary repair of the ends with submucosal or Cornell sutures along with associated soft tissue injuries and all such wounds should be drained after repair. If the diagnosis is after 12 h of the injury, then it may cause an increase in morbidity and even mortality and the primary repair of such wounds is less likely to be successful. All these patients should ideally undergo debridement and drainage of the wound and should be followed by a planned repair when signs and symptoms of mediastinitis are controlled. There should be a closed monitoring of all the patients with neck injury and immediate intervention with repeat exploration should be sought if signs of infection develop.

References

1. Vishwanatha B, Sagayaraj A, Huddar SG, et al. Penetrating neck injuries. Indian J Otolaryngol Head Neck Surg. 2007;59:221–4.
2. Saito N, Hito R, Burke PA, Sakai O. Imaging of penetrating injuries of the head and neck: current practice at a level I trauma center in the united states. Keio J Med. 2014;63:23–33.
3. Monson DO, Saletta JD, Freeark RJ. Carotid vertebral trauma. J Trauma. 1969;9:987–99.
4. Low G, Inaba K, Chouliaras K. The use of the anatomic "zones" of the neck in the assessment of penetrating neck injury. Am Surg. 2014;80:970–4.
5. Sperry JL, Moore EE, Coimbra R, et al. Western Trauma Association critical decisions in trauma: penetrating neck trauma. J Trauma Acute Care Surg. 2013;75:936–40.

12 Battered Baby Syndrome: Diagnosis and Management

Rakesh Mishra, Nityanand Pandey, and Amit Agrawal

12.1 Introduction

Battered baby syndrome (BBS) or child abuse has been known by various terms for many decades. This is often an under-examined entity. These laws were designed to protect the rights of children in Western and developed countries. However, in many developing countries, including India, the laws on the protection of the child from abuse and trauma at the hands of the caregiver are not well placed. This is because of cultural differences and the fact that the difference between the practice of inculcating discipline and maltreatment is blurred. The degree of trauma that a child is subjected to can vary from minor or mental alone to severe or fatal. In several reports from developed nations, BBS has been identified as a major public health problem leading to disability and death in children, particularly in infants. In this chapter, we present an overview of BBS and the clinical aspects of BBS. The psychological aspects of BBS and rehabilitation are too broad to be covered in this chapter, and readers are directed to the reference at the end of this chapter for a detailed reading.

R. Mishra (✉)
Department of Neurosurgery, Institute of Medical Sciences, Banaras Hindu University, Varanasi, India

Department of Neurosurgery, All India Institute of Medical Sciences, Bhopal, Madhya Pradesh, India

N. Pandey
Department of Neurosurgery, Institute of Medical Sciences, Banaras Hindu University, Varanasi, India

A. Agrawal
Department of Neurosurgery, All India Institute of Medical Sciences, Bhopal, Madhya Pradesh, India

© The Author(s), under exclusive license to Springer Nature Singapore Pte Ltd. 2024
A. Agrawal et al. (eds.), *Special Considerations in Trauma Care*,
https://doi.org/10.1007/978-981-99-9662-9_12

12.2 History of the BBS

BBS is also known as shaken baby syndrome. John Caffey first described what he identified as "whiplash shaken infant syndrome" in 1946 [1].

He was a radiologist who identified a cluster of infants and small children with subdural, subarachnoid, and retinal hemorrhages and traction injury of the periosteum of long bones in the absence of external injury, skull fracture, and long bone fracture. In his landmark report, he described 6 infants who had a subdural hematoma and 23 fractures of the long bones, of which 14 had metaphyseal fractures and 9 had diaphyseal fractures. Surprisingly, he noted no history of trauma or comorbidity which could explain the severe injuries in these cases. At that time, he concluded that long bone fractures were traumatic and appeared to be an associated complication of infantile subdural hematoma (SDH); however, the mechanisms were not clear. Later, he continued to build upon his work; in 1974, he identified the diagnostic features of "Whiplash shaken infant syndrome" as intracranial and intraocular hemorrhages in the absence of skull fracture, long bone metaphyseal fracture with no signs of external injury, and history of trauma. He further suggested that an infant with unexplained seizures, irritability, bulging fontanelle, forceful vomiting, and paralysis should be carefully managed with caution for the possible diagnosis of whiplash-shaken infant syndrome.

He further described that prolonged and habitual whiplash shaking leads to chronic insult, resulting in idiopathic mental retardation or cerebral motor defects. Some children may later develop decreased hearing or vision. Dr. Caffey associated morphological differences, such as a larger head size to body ratio, weaker neck muscles, weaker tone, and increased water content of the brain in infants with increased susceptibility to injuries from casual violent shaking.

With the advent of computed tomography (CT), the ease of diagnosis has increased. Later, researchers also identified that there was an impact in some of these cases, in contrast to Caffey, who suggested no history of trauma. Over time, the terms BBS, shaken baby syndrome, or shaken infant syndrome became synonymous with Caffey's "Whiplash shaken infant syndrome." The term shaken infant syndrome comprises severe head injury in an infant attributable to both shaking and impact. In the last decade, non-accidental trauma (NAT) in children has been used to describe these injuries because it has fewer negative connotations.

Dr. Caffey probably provided the first description of BBS as stated above; it was not recognized as a separate entity till 1960 when Henry Kempe coined the term "Battered Baby Syndrome" [2].

Child abuse is an umbrella term that includes several variants such as shaken baby syndrome, battered child syndrome, BBS, and non-accidental injuries in children. The World Health Organization (WHO)'s regional office in Southeast Asia in New Delhi states that these variants are called by different names but have the same outcome: the child gets harmed at the hands of the caretaker, who is frequently a close relative [3].

12.3 Presentation of a Child With BBS

It is relatively easier to identify a case of BBS when the parents bring the child to the hospital during the acute phase of the injury. However, this scenario becomes complicated when a child is neglected and battered. When the child is both neglected and battered, the parents may not insist on hospital admission; rather, the child is brought to a very late stage. There are several reports where parents brought the child with a lump that showed a well-developed callus around the fracture site.

The principal identifying feature is that the child who has suffered abuse in the hands of the caregiver is brought to the hospital by parents and relatives with injuries inconsistent with the history provided. These children may present with injuries at different stages of healing or with intracranial infection-like presentations. It is not surprising that many of these children were initially treated for these disorders by primary healthcare providers [4]. Therefore, healthcare providers and the public must be aware of how to recognize and report BBS. There are well-established guidelines in Western and developed countries; however, guidelines and practice recommendations are lacking in most developing countries, including India. In India, the National Commission for Protection of Child Rights and the Indian Academy of Pediatricians have recently formulated guidelines on reporting child abuse.

12.4 Epidemiology

The WHO Club BBS in child maltreatment is defined as any mental, emotional, or physical trauma to a child between 0 and 18 years of age with long-term functional sequelae. In this chapter, we restrict our discussion to the neurological aspects of BBS [5]. As per WHO, nearly 3 in 4 children of approximately 300 million children aged 2–4 years suffer some form of physical or psychological abuse at the hands of the caregiver [5]. Child maltreatment has long-term adverse effects on the physical and mental health of the child, and the resultant social and occupational outcome reduces the country's growth [5].

A literature search identified only a few case reports, suggesting that there are no formal guidelines on surveillance and reporting BBS. Therefore, the exact burden of the disease, patients, and societal risk factors has not been established. There is a need for increased awareness among policymakers to recognize and reduce the incidence of child abuse in developing countries. The only study conducted to date in India was in 2007 labeled "The national study on child abuse." The study comprised a sample of 12,447 children studied by the Ministry of Women and Child Development, India across 13 states, and concluded that two out of every three children suffered from child abuse in this sample. However, this study was not error-free and did not provide a precise burden on the problem. The main criticism of this cross-sectional survey study was the use of purposive sampling, non-probability sampling methods, arbitrary selection, non-objectivity of the respondents, and other statistical errors in the methodology.

In a population-based study, it was reported that the incidence of abusive head trauma was higher in infants than in older children with 21 in 100,000 infants suffering abusive head trauma every year with an associated mortality of 33% and morbidity of 50% among the survivors [6]. Child abuse can be seen at any age but is commonly reported in children less than 2 years of age and is most frequently seen in children under 1 year of age. When a child grows, they can run away from complaining and gain security.

12.5 Clinical Aspects

A child with the BBS is likely to be malnourished and appears neglected with general health below par of the peer group. The child is likely to have evidence of neglect including poor skin hygiene, hair growth, multiple soft tissue injuries, skin bruises of different ages, malnutrition, and a history of parental neglect and trauma. It was found in one study that BBS children with abusive head trauma have other pre-existing comorbid neurological ailments in the form of cerebral atrophy and ex vacuo ventricular dilatation [7]. This suggests multiple incidences of trauma and chronic traumatic encephalopathy kind of neuroimaging in these children. Studies on the long-term behavioral and cognitive sequelae in these patients are lacking.

Clinicians should suspect BBS when there is unsuspected or unrecognized trauma, mild or moderately severe trauma with doubtful history, evidence of neglect, evidence of multiple injuries to the soft tissue and skeleton, and injuries of different periods.

12.6 Radiological Aspects

Clinicians should not hesitate to ask for radiology imaging and advanced imaging techniques based on the body regions involved if there is suspicion of BBS. To accurately interpret the radiology related to BBS, the clinician should precisely know the child's age, the nature of the injury, and the time interval between the injury and radiology. Subperiosteal hematoma is a significant radiographic finding indicative of child abuse because the periosteum of infants can be easily stripped with trauma compared to older children. If the initial films are not confirmatory, repeat imaging should be performed at an interval of 2–3 weeks because there may not be any findings on the initial examinations of the long bones. The pattern of bony injuries commonly seen in BBS includes shaft fracture due to direct blow or compression force, epiphyseal separation, and periosteal shearing due to torsional and tractional forces in grasping the extremities, as handled by adults. The key skeletal injuries physicians should look for in the diagnosis of BBS are predilection for epiphysis, periosteal injury, irregularity of mineralization, multiple callus, different stages of healing, subperiosteal hemorrhage in metaphyseal and epiphyseal regions, and subdural hemorrhage in absence of skull fracture.

12.7 Abusive Head Trauma

Head injury is one of the most common injuries sustained by a child in BBS and contributes to morbidity and mortality. Abusive head trauma may present with multiple subdural, interhemispheric, epidural, hypoxic-ischemic, and brain edema [8, 9]. In a systematic review of 2353 patients with abusive head trauma, researchers found that the odds ratio of having subdural hemorrhage was 8.2 (95% confidence interval 6.1–11; p-value <0.0001), while the odds ratio for subarachnoid hemorrhage was 0.98 and extradural hemorrhage was 0.1 [9]. In the same study, it was reported that the odds of sustaining multiple intracranial hemorrhages and interhemispheric hemorrhage were highest among other patterns of intracranial hemorrhage in abusive head trauma [8]. Subdural hemorrhage over the convexity and supratentorial region was more likely with abusive head trauma than at the infratentorial location [2]. Another key characteristic of neuroimaging of these extra-axial lesions was the presence of multiple attenuations in different lesions or the same lesion at the same time. Low attenuation of subdural hemorrhage was more likely in abusive head trauma than in non-abusive head trauma [9]. Wells et al. created a multiple logistic regression model with four variables, namely, convexity SDH, interhemispheric SDH, low attenuation SDH, and absence of skull fracture, and reported the predictive sensitivity of 84% and specificity of 83% for abusive head trauma at cutoff >0.45 [10]. Cobbs et al. reported in their study of 30 children that multiple convexity subdural hemorrhages, interhemispheric hemorrhage, and a combination of subarachnoid hemorrhage with subdural hemorrhage were more common in abusive head trauma, while intraparenchymal hemorrhage and skull fracture were more common in the non-abusive head trauma [11]. Ichord et al. published their study on children aged 0–36 months about the relationship between the clinical features and hypoxic-ischemic changes identified on diffusion-weighted imaging [7]. In this study, the authors reported frequency of four different combinations: noncontiguous intracranial injury (SDH, subarachnoid hematoma, or contusions) and Hypoxic-Ischemic Injury (HII), contiguous intracranial injury and HII, traumatic lesions without HII, and nondiscriminatory traumatic lesions [7]. The authors reported that the combination of HII with intracranial traumatic lesions at noncontiguous and non-co-localizing regions were more characteristics of abusive head trauma [7]. They further reported that patients with HII in abusive head trauma had higher risk of seizures at presentation, requiring intubation, requiring neurosurgical intervention and in-hospital rehabilitation [7].

12.8 Management

The primary management of BBS is prevention through education and increasing awareness so that the incidence of further child abuse can be minimized to the same child or different in society. The involvement of pediatricians with awareness of child abuse and education of clinicians, including neurosurgeons catering to pediatric patients in large-volume centers, is of paramount importance. Patients with BBS should be actively admitted and managed according to the required specialty. In addition, there is an important window of intervention for the family that clinicians should not miss. As the parents of child abuse are likely to have been used in their childhood and have schizoid or depressive personalities, the involvement of a family therapist, counselor, social service volunteer, psychiatrist, and psychologist is critical to comprehensive care in the child abuse case. The legal aspects of the region should be adhered to and authorities should be notified. When a child is discharged from the hospital, a follow-up period is essential. As these children are likely to have neurological comorbidities, they should be followed up with adults to assess the behavioral and cognitive symptoms that arise later in life.

The system should be involved at all levels, from the government to society, as a unit and at the individual level. The level of awareness of the treating physician has to be of the highest standard because 25–50% of these children will either die or be permanently injured within a year. National organizations should create programs for the follow-up and rehabilitation of these families, and there should be helpline numbers for caregivers to reach out for appropriate notification and registration of patients with BBS.

12.9 Future Directions

In the case of a battered baby, the doctor performs his professional duties by providing appropriate treatment and societal duties by informing the authorities. As many such patients often belong to well-to-do families, neglected babies may not even come to the attention of the hospital. Therefore, a natural question arises as to why the authorities have an outlook and surveillance of hospital cases only. There is a need for greater integration of child welfare organizations at the societal level by involving and educating community members, ASHA workers, Anganwadi workers, and panchayats. Therefore, the role of primordial prevention by education and preventive medicine is highlighted and active participation of the community, healthcare workers, policymakers, non-governmental organizations (NGOs), child welfare organizations, and law-enforcement agencies should be aspired to.

The understanding of BBS is minimal among primary healthcare workers and pediatricians attending to these babies. The integration of education into the medical curriculum will be a fruitful strategy to address this issue. It has to be realized that medical professionals have unique expertise to understand the troublesome situation of parents and children in the case of BBS. Therefore, this potential of healthcare workers should be nurtured to identify means to mitigate the trouble of both parents and children. In a family where a BBS child with BBS is found, the child is in a constant state of threat to health and safety. The job of a medical professional is twofold: one is to bring the child to safety by admitting and treating them in the hospital, and the other is to actively rehabilitate the parents. John Caffey [1], who first identified BBS, proposed a nationwide educational campaign in 1974 with a song slogan.

References

1. Caffey J. The whiplash shaken infant syndrome: manual shaking by the extremities with whiplash-induced intracranial and intraocular bleedings, linked with residual permanent brain damage and mental retardation. Pediatrics. 1974;54(4):396–403.
2. Kempe CH, Silverman FN, Steele BF, Droegemueller W, Silver HK. Battered child syndrome. JAMA. 1962;181(1):17–24.
3. De Silva DH, Hobbs CJ. Managing child abuse: handbook for medical officers. Geneva: World Health Organization; 2004.
4. Jayakumar I, Ranjit S, Gandhi D. Shaken baby syndrome. Indian Pediatr. 2004;41(3):280–4.
5. Purkait S, Mahajan S, Sharma MC, Sarkar C, Suri V. Pediatric-type diffuse low grade gliomas: histomolecular profile and practical approach to their integrated diagnosis according to the WHO CNS5 classification. Indian J Pathol Microbiol. 2022;65:42–9.
6. Jayawant S, Rawlinson A, Gibbon F, Price J, Schulte J, Sharples P, et al. Subdural haemorrhages in infants: population based study. BMJ. 1998;317(7172):1558–61.
7. Ichord RN, Naim M, Pollock AN, Nance ML, Margulies SS, Christian CW. Hypoxic-ischemic injury complicates inflicted and accidental traumatic brain injury in young children: the role of diffusion-weighted imaging. J Neurotrauma. 2007;24(1):106–18.
8. Arhami Dolatabadi A, Baratloo A, Rouhipour A, Abdalvand A, Hatamabadi H, Forouzanfar M, et al. Interpretation of computed tomography of the head: emergency physicians versus radiologists. Trauma. 2013;18(2):86–9.
9. Kemp AM, Jaspan T, Griffiths J, Stoodley N, Mann MK, Tempest V, et al. Neuroimaging: what neuroradiological features distinguish abusive from non-abusive head trauma? A systematic review. Arch Dis Child. 2011;96(12):1103–12.
10. Wells RG, Vetter C, Laud P. Intracranial hemorrhage in children younger than 3 years: prediction of intent. Arch Pediatr Adolesc Med. 2002;156(3):252–7.
11. Ewing-Cobbs L, Prasad M, Kramer L, Louis PT, Baumgartner J, Fletcher JM, et al. Acute neuroradiologic findings in young children with inflicted or noninflicted traumatic brain injury. Childs Nerv Syst. 2000;16(1):25–33; discussion 4.

13 Military Injuries: Special Considerations

M. S. Sridhar and Krishan K. Yadav

13.1 Introduction

Injuries sustained in the battlefield need special consideration as the mechanism of injury, circumstances, the facilities available to manage these injuries, and the aim of management are different from the injuries sustained in a civilian setup. Management of these injuries requires an intimate knowledge of the ballistics to understand the full nature of injuries that a surgeon is likely to encounter. To understand the circumstances in which these injuries occur or to grasp the facilities available and the conditions under which these injuries are to be managed cannot be fully elucidated. However, it is the responsibility of all surgeons and emergency physicians to be essentially aware of the basics of missile injuries of all types.

13.2 Ballistics

Ballistics is the science **of the propulsion, flight behavior, and impact of projectiles such as bullets and unguided bombs**. It is divided into i**nternal ballistics**, which is the behavior of the projectile from the firing till it leaves the muzzle, **external ballistics,** which is the behavior of the projectile after it leaves the muzzle, and **intermediate ballistics,** which studies the transition from internal to external ballistics [1, 2]. A basic knowledge of ballistics is important for the surgeon to comprehend the amount of tissue damage that is likely to occur or to anticipate the amount of tissue damage that has already occurred to effectively manage these cases.

M. S. Sridhar (✉) · K. K. Yadav
Command Hospital Air Force, Bangalore, Karnataka, India

© The Author(s), under exclusive license to Springer Nature Singapore Pte Ltd. 2024
A. Agrawal et al. (eds.), *Special Considerations in Trauma Care*,
https://doi.org/10.1007/978-981-99-9662-9_13

13.3 External Ballistics

An object propelled through space at high speed is subject to various forces. These forces interact which results in the final trajectory of the missile. These forces are as follows:

1. The various forces acting due to the bullet motion
   (a) Velocity:
      Forward (speed and direction)
      Rotational: It varies depending on the length of the barrel of the gun or rifle.
   (b) Velocity of the bullet at the muzzle end for various firearms is as follows:
      Revolver: 600–900 ft/s
      Pistol: 1200–1440 ft/s
      Rifle: 2000–3500 ft/s
2. Forces that are present in the medium through which the missile travels
   (a) Air resistance
   (b) Gravity

The final force with which the missile strikes the person depends on these forces and also on the distance which the missile travels—which determines the amount of kinetic energy expended by the missile in reaching the person with the residual kinetic energy in the missile, which is dissipated within the tissue around the point of entry of the victim. This is expressed as the kinetic energy formula:

$$\mathrm{KE} \propto \mathrm{W} \times \mathrm{V}^2$$

That is the kinetic energy (KE) is proportional to the product of the weight of the missile (W) and the *square* of its velocity (V).

More importantly, the surgeon should be aware of the amount of kinetic energy dissipated to the tissues after the impact, which is expressed mathematically as

$$\mathrm{KE} = \mathrm{W} \propto (\mathrm{Ven} - \mathrm{Vex})^2$$

where Ven is the velocity of the missile at impact and Vex is the velocity of the missile at the exit. If the missile does not exit the victim, then Vex becomes zero and the entire kinetic energy is dissipated in the tissues of the victim.

Four patterns of movement of the missile occur, in the air along its trajectory, before it strikes the target. This is more pronounced when the velocity of the missile approaches and exceeds 3000 feet/s. The patterns of movement are enumerated below and are represented in Fig. 13.1 [3]:

(a) Yaw—Yaw is an oscillation of the bullet on its longitudinal axis while in flight.
(b) Tumbling—Tumbling is a forward rotation about the center of the bullet.
(c) Precession—Precession is a circular yaw.

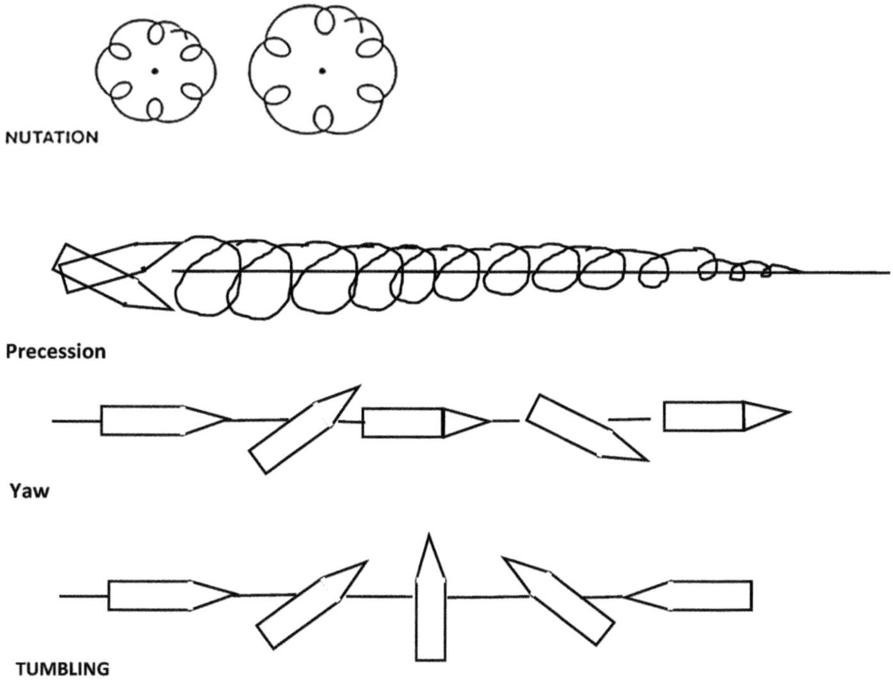

Fig. 13.1 Diagrammatic representation of yaw, precession, nutation, and tumbling

(d) Nutation—Nutation is a forward rotation in the long axis of the bullet in a rosette pattern of small circles about a larger circle.

13.4 Mechanism of Injury

The mechanism of the injury and the final outcome of the damage depend primarily on the mode and amount of kinetic energy transferred to the tissue. The energy transferred is dependent on the angle by which the missile strikes the individual, the site of impact, and the tissues under the site of impact, in addition to cavitation and secondary missile injury [3–6].

The mechanism of wound production is primarily by

(a) Laceration and crushing
(b) Shock waves
(c) Cavitation

The sequence of events that occur when the missile strikes a target is as follows:

Missile strikes soft and elastic tissue.
Pushes and stretches the skin and underlying tissue.
Rotates upon its axis.
Indentation is produced.
Perforation of the tissue.
Passage of the bullet.
The energy of the bullet is dissipated to the tissue.
Damage is proportionate to the diameter/velocity of the bullet.

13.5 Laceration and Crushing

Laceration and crushing effects are produced by the direct effect of bullet/missile on the tissues. There are a few terms that are used traditionally in describing the wounding potential of missiles, these are as enumerated below, with explanation:

1. Frontal area: Frontal area refers to the area of the projectile where it strikes the tissue. This is affected by expansion, tumbling, and fragmentation.
2. Fragmentation: Bullet fragmentation occurs either spontaneously or when a bone is struck and produces secondary missiles. Among all factors, fragmentation is responsible for the greatest wounding potential.
3. Velocity: The velocity of the missile is the most important factor determining the amount of energy transferred to the tissues and subsequent resultant tissue damage.

Alteration in the angle of incidence causes additional dissipation of kinetic energy. If a missile strikes a target at any angle other than 180°, that is other than its point, the angle of incidence of the missile is altered, which leads to additional tissue contact and more injury at the point of entry.

13.6 Shock Waves

When the missile strikes the tissue, kinetic energy is transferred to the tissue. The kinetic energy transferred is higher if the missile is of a high velocity ($KE = ½ M \times V^2$). The tissue in front and around the missile after entry into the tissue is compressed by the missile. The region of compression moves as a shock wave in a spherical form along the tract of the missile, with progressively reducing shock waves as the energy keeps dissipating. Pressure changes remain for a fraction of a second and may reach up to 100 atm. This results in tissue damage at a distance from the wound track. Therefore, muscles, bones, blood vessels, nerves, and various internal organs, which are at a distance, may be damaged despite the fact that they had no direct contact with a missile. The extent of damage in these tissues is proportional to the tensile strength of the tissue and is extensive in tissues such as skeletal muscle. This resultant damage requires extensive debridement of the injured tissues and changes the priorities in the management of the patient. The saving of life is the primary aim, followed by the salvage of limb and finally attempt at salvage of limb function.

13.7 Cavitation

Cavitation is a ballistic phenomenon that results from the spreading shock wave. As the tissues along the path of the missile move away due to the shock wave, they move forward and laterally along the path of the missile—*at about the speed of sound in water*—4800 ft/s, a transient, water-vapor-filled cavity is produced. This cavity is initially at sub-atmospheric pressure because of the speed with which it is created and this cavity collapses within microseconds in response to atmospheric pressure and tissue pressures around the cavity [5–7].

Energy from the bullet is dissipated forward and laterally away from the bullet and tract. If the missile is of a high velocity—>3000 ft/s—the cavity continues to enlarge even after the bullet has passed. The cavity that is created is sub-atmospheric, and since it has negative pressure, it sucks air and debris from both ends.

This cavity is temporary, and it reforms and collapses several times with diminishing amplitude due to oscillations of the shock waves along the path of the missile, this occurs till all motion ceases. This phenomenon results in greater tissue damage to inelastic tissues (liver, spleen) than elastic tissues (e.g., lung). In tissues with low-tensile strength (organs), cavitation develops more rapidly and extensively (*muscle is intermediate in tensile strength; bone and tendon have high-tensile strength*). The missile path/tract remains back as a permanent cavity (Fig. 13.2).

Organs most susceptible due to cavitation are as follows:

Brain and brainstem
Heart and aorta
Other great vessels of the chest
Lung, specifically tension pneumothorax
Abdominal
Peripheral arterial tree

If the path of the missile is short, that is if the target is closer to the gun, the missile may exit the tissues as degradation of the energy from the missile to the tissues is incomplete and is probably beginning to increase; secondary to yaw and deformation of the bullet, this results in large exit wounds as shown in the figure.

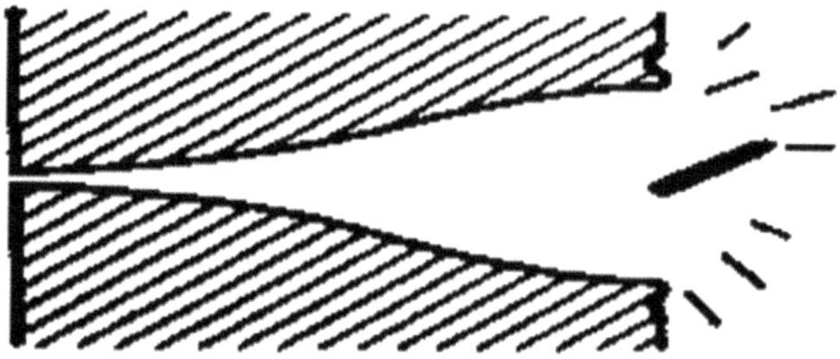

If the path of the missile is long, then energy degradation occurs deep in tissues; this results in a large amount of damage through cavitation, and the entrance and exit wounds may be small, in such a scenario as shown in the figure.

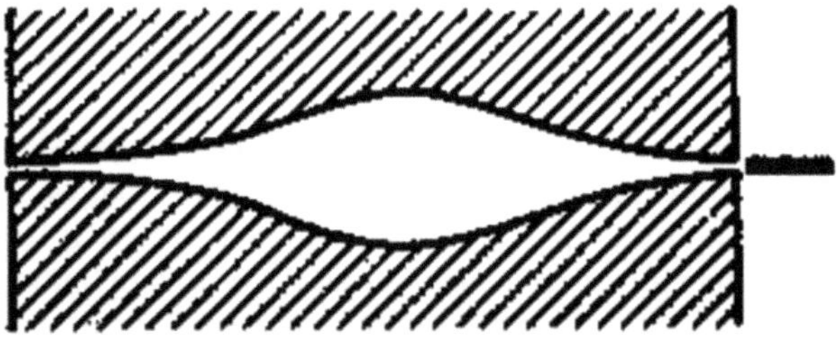

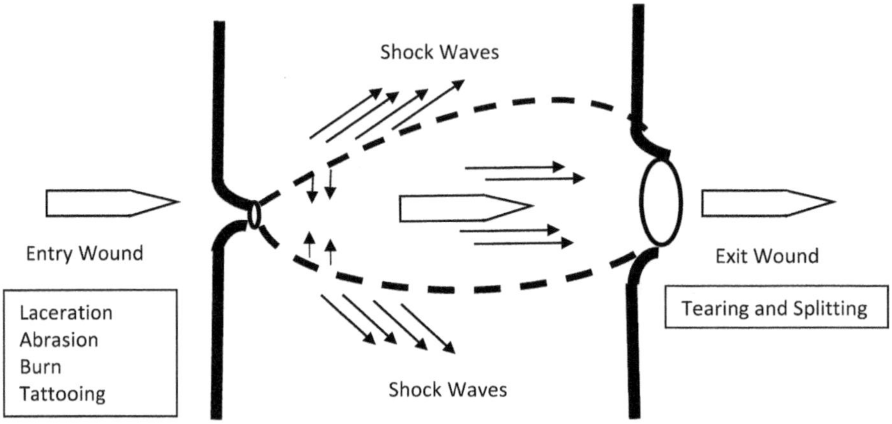

Management Principles of Missile Injuries

Fig. 13.2 Diagrammatic representation of the effect of a missile on tissues

13.8 Management Principles of Missile Injuries

13.8.1 General Principles

Initial management of any victim of a missile injury does not differ from a victim of a polytrauma. Resuscitation by a multidisciplinary team should be based on the principle of resuscitation in the "golden hour of shock," of the injuries which would be fatal, if not untreated in the initial few minutes to few hours after trauma. A minimum of two large-bore intravenous lines, nasogastric tubes, and a urinary catheter should be inserted. They should be managed using standardized diagnostic algorithms and therapeutic concepts according to the Advanced Trauma Life Support (ATLS)® guidelines. Broadly, it includes primary survey and, simultaneously, clearing and securing the airway, ensuring adequate respiratory effort, if necessary endotracheal intubation/cricothyroidotomy/tracheostomy may need to be done, control of external hemorrhage, ensuring adequate perfusion of tissues by maintaining adequate blood pressure should be the immediate response. A brief history should be obtained, with importance being given to the type of firearm/explosive; this may, however, be sketchy or even unobtainable. This is followed by a secondary detailed survey to assess the extent of damage [8–10].

After the threat to life by asphyxiation or bleeding and shock, the next priority in trauma management should be the victim's central nervous system. The entire spine should be carefully examined along with a neurological examination for possible fracture/dislocation. Neurological examination should be done only when the patient is hemodynamically stable and should always include an assessment of level of consciousness, pupillary size, light reflex, movement and sensation of extremities, and deep tendon reflexes.

13.9 Management Specific to Missile Injuries

All clothing worn by the victim should be removed, and a careful search should be made for all the entrance and exit wounds. It should be kept in mind that these may be hidden by hair on scalp, face, axillae, and groin. The identification of the entry and exit wounds is critical since it directs the subsequent radiological examination of the body region where an entrance or exit wound is identified. It is better to obtain a whole-body radiological screening. Metallic fragments within the body are indications for surgical exploration and debridement when high-velocity injury is sustained by the patient. It should be kept in mind that high velocity/low velocity/close or distant range/shotgun wounds always need debridement—*gunshot wounds need debridement*.

It is an old myth that bullet and missile injuries are sterile from the heat they generate. This has been conclusively proved by Wolf et al. that it is not so. They experimentally proved that bullets coated with *Staphylococcus aureus* and shot into a sterile gelatin block subsequently grew positive cultures of *Staphylococcus aureus*, from the gelatin block [11]. It is always prudent to start broad-spectrum antibiotics in all cases of missile injuries.

13.10 Broad Guidelines for Managing Missile Injuries

1. Prompt and multidisciplinary resuscitation and neurological examination is extremely essential.
2. Strip the patient and carefully search for all entrance/exit wounds thoroughly.
3. It is always better to screen the entire body radiologically and perform a whole-body CT scan.
4. Debride all high-velocity wounds and always practice delayed primary closure in all cases.
5. Craniocerebral missile injuries always require craniectomy and debridement.
6. Missile injuries in the maxillofacial regions will require tracheostomy/cricothyroidotomy to secure the airway; they may also require external carotid arterial ligation for hemostasis.
7. Orbital missile injuries may require enucleation.
8. All penetrating neck wounds should be explored surgically and repair of carotid artery/jugular venous/esophageal injuries should be done. Tracheal injuries will require a tracheostomy.
9. Most missile injuries to the chest can be managed with a chest tube without any thoracotomy. The color of the chest drain should be monitored closely till the patient is stable. If it is continuously bloody, then a thoracotomy is indicated.
10. Abdominal missile injuries always require exploratory laparotomy and appropriate organ management.
11. Missile injuries of the urinary tract usually manifest with gross hematuria the extent of the injury can be assessed by intravenous urography/CT scan/MRI.
12. Missile of the limbs that are close to a major vessel or /and that are accompanied by a compound fracture of the long bones requires exploration, stabilization of the fractures, and repair of arteries and veins.

13.11 Conclusion

The most important underlying principle of management of missile injuries is not to cause more damage in extracting the shrapnel than the primary damage that has already occurred. The wounds debrided should always be left open and delayed primary closure should be practiced in all missile injuries. Specific organ management is dictated by the extent of injuries. Damage control surgery should be practiced in all patients who have sustained missile injuries.

References

1. Barach E, Tomlanovich M, Nowak R. Ballistics: a pathophysiologic examination of the wounding mechanisms of firearms: part I. J Trauma. 1986;26:225.
2. Ragsdale BD. Gunshot wounds: a historical perspective. Mil Med. 1984;149:301–15.
3. Finck PA. Ballistics and forensic pathologic aspects of missile wounds. Mil Med. 1965;130:545.
4. Heaton LD, Hughes CW, Rosegay H, Fisher CW, Feighny RE. Military surgical practices of the United States Army in Vietnam. Curr Probl Surg. 1966;1:59.
5. Whelan TJ, Burkhalter WE, Gomez A. Management of war wounds. In: Advances in surgery, vol. 3. 1st ed. Chicago: Year Book Medical; 1968.
6. Rich NM. Weapons and wounds. J Trauma. 1975;15:464.
7. Swan KG, Swan RC. Gunshot wounds: pathophysiology and management. Paris: PSG Publishing Company; 1980.
8. American College of Surgeons Committee on Trauma. Advanced trauma life support (ATLS) for doctors. 7th ed. Chicago: American College of Surgeons Committee on Trauma; 2004.
9. Scharplatz D, Sutter PM. 5 years ATLS (Advanced Trauma Life Support) courses in Switzerland. Swiss Surg. 2003;9:263–7.
10. Bouillon B, Kanz KG, Lackner CK, et al. The importance of advanced trauma life support (ATLS) in the emergency room. Unfallchirurg. 2004;107:844–50.
11. Wolff AW, et al. Autosterilisation in low velocity bullets. J Trauma. 1978;19:63.

14 Algorithm for the Management of Craniocerebral Injuries

Rewati Raman Sharma, Apollina Sharma, and Kalpana Devi Kariyappa

14.1 Introduction [1–6]

The normal functioning brain is the master of the consciously productive meaningful life where lack of brain functions results in a vegetative life. Traumatic injury to the brain may leave the victims anywhere in this spectrum between the conscious active life and the vegetative life.

Therefore, brain injury is the ultimate concern of head injury for which prevention is the only realistic cure. It occurs in split seconds, and by the time it happens, it is already a history leaving ahead consequences to be managed, by the medical profession, family, and society in general with whatever resources are available at their hands.

In general, one-third to one-half of all trauma deaths occur due to severe head injury (SHI). Among the survivors, there is a large percentage of patients with disabilities needing continuation of care with great magnitude of stress and strain, on the trauma care workers. The evidence-based timely management strategy is of paramount importance. A well-planned systematic clinical approach with well-trained medical staff members is necessary for initial acute trauma management while making the possible diagnosis, requesting an appropriate investigation and the rational use of NICU facility as well as choosing problem-solving neuro-surgical procedures wherever needed with careful postoperative management and thereafter the use of rehabilitation services to improve the overall outcome. The determination of the management priorities is of utmost value.

R. R. Sharma (✉) · K. D. Kariyappa
NMC-Ghubra Hospital, Muscat, Oman

A. Sharma
McGill University, Montreal, QC, Canada

© The Author(s), under exclusive license to Springer Nature Singapore Pte Ltd. 2024
A. Agrawal et al. (eds.), *Special Considerations in Trauma Care*,
https://doi.org/10.1007/978-981-99-9662-9_14

14.2 Special Considerations in Head Injury

14.2.1 Epidemiology Statistics of Head Injury [6–11]

The majority of traumatic incidences result in poly-trauma with various combinations of multiple organs with varied extent and severity. Therefore, the responses of these patients vary according to the organ systems injured and the severity of their injuries. Race, age, sex, and geographical sites are not immune to injuries, although it is less common in children, females, and in rural areas. In general, the incidence of head injury is 300–400/100,000 population, more in the urban areas 600–700/100,000, and in rural areas around 200/100,000 population. The great majority of patients are young males (20–45 years). In India, there is one head injury per minute, and every 6–8 min, there is one death related to severe head injuries.

In the USA, there is one head injury per 15 seconds and a trauma patient dies of SHI every 10–12 min. In India, poorly designed and badly maintained roads, an increased number of vehicles, and driving under the influence of alcohol and controlled medications are largely responsible for road traffic accidents. Among the patients who reach hospital facilities, the great majority of head injuries (80%) are minor, 10–15% of cases are moderate, and 5–10% of cases are SHI. In modern times, a unified safe evidence-based approach is the best way forward in initial care, transportation, and definitive care. This helps in the triage of the patients and indicates the needs of the patients requiring to be transferred to a specialized center. In India, the annual mortality due to road traffic accidents is about 60,000–80,000 cases. About 5–10% of cases of all traffic accidents result in fatality (Fig. 14.1a, b). In cases of SHI in general, a third of the patients die, a third have a varying degree of disability, and a third have reasonably good outcomes. The financial losses due to road traffic accidents across the globe are billions of dollars.

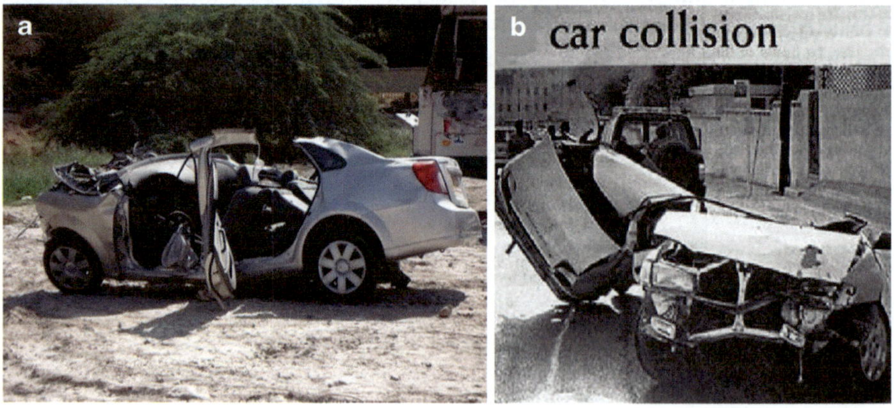

Fig. 14.1 (**a**, **b**) Automobile accidents with vehicular damages

14.2.2 Craniocerebral Anatomico-Physiological Considerations [12–15]

1. *Anatomically*, covered with a soft scalp, the bony hard shell of the skull/cranium uniquely protects the delicate functioning brain. The brain and its blood vessels are well covered within three meningeal layers (dura mater, arachnoid membrane, and pia mater) and float in the spongy cerebrospinal fluid (CSF) cushion all around it to prevent injuries from the day-to-day jerks, impacts, trauma. Head injury is defined as an injury to the region of the head consisting of the scalp, skull, and brain with its coverings and neurovascular structures. These five structures of the head are damaged in various combinations with varying extent and severity at the time of presentation.

   However, the main factor that determines the eventual outcome is the traumatic brain injury per se. The brain occupies an intracranial compartment that is further divided by the tentorium cerebelli into supra-tentorial compartment (harboring the cerebrum which is divided into two equal halves called cerebral hemispheres, by the falx cerebri, and each cerebral hemisphere is made up of four lobes-frontal-parietal-temporal and occipital as well as basal ganglia) and an infratentorial compartment (containing the cerebellum and brain stem).

   The brain is enclosed in its three meningeal coverings, the outer dura mater (lining the cranial cavity internally and containing venous sinuses), arachnoid mater (containing circulating extra-cerebral CSF and forming arachnoid granulations to filter and drain CSF back into the blood circulation via dural venous sinuses), and the intimate surface lining of the brain called the pia mater. The subarachnoid spaces between the inner two layers contain circulating CSF and are named cisterns according to their intracranial locations—superolateral cortical cerebral cisterns, suprasellar, and brain stem cisterns (interpeduncular, ambient, collicular, prepontine, premedullary cisterns, etc.), cerebellopontine and cerebello-medullary cisterns, cisterna magna, and spinal cisterns. The CSF spaces within the brain are named ventricles (two lateral ventricles, a third ventricle, and a fourth ventricle). The CSF spaces communicate via foramina-Munroe (between the lateral and third ventricles), aqueduct of Sylvius (between the third and fourth ventricles), and foramen of Magendie (midline) and Luschka (lateral)—between the fourth ventricle and cisterna Magna (midline) and cerebello-medullary cistern (laterally).
2. *Physiologically,* in adults, about 150 mL of the CSF is present in the craniospinal CSF Spaces—the cerebral ventricles and subarachnoid cisterns and is replaced every 8 hourly via CSF production (Choroid plexus of the ventricles) and equal absorption (arachnoid granulations in relation to the venous sinuses especially the superior sagittal sinus). The Choroid plexus in the lateral ventricle (main), third ventricle, and fourth ventricles are involved in the CSF production.

   Providing effective therapeutic measures especially to avoid or to treat ischemia and hypoxia is the main therapeutic objective to achieve the goal of better clinical outcomes in patients with brain injury. The maintenance of cerebral perfusion pressure (CPP) within the normal range is the primary goal in the management of traumatic brain injury for the prevention of secondary brain injuries. CPP is the main auto-regulated driving force for the cerebral blood flow (CBF) and is measured as: CPP = MAP (mean arterial pressure which should be more than 90 mmHg)—ICP (intracranial pressure which is normal in the range of 5–15 mmHg) and is about 54 mL/100 g of the cerebral tissue/min. The need-based increase in CBF (with dilated cerebral vasculature) occurs in conditions such as hypercarbia, hypotension, hypoventilation, and low blood pH, whereas hypertension, hypocarbia, and alkalosis cause vaso-constriction with reduced CBF. The CBF is auto-regulated within a range of 50–150 mmHg MAP. Brain injury disturbs the auto-regulatory mechanisms; hence, the key management of brain injury is to achieve a sufficient CPP with therapeutic measures by normalizing the MAP and ICP. The MAP is manageable with medications and fluid therapy, and the ICP is measured with ICP devices and therapeutic measures taken to normalize it.

3. ICP: The intracranial space has a fixed volume occupied by cerebral parenchyma (80%), blood volume (10%), and CSF (10%). The ICP is dependent on the Monroe-Kelle doctrine: if one intracranial component increases in its volume, then the other components are getting reduced in their volume to accommodate the expanded component so as to keep the ICP within normal range. Intracranial compliance prevents a sustained increase in ICP until the Monroe-Kelle mechanism is exhausted. Therefore, as the volume of one component is increased, another component reduces itself to accommodate/compensate or else the ICP must go up. If the ICP is not controlled effectively, then a lethal vicious circle sets in. These inter-relations and interactions outline the importance of the cardiovascular and respiratory systems governing the ICP. Therefore, these parameters must be monitored effectively in the NICU unit and treated as per the needs.

14.2.3 Pathophysiology of Head Injury [16–27]

14.2.3.1 Primary and Secondary Brain Injuries

Traumatic brain injury is basically classified into primary injury (acute neuronal damage and cell death resulting directly due to traumatic force) and secondary brain injury (cascades of intracranial events, minutes, hours, days, or weeks following acute trauma, causing secondary brain damage).

The role played by the mechanism of trauma cannot be overemphasized as there may be more than the local injuries and a continuum of damages occurs in high-velocity injuries. Therefore, a high index of suspicion should be maintained to diagnose in high-velocity vehicular accidents, falls from height, and gunshot injuries.

The head injury is a dynamic process. At the time of the primary traumatic event, the force of direct impact (direct strike or penetrating injuries) causes localized focal brain damage at the site of impact on the head, whereas indirect injuries occur due to acceleration and deceleration shearing waves, generated by the traumatic force, diffusely in the brain around the initially damaged brain area. In many cases, both mechanisms are contributory. The primary brain lesions are cerebral concussion, cerebral contusion, cerebral laceration, and diffuse axonal injury (DAI)—ischemia and infarction. The neurovascular structures may be ruptured/lacerated with serious consequences.

The brain is also secondarily injured when the neuronal damages occur due to compressive effects of cerebral swellings/ cerebral edema and mass effect-producing lesions (epidural, subdural and intracerebral hematomas, cerebral contusions, hydrocephalus, etc.) needing decompression/evacuation. Also, systemic problems such as shock, hypotension, hypoxia, hyperglycemia, hyperthermia, etc., cause more generalized secondary brain damage and therefore, it is necessary to identify, prevent, and correct if these are present.

14.2.3.2 Dynamic Events Following Brain Trauma

In high impact-high energy traumatic events, the primary brain damage results in less than 200 ms which cannot be reversed. Thereafter, the dynamic events at the cellular and molecular levels cause further brain damage. The brain is about 2% of the body weight but consumes 15–20% of the cardiac output and 20% of the total oxygen consumption of the body. The traumatic inflammatory responses with ischemia/hypoxia result in further serious effects on the functioning of the brain. There is **expansion in the brain volume** due to cerebral edema or traumatic swelling, etc.

The increased brain volume due to cerebral edema and swelling within the fixed intracranial space is **initially accommodated/compensated by effective compression of the intracranial blood vessels/volume** and later with the compression/displacement of the CSF spaces: first the reduction of the ventricular volumes and basal CSF cisterns and later the effacement of supero-lateral convexity subarachnoid spaces. Interestingly, to help the situation, there is an increased CSF absorption and reduced CSF production as well within the compensatory state.

When the available compensatory mechanisms are exhausted, then the ICP rises precipitously with only a very small increase in the intracranial volume of CSF. When ICP is not controlled effectively, then **a lethal vicious circle sets in**. When the ICP is not uniform within the intracranial cavity, **pressure gradients can develop across intracranial compartments** within the skull. When the pressure gradient exceeds the plasticity of the brain, the brain herniates from one compartment to another compartment in the intracranial cavity. **Herniation of the brain** tissue causes compression of the part of the brain normally present there along the dural edges of the falx cerebri (medial cerebral compression) or tentorial cerebelli (mesencephalic compression) or foramen magnum (medullary compression), which results in acute ischemia and necrosis of the compressed brain tissue (sub-falcine herniation, uncal herniation, tonsillar herniation, etc.). Mid brain compression leads to **Cushing's reflex (hypertension, bradycardia, and bradypnea)** prompting immediate active management.

When the ICP is outside its normal range, the auto-regulation of CBF is lost and the CBF flows in a more linear passive pressure relationship to CPP. In such conditions, normal CBF is restored when CPP is greater than 90 mmHg. However, when the ICP is in normal range, the CBF is maintained when the CPP is above 60 mmHg.

Within a Golden hour, when the secondary insults develop due to disturbed homeostasis and damaged cerebral tissues and need support to deal with these to have chances of survival and recovery; otherwise, the mortality rates increase.

The secondary insults such as intracranial hematomas and disordered autoregulation of CBF resulting are ischemia or cerebral congestion, disordered blood–brain barrier resulting in cerebral edema, raised ICP, and cerebral ischemic or compressive infarctions of the brain tissues. This is the main stage when patients with craniocerebral trauma require protocol-based—algorithmic—management in the NICU units to primarily deal with ischemia, hypoxia, and raised ICP.

The clinical outcomes with significant morbidities and mortality are associated with serious, severe, moderate, and even mild head injury patients. The prevention of head injury is the safest deal (Fig. 14.2a, b).

The role of modern neuro-rehabilitation services cannot be overemphasized to provide nursing care, physiotherapy, occupational therapy, speech therapy, orthotics, and general rehabilitation services. The entire management is therefore challenging. Patients with severe traumatic brain injury also have a 50% incidence of other associated musculoskeletal and other organ-system injuries with increased morbidities and mortalities, and the overall cost of management is enormously high.

14.2.4 Classification of Craniocerebral Trauma [28–33]

Considering the clinical severity of the head injury, the head injuries are classified as per GCS: Minor (GCS-14–15), Moderate (9–13), and Severe (GCS 8 or less). Taking the duration of loss of consciousness (LOC) into consideration, the head injuries are classified as minor (LOC less than 30 min), moderate (more than 30 min to 6 h), and severe (LOC more than 6 h). The mortality in minor HI is less than 1%, in moderate HI about 2.5%, and in severe HI about 40–50% within 24–72 h. Up to 20% of the patients with SHI die at the site of an accident or during transportation.

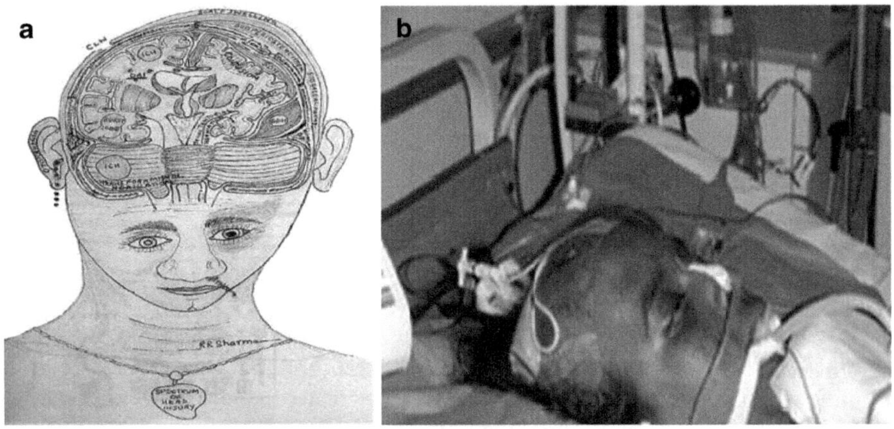

Fig. 14.2 (**a**, **b**) Spectrum of head injury and ICU care

Recognition of the life-threatening potential of each type of head injury is important to provide optimum care in "the Golden Hour and thereafter."

Considering anatomical factors in clinical neurosurgical care, the primary head injuries are classified as follows.

1. Scalp injuries
   (a) Abrasions
   (b) Friction
   (c) Burns
   (d) Contusions, sub-galeal and sub-periosteal hematomas, incised wounds, contused lacerated wounds, avulsions, degloving injury, scalp swellings, etc.
2. Cranial and adnexal injuries
   (a) Calvarial injuries:
   Ping-pong depression, hairline fractures, stellate fractures, comminuted fractures (Fig. 14.3), elevated fractures, compound (intracranial space open to the environment), growing skull fractures, etc.
   (b) Cranial base injuries:
   Anterior, middle, and posterior cranial fossa fractures manifesting as Raccoon's eyes, nasopharyngeal bleed, temporal boggy swelling, Battle's sign, bleeding from the external auditory meatus, CSF otorrhea-rhinorrhea, pharyngorrhea, injuries to the paranasal and mastoid air sinuses, and orbital injuries.
3. Intracranial injuries (Fig. 14.4)
   (a) Meningeal (dural-arachnoial) injuries:
   Incised wounds, dural tears, lacerations and avulsions, pneumocephalus, extradural hematoma, sub-dural hematoma, subdural hygroma, etc.
   (b) Meningo-vascular injuries:

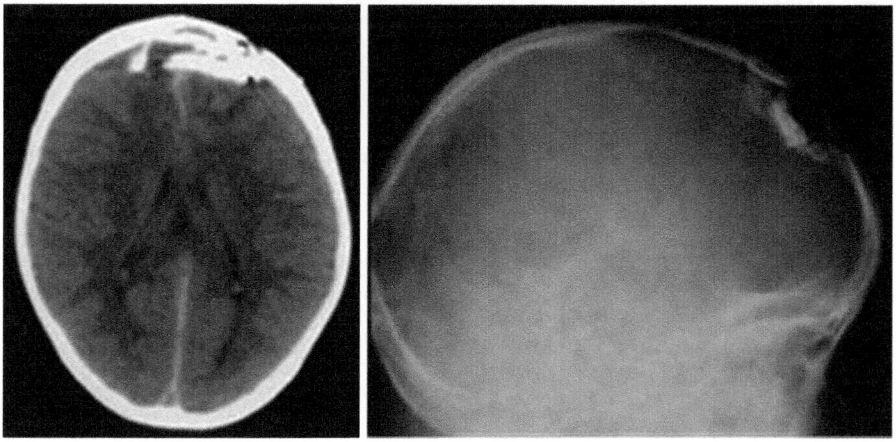

Fig. 14.3 Compound depressed skull fracture with associated extracranial and intracranial injuries

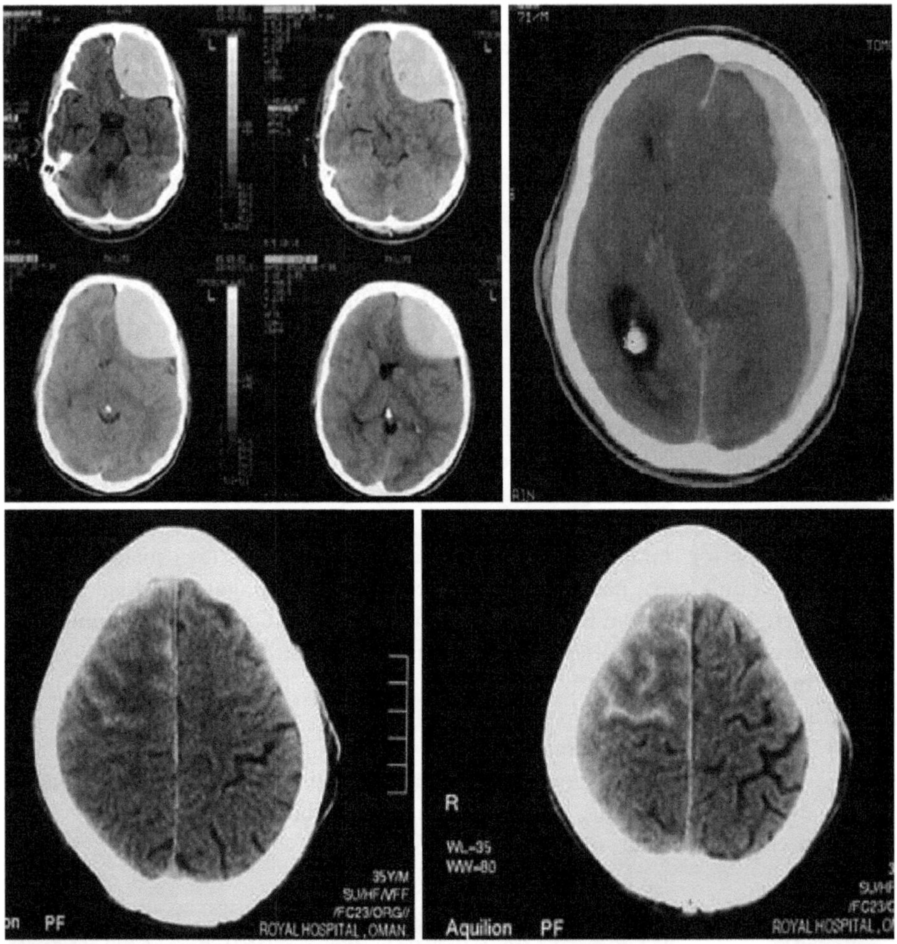

Fig. 14.4 Intracranial–extracerebral lesions: Extradural hematoma (EDH), Subdural hematoma (SDH), and Subarachnoid hemorrhage (SAH)

Sub-arachnoid hemorrhage, traumatic lesions, carotid and vertebra-basilar systems, dural venous sinus injuries, etc.

(c) Encephalic (brain) injuries:

Diffuse brain injuries (Fig. 14.5)

Concussion

DAI and diffuse brain swelling

Focal brain injuries contusion

Contusion-hemorrhage (Fig. 14.6)

Hemorrhage: Subdural, sub-arachnoid, intracerebral, and intraventriclar

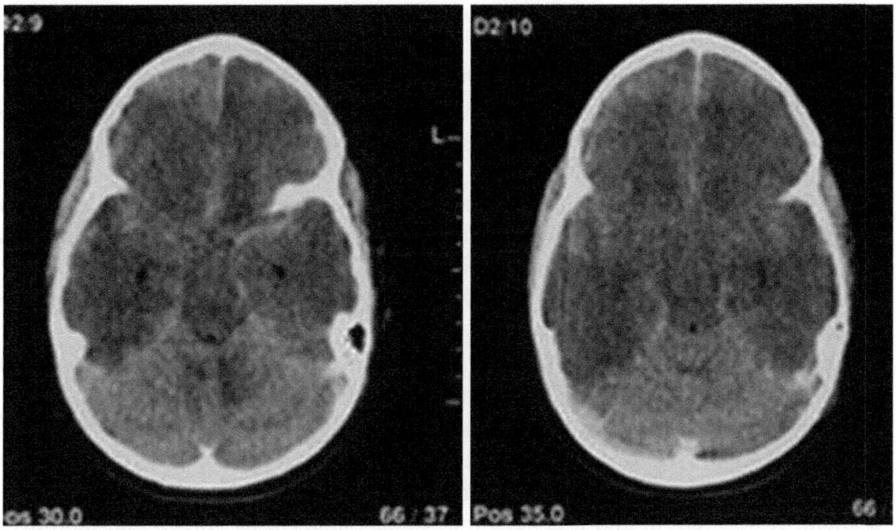

Fig. 14.5 Diffuse brain injuries

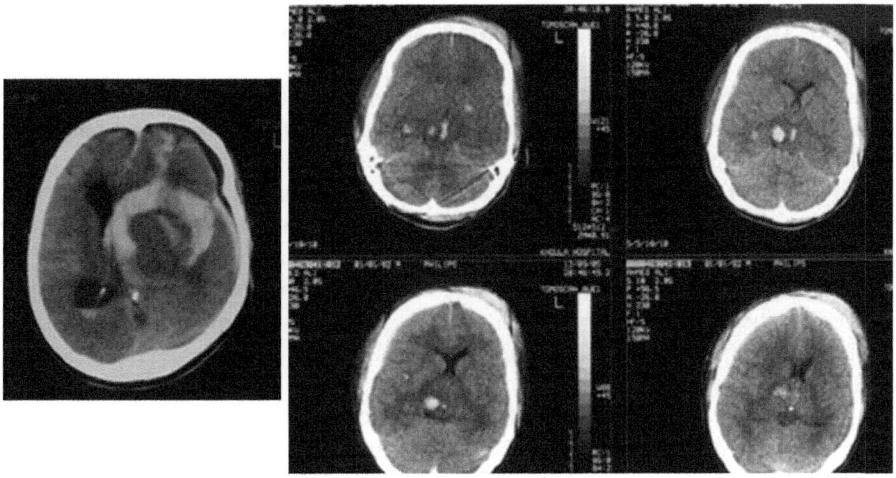

Fig. 14.6 Focal and multifocal cerebral injuries: contusions, laceration, and hemorrhages

14.2.5 The Impact of ATLS Program [34–39]

In current practice, there are positive radical changes in the care of trauma patients due to innovative management strategies leading to better outcomes as compared to before. Since 1976 onwards, the American College of Surgeons has tirelessly worked hard to improve trauma care and its Committee on Trauma has established the Guidelines for the Care of Injured Patients and has developed a highly professional didactic system of care program called the ATLS program which is globally practiced. A systematic concise approach to the early care of trauma patients is the hallmark of the ATLS program. In this program, there is a concise frequently repeated approach for assessing and managing multiple injured patients that is safe and reliable in a planned priority-based manner:

1. Primary survey (ABCDEs)—Rapid accurate assessment of the clinical condition
2. Simultaneously with the primary survey-immediate priority-based resuscitation and stabilization of life-threatening injuries
3. A quick clinical determination of whether a patient's needs exceed the on-site available resources and skills
4. Rapid safe transfer from the on-site to the facilities where the needs of the patient will be reliably met: hospital, inter-hospital, intra-hospital, etc.
5. Secondary survey (head-to-toe examination and patient's history) with optimal care is the main Moto at this stage and therefore providing continued appropriate care and ensuring no deterioration in the care occurs during the initial assessment, resuscitation, and transfer process, secondary assessment, and definitive care to achieve the best possible clinical outcome

14.2.6 The Initial Evaluation and Management [40–45]

Trauma patients are usually present to the medical staff—trauma team—in three different scenarios: pre-hospital settings, accident emergency department, and within the hospital.

In the pre-hospital scenario, the key points, including a minimized scene time, which matters are the importance of maintenance of the airway with protective immobilization of the cervical spine and adequate breathing, control of external bleeding, maintenance of blood pressure to control shock, and immobilization to prevent further spinal/limb injuries as well as a clear vision to immediately transport to the closest appropriate trauma care facility.

1. Patients with altered GCS, low BP, and inadequate breathing efforts are obvious candidates to be transported to the higher trauma centers.
2. The following types of patients with normal GCS and vital signs have a higher potential for deterioration and therefore also transported to the trauma center:
   (a) Despite normal GCS and vital signs, the following types of injuries need facilities of the trauma care center: severe penetrating injuries, open and depressed skull fractures, flail chest-instable chest wall, pelvic fractures, proximal limb fractures, and with an extremity in a serious state, that is, crushed, degloved, mangled, pulseless, paralyzed, etc.
   (b) Patients with normal GCS and vital signs, but with the h/o a mechanism of high energy impact injury such as falls, motor vehicular injuries/crush, and high impact pedestrian and cyclist injuries are also the candidates for transportation to the higher trauma center.

(c) Patients with normal GCS and vital signs, but in the category of extremes of ages (children and elderly above the age of 65 years) pregnant ladies, burn injuries, and medical conditions such as bleeding disorders, or already on the anticoagulant therapy.
(d) When in doubt, transport to a trauma center.

In-hospital scenario, at a designated resuscitation area, the trauma team leader with the team members, using standard precautions (face mask, eye protection, and water-impervious gown and gloves), ensures detailed patient information, proper functioning equipment, resuscitation fluids, additional assistance, and facilities—laboratory and radiology.

In the resuscitation area, trauma patients are brought by the Emergency Medical Service Personnel, relatives/bystanders, or transported from the in-hospital services.

As soon as the patients are received, a prompt assessment of trauma patients is performed and their treatment priorities are formulated. The main determinants are the measures of vital signs (airways, breathing-respiratory rate, circulation-blood pressure), GCS (level of consciousness), pupillary responses, as well as neurological and general examination, in that order of priority.

A rapid primary survey with concurrent resuscitation of vital functions in a logical and sequential manner identifies life-threatening conditions and treats them in a prioritized manner to normalize vital functions.

The priority-based sequential steps (detailed elsewhere in the book) in the primary survey are as follows:

1. The airway with cervical spine control is the first priority: Airway maintenance with cervical spine immobilization.
2. The second priority is to ensure that breathing is adequate: Breathing and ventilation care.
3. The third priority is assessment and management of circulation: Circulation with hemorrhage control.
4. The fourth priority is assessment of neurological examination (Table 14.1): disability (assessment of neurological status).
5. The fifth priority is exposure and environmental control.

Table 14.1 GCS scores

Eye opening		Best verbal response		Best motor response	
Spontaneous	4	Oriented	5	Obeys commands	6
To speech	3	Confused	4	Localizes to pain	5
To pain	2	Inappropriate	3	Flexion to pain	4
None	1	Incomprehensive sounds	2	Abnormal flexion	3
		None	1	Extension to pain	2
				None	1

Minor HI (GCS score: 13–15); Moderate HI (GCS score: 8–12); Severe HI (GCS score: 3–8)

14.2.7 Neurological Assessment in Fully Resuscitated HI Patients [19, 46–50]

The following examination is periodically/repeatedly performed in patients with head injury:

1. Level of consciousness-as assessed by GCS: categorizing mild, moderate, and severe HI (Table 14.1)
2. Pupillary examination to assess the laterality of cerebral trauma with potential mass effect
3. Fundal examination if possible
4. Motor-sensory neurological examination to find out neurological deficits:
   (a) Cranial nerve examination: brain stem (laterality of facial paresis)
   (b) Limb examination: motor-sensory-reflexes (laterality of hemiparesis of limbs and plantar response)
   (c) Sphincter functions (fullness of bladder)

Periodic neurological assessment is undertaken to make sure whether the patient remains stable (needing observations) or is deteriorating (needing further interventions) as in cases of intracranial expanding, that is, extradural hematoma. The classical warning signs are such as deterioration in GCS, pupillary changes, focal deficits, bradycardia, secondary hypertension, and bradypnea (Cushing's syndrome). Unconscious patients with one-sided dilated unreactive pupil may indicate an ipsilateral intracranial hematoma (extradural hematoma) with focal herniation needing immediate operative actions.

14.2.8 Diagnostic Investigations in Head Injury [51–59]

During the resuscitation, the following investigations are done concurrently:

(a) Plain X-rays of the chest (PA view), cervical spine (lateral view), and pelvis (AP view) to find fractures, instability, and assessment of blood losses
(b) Blood tests—CBC, blood grouping and cross matching (as needed), blood sugar, G6PD, alcohol and drug levels, as well as liver and renal functions with care and corrective actions
(c) Periodic CT head and CT angiography as needed (Table 14.2): Following resuscitation, the patient with a significant head injury is routinely undergoing a CT scan of the head and, in some institutions, head-to-toe CT screening wherever possible. Moreover, the CT head must be done in clinical conditions pointing to deterioration in functions/structure—such as deterioration in the level of consciousness, pupillary abnormalities, focal neurological deficits, penetrating HI, orbital–nasal–skull base injuries, intoxications, drug overdose, infants-children, old ages, etc.

Table 14.2 The criteria for the CT scan after a recent head injury

Serial No.	The clinical condition
1.	Minor head injury (GCS 15/15): H/O concussion (LOC), Amnesia particularly if posttraumatic amnesia, seizures, focal neurological deficits-symptoms-signs, unremitting headaches, persistent vomiting, giddiness, transient blindness, extensive lacerations of the scalp involving the skull
2.	GCS 3-14/15: Minor, Moderate, and SHI patients
3.	Cranial vault or skull base fracture: CSF leak, bleeding ENT, herniation of brain matter.
4.	Alcohol/drug intoxication, bleeding disorders, anticoagulant therapy, coagulopathy
5.	Difficulty in assessing the patient, high energy impact, cerebral irritation phenomenon, etc

The periodic assessment of the patients continues in the ICU and if needed the CT head is repeated as needed as intracranial hematomas may gradually enlarge over a short period of time and changes in the clinical status dictate the need again to repeat a CT scan of the head. Medically treatable conditions such as cerebral concussion (normal brain scan and DAIs), multiple small cerebral contusions, generalized cerebral edema, and generalized cerebral swelling are well diagnosed as well as the conditions which may need surgical interventions such as large cerebral contusion, contusion hemorrhage, cerebral lacerations, and hematomas—EDH, SDH, ICH, IVH, etc. These patients are routinely cared for in the NICU with a plethora of tests and radiological services.

14.2.9 Standardized Didactic Algorithmic Management of Head Injury [56–64]

In January 2017, the Brain Trauma Foundation's New Guidelines for the Management of Severe Traumatic Brain Injury were published in the *Journal of Neurosurgery*. These guidelines have evolved from the initial one in 1995 with revision in 2000 and updated in 2016 and finally the new guidelines as evidence-based management protocols in 2017. Experiences were accumulating as to why some of the minor head injury patients have deteriorated and some of the SHI patients recovered well [34–39].

Therefore, intensive treatment, algorithmic care, and vigilant reassessments to prevent deterioration are the central core of head injury management. The neural tissues (neurons, glial cells, and cerebral blood vessels) are vulnerable to the primary traumatic injury which initiates the cascade of metabolic derangements and exposes the brain to secondary injuries with hypoxia, hypotension, raised ICP, cerebral arterial spasm, ischemia, and decreased CBF and CPP. Systemic insults such as hypovolemic state, disseminated intravascular coagulopathy, hyperglycemia, severe loss of blood and anemia, electrolyte imbalance, renal failure, cardiopulmonary arrest, and adult respiratory distress syndrome lead to secondary cerebral insult that is called second accident [16, 65–70].

An internationally accepted, standardized, reliable, didactic system of objective assessment that leads to the categorization of the severity of traumatic brain injury is the GCS, and this is currently practiced routinely around the world, practically in all medical facilities/institutions with inter-observer reliability. Morphology of traumatic head injury is an unreliable predictor of the clinical outcome, whereas the GCS is the objective assessment of the real-time functionality of the central cerebrospinal neuraxis, and therefore, it is a better predictor of the clinical outcome. The cerebral functionality may be low due to various factors in the initial assessment of TBI. Therefore, there is unreliability of GCS at that time, and to be reliable, it must be post-resuscitation, non-sedated, and non-intubated GCS (Table 14.1). Considering three factors: eye opening (1–4), verbal response (1–5), and motor response (1–6), the overall best GCS response score will fall between 3 and 15 numerical values. The score 13–15 is categorized as mild HI, the score 9–12 as moderate HI, and the score 3–8 as severe HI. Further management is based on the algorithmic didactic protocol for the best outcome.

14.2.9.1 Algorithm 1: Management of Minor Head Injury (MI HI) [16, 59–70]

Post-resuscitation, non-sedated, and non-intubated patients with GCS of 13–15 are categorized as minor head injury or mild traumatic brain injury (Table 14.3). The word minor is synonymous with the word mild in the context of head injury management. Among all head injury patients, about 80% of cases are of minor HI presenting in the A/E department. The central point of the management strategy is to have a close monitoring of their clinical /behavioral condition for 24–72 h following trauma either in the hospital or at the residence depending on the available facilities such as hospital bed, family, friends, house location nearer to hospital, easy accessibility to the hospital, mechanism of injury-low velocity injuries, no use of alcohol or drugs by the patient, etc., along with supportive care as needed.

Table 14.3 Mild head injury (GCS 15/15) with no symptoms and signs of brain injury: discharge instructions

Serial No.	Development of new clinical features: symptoms /signs	Action by the responsible companion
1.	Altered consciousness, drowsiness, confusion, transient Amnesia, seizures, focal neurological deficits (pupillary inequality, weakness of loss of sensations in any part of the body limbs)—other symptoms—signs, unremitting headaches, persistent nausea/vomiting, giddiness, transient blindness, extensive lacerations of the scalp involving the skull, CSF leak, bleeding ENT, etc.	Please bring back the patient to the hospital in the A/E department for review and sos CT head and possible admission
2.	A very slow or very rapid pulse, or an unusual breathing	
3.	Agitation, aggression, altered behavior	
4.	The patient doing clinically/observationally well at home	To continue the same observations and follow-up in NS OPD or in local health center

These patients may have h/o one or more of the following "risky" symptoms such as LOC, disorientation, confusional state, emotional labiality, headaches, persistent vomiting, giddiness, seizures, posttraumatic amnesia, amnesia of event, retrograde amnesia, transient/persistent focal neurological deficits, CSF leaks, osteo-plastic morphological injuries, etc. Patients with these conditions may deteriorate further with increased morbidity and mortality.

Therefore, these patients with mild head injury are clinically further subdivided into three classes/categories according to the degree of clinical risks (Algorithm 1).

1. Low Risk—Minor HI: The great majority of patients are asymptomatic GCS of 15/15 without any of the aforementioned "risky" symptoms. Therefore, patients with GCS 15/15 without aforementioned co-existing symptoms or any other "risky" presenting symptom are categorized as low risk—mild HI. There is an expected low risk of further clinical deterioration and a low risk of developing intracranial hematoma requiring neurosurgical intervention in less than 0.1–0.5% of such cases. The overall prognosis is excellent.

   Only 10% of GCS 15/15 have positive CT scan of the head and about less than 1% need neurosurgical intervention. After 2–4 h of observations in the A/E, these patients even with scalp or facial injuries without any associated craniocerebral injuries can be discharged home under the care of a responsible individual with an appropriate head injury written observation-instruction-guidance sheet along with an OPD follow-up date and in case of deterioration then to attend A/E department immediately (Management—Algorithm 1).

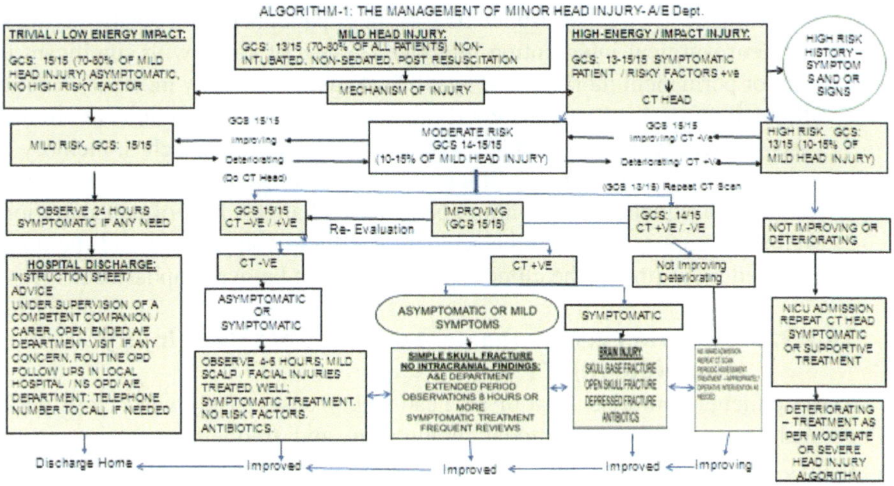

2. Moderate Risk—Minor HI: Patients with GCS of 15/15 with "risky" symptoms as mentioned before and patients with GCS14/15, both, comprise moderate risk—minor HI. These patients with risky symptoms are carefully observed in the A/E department with repeated primary surveys and subjected to CT scans of the head (plain X-rays of the head only if a CT facility is not available).

If the CT head scan shows only normal findings without skull fracture or any intracranial abnormality, then they will remain admitted in the hospital only till the subsidence of their symptoms with satisfactory observations and symptomatic treatment usually for 24–48 h. The risks of delayed intracranial hematoma needing neurosurgical intervention are 0.5–1.0%. Alternatively, these patients with CT negative moderate risk—minor HI may be allowed to return to their residence at the special request of a responsible family member who will keep a very close watch for increasing headaches, repeated vomits, worsening obtundation, and development of other risky symptoms. The patient will have quick access to the A/E department if and when it is needed for the patient to come to the hospital within a short period of time. The overall management outcome is excellent in these cases. The patients placed in the initial category of moderate risk—minor HI; later, if found to have a positive CT scan finding, then they are considered as high risk—minor HI and treated according to the protocol of high risk—minor HI.

3. High risk—minor HI: The patients with GCS of 13/15, as well as the patients with GCS 14–15 having continued risky symptoms and or having positive CT findings are categorized as high risk—minor HI. The patients with normal initial CT scan findings with continued symptoms must be carefully observed as they require early repeat CT scans within or at the 24-h period for further evaluation.

   These cases are always admitted to the hospital along with the patients having coagulopathy, drug or alcohol abuse, previous neurosurgical interventions, and age above 60–65 years. These patients are carefully and repeatedly observed clinically, with periodic neuro-radiologically investigated and algorithm-based symptomatically treated. About 10% of these patients have a positive brain scan and neurosurgical intervention in about 1.5–8% of cases with significant transient or permanent morbidity in 10–30% of cases and rarely mortality. The overall outcome in these cases is good (about 80–90%) but a significant number of cases present with posttraumatic syndrome, recurrent headaches, memory deficits, emotional disturbances, difficulty in performing employment tasks, psychological consequences in attention, behavioral changes, lack of concentration, as well as litigation related to the accident itself and compensation of the injuries. Detailed recording of the clinical findings cannot be overemphasized.

14.2.9.2 Algorithm 2: Management of Moderate Head Injury (Moderate HI) [71–78]

These patients comprise 10% of all head injury cases. They need close periodic clinical observations, multimodal monitoring, and frequent neuro-imaging (CT scans). These patients are managed in high-dependency or NICU facilities. In about 40% of moderate head injury cases, the CT scans show significant intracranial findings in the form of intracranial hematomas, cerebral contusions, subarachnoid hemorrhage, intraventricular hemorrhage, etc.

They have a great potential to deteriorate due to combinations of pathophysiological mechanisms of head injury and secondary insults (Algorithm 2) and therefore need high degrees of awareness for the detection of the causative mechanism of deterioration and its rectification in time. Nearly about 8–10% of moderate head injuries need neurosurgical intervention. The overall mortality is in the range of 10–20% and morbidity is as high as 50% of cases. These patients are therefore monitored very carefully and given needed supportive care in high dependency or in intensive care units so as to try to prevent their deterioration and progress to SHI.

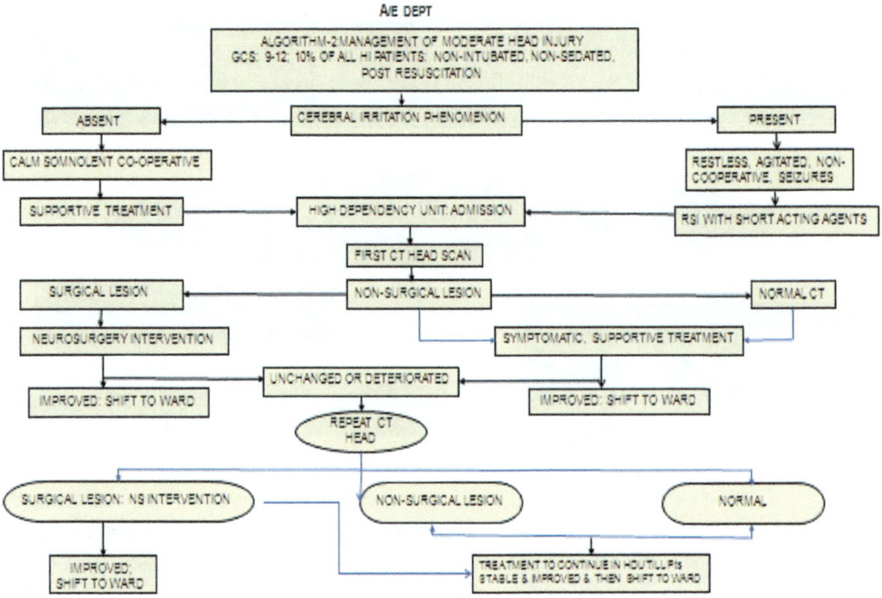

14.2.9.3 Algorithm 3: Management of Severe Head Injury (GCS: 3–8) [79–86]

Patients with SHI(in coma) after adequate resuscitation (correction hypoxia, hypoxemia, and hypotension) are electively sedated, paralyzed, intubated, and ventilated. These patients (Algorithm 3) require stable vital parameters within normal range before transferring to another hospital or shifting to a CT suite in the same hospital. The monitoring of blood pressure and tissue oxygenation continues during transport so that problems can be identified and corrected early.

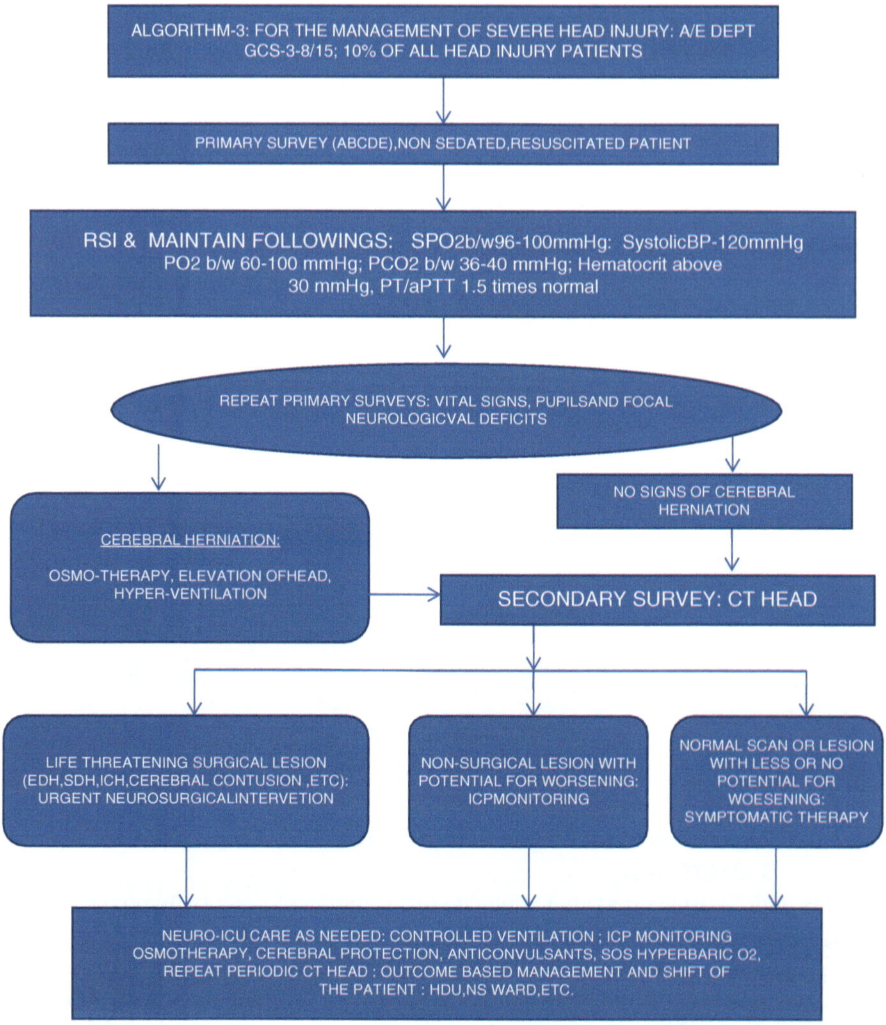

Current Neurosurgical Practice

A general outline of the current neurosurgical practice in head injury is as follows:

Acute Scalp Injuries [87]

Traumatic scalp swellings are treated conservatively except in rare instances where an aspiration may have to be done for clinical or social reasons.

1. Traumatic scalp swellings are treated conservatively:
   (a) Caput succedaneum
   (b) Subgaleal hematoma
   (c) Subperiosteal hematoma

2. **Lesions without full-thickness breach in the continuity of the scalp are treated conservatively**: Abrasions and contusions.
3. Lesions with full-thickness breach in the continuity of the scalp are best treated surgically:
   (a) Lacerations—(1) partial thickness and (2) full thickness
   (b) Contused laceration
   (c) Contused laceration with minimal tissue loss
   (d) Complicated contused lacerated scalp wounds with greater tissue loss
   (e) Scalp avulsions

Acute Cranial Injuries: Skull Fractures [87–90]

In the presence of an intact scalp or an intact mucosal barrier at the cranial base in the regions of the paranasal or mastoid sinuses, a skull fracture is termed a closed skull fracture because there is no communication between the fracture and the external environment (air).

When the scalp and periosteal mucosal skull base barriers are not intact and the fracture site or intracranial cavity is directly exposed to the external environment, then the fracture is termed open (or compound) skull fracture. The risks of complications such as infections are more common in open fractures than in closed ones.

The former is therefore managed with surgery (where indicated) and the latter is mostly managed conservatively. Skull fractures are grouped under the following categories, shown along with their most common mode of management:

(a) Ping-pong fracture—managed conservatively
(b) Linear skull fracture—managed conservatively
(c) Diastatic fractures—managed conservatively
(d) Stellate fractures—managed conservatively
(e) Comminuted fractures—managed conservatively
(f) Depressed or elevated fractures are managed conservatively if closed, and surgical therapy if open skull fracture.

An open depressed skull fracture is an emergency because of the risk of bacterial infection of the intracranial compartment. Surgery is performed within 6 h following an accident, under antibiotic cover and tetanus prophylaxis.

Surgical objectives in an open depressed fracture are as follows:

1. Thorough inspection
2. Saline irrigation and cleansing
3. Debridement of the devitalized tissues
4. Water-tight dural closure
5. Cosmetic corrections: immediate or later.

Acute Intracranial Injuries [91–100]

These are subdivided into focal and diffuse injuries.

Focal Injuries [101–105]

Intracranial Bleeding with and Without Significant Cerebral Contusions

1. Meningeal hemorrhage (EDH/SDH/SAH):
   Significant EDH and SDH are best treated with conventional neurosurgical approaches. SAH is treated by conservative medical therapy.
2. Cerebral hemorrhage (ICH/IVH):
   (a) Superficial cortical and subcortical hematomas with and without contusions are best managed with emergency neurosurgical techniques.
   (b) Deep subcortical, basal ganglionic, thalamic, and brain stem hematomas are best approached by stereotactic or endoscopic procedures.
   (c) IVH is best treated with external ventricular drainage.

Cerebral Contusions/Lacerations
These are best managed by conventional neurosurgical techniques.

1. Impalement injuries are best treated with conventional neurosurgical approaches and only a select subset may need stereotactic surgery.
2. Bullet injuries are best treated by conventional neurosurgical approaches and only a select subset will need stereotactic surgery.

Diffuse Injuries [106–112]
The majority of these patients are on the ventilator in the NICU, with ICP monitoring and measures to control high ICP.

(a) Concussion—intensive neurosurgical observations
(b) DAI—neurointensive care
(c) Diffuse cerebral edema—neurointensive care
(d) Diffuse cerebral swelling—neurointensive care
(e) Diffuse hypoxic encephalopathy—neurointensive care

14.2.10 Neurointensive Care Unit

Patients with significant head injuries are cared for in the NICU routinely with a combination of medical-anesthetic and neurosurgical measures to effectively manage these patients and prevent irreversible ischemic and hemorrhagic damage to the brain.

The NICU, liaising closely with neurosurgical operation theatres and the neuroradiological department, is equipped with modern facilities for controlled ventilation and normalization of circulation, ICP monitoring, cerebral protection, and medications including anti-convulsant medications. There are many aspects of ICU management that need consideration; however, the most concerned ones are described here in brief.

14.2.10.1 Managing Adequate Oxygenation and Circulation [113–117]

In SHI patients, intubation and ventilation initially with 100% oxygen are of paramount importance in reducing morbidity and mortality. The presence of hypoxia and hypotension doubles the mortality rate, and hence secured airways and breathing are essential along with the maintenance of blood pressure to achieve the best outcome. One episode of hypotension increases mortality by 27–50% and multiple episodes of hypotension by 75%. Therefore, the loss of blood is minimized by controlling bleeding effectively. Hypoxemia due to any cause must be treated whether due to bleeding in any organ system, spinal cord injury, and oligemic shock. The correction of the hypoxemia concurrently with resuscitation takes priority over the head injury with fluid resuscitation (first corrective measure), blood transfusion (second corrective measure), and vasopressor agents (last corrective measure) along with oxygenation. The MAP is kept at or above 90 mmHg to maintain CPP around 70 mmHg. The hematocrit should be maintained above 30%. Hypertension secondary to raised ICP is best treated by measures lowering the ICP. In cases of SHI, controlled ventilation (aimed to keep $PaCO_2$ between 3.3 and 3.9 kPa and PaO_2 between 13 and 20 kPa) with X-ray chest, arterial blood gas analysis, ICP monitoring, periodic CT head, cerebral protection, and posttraumatic seizures management go hand in hand.

14.2.10.2 Intracranial Pressure (ICP) Management [118–122]

Maintenance of the CPP at around 70 mmHg as stated earlier is the central point of managing ICP and MAP (CPP = MAP–ICP). Normally, the ICP fluctuates between 10 and 15 mmHg. Severely raised ICP (above 40 mmHg) is associated with more than 50% of deaths in cases of severe HI, whereas moderately raised ICP (25–40 mmHg) increases mortality and morbidity, and therefore, "ICP monitoring & its effective management" is an important measure undertaken in cases of significant HI. Maintenance of MAP, ICP, and CPP within their acceptable ranges is of paramount importance. Nowadays, there are many reliable ICP measuring devices—Camino, Codman, and others. The catheter tip transducer may be placed anywhere from extradural space to intraventricular locations. The intraventricular catheter tip is used to drain ventricular CSF to lower the ICP and improve the CPP. The intracranial compliance is also measured. On injecting 1 mL of the saline intraventricular if the ICP is raised more than 2 mmHg, then the cerebral compliance is significantly reduced. Lundberg (1960) reported three main waveforms: A-wave or plateau wave (above 40–50 mmHg) indicates highly raised ICP due to an acute intracranial event (and persists usually for 5–20 min as compensation mechanisms become operative but if continued beyond this period then the compensation mechanisms may already be exhausted) and manifests clinically with severe headaches, pupillary changes, bradycardia, bradypnea, secondary hypertension, decerebrate posture, etc. The clinically insignificant, B-wave (related to breathing efforts, 0.2–2 cycles/min) and C-wave (cardiac cycle-systemic pulse related 4–8 cycles/min) were also noted.

The focal or generalized raised ICP, especially the plateau waves, are best managed with the following measures:

1. Head elevation to 30° to help drain intracranial venous blood
2. Maintenance of normal vital parameters—including normothermia
3. Agitation control with narcotics/sedatives
4. Intubation and controlled ventilation (up to hypocapnia levels between 25 and 33 PCO_2).
5. CSF drainage up to the point to bring down ICP from above to 15 mmHg
6. Diuretics: Osmotic (mannitol in the dose of 0.2–1 mg/kg IV periodically) and Loop diuretics (furosemide), keeping serum osmolality below 320 mosmol/L
7. The CT head to look for the cause of increased ICP—hematoma, hydrocephalus, edema, etc.
8. Neurosurgical intervention wherever indicated in cases of raised ICP (Fig. 14.7a, b) and if no neuro-surgical intervention is indicated, then to lower the intractable high ICP, barbiturate therapy is an option to be instituted strictly in NICU with supportive services. Under EEG control reaching burst suppressing pattern while maintaining MAP above 100 mmHg and CPP around 50 mmHg, pento-barbitone infusion (50–100 mg to start with and then the monitored doses given) is given for a period of 24–72 h only till ICP reaches below 20 mmHg, before weaning off from the pento-barbitone therapy.

14.2.10.3 Cerebral Protection [123–125]

The dynamic functionality of the brain cell mainly depends on aerobic respiration (3–5 mL of O_2/100 g/min) with negligible available oxygen stores, and therefore significant ischemia/hypoxemia or low CPP threatens the survival of the active brain cells. Neuro-protection means enhancing the tolerance of the brain cells against ischemia/hypoxemia. The therapeutic measures increasing the ability of the

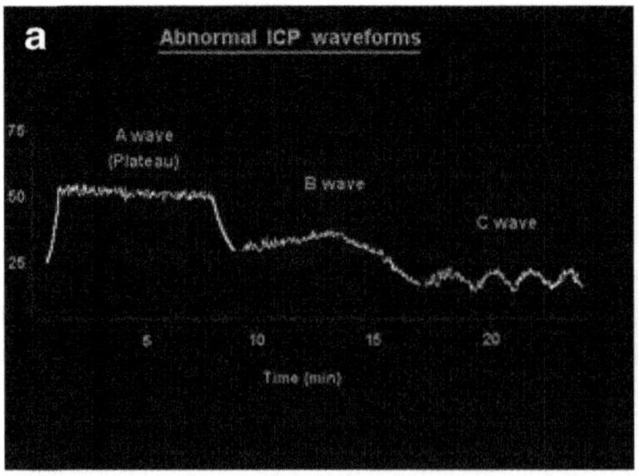

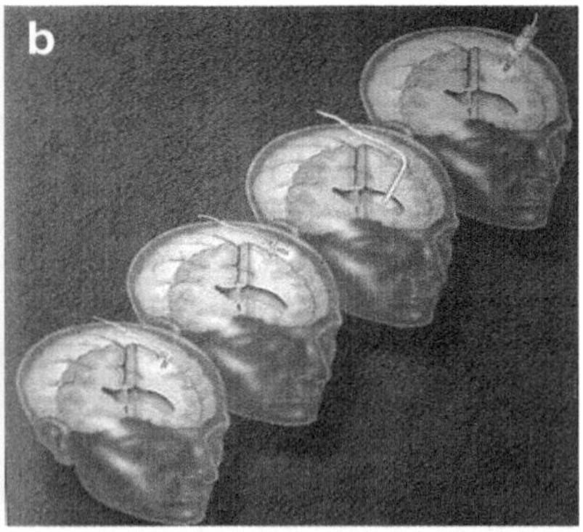

Fig. 14.7 (a, b) Intracranial pressure monitoring with ICP waveforms

brain/neuronal cells to tolerate or survive adverse ischemic/hypoxemic conditions are called cerebral protective measures or simply cerebral protection. Inadequate blood supply (lack of oxygen and energy substrates) leads to anaerobic metabolism, and thereby, lactic acidosis and oxygen free radicals which in turn damages neuronal membranes with cellular hypoxia, ischemia, and edema.

The cerebral protective measures improve aerobic respiration, microcirculation, and cellular edema, help in scavenging free radicals, and prevent lipid peroxidation. These measures to improve oxygenation include controlled ventilation with high FiO_2, controlled use of vasopressors for hypertensive therapy, hypervolemic therapy, blood transfusion, perfluoro-carbons, and anti-coagulants. On the contrary, the measures to lower the neuronal metabolic demand are barbiturate coma, moderate hypothermia, and drugs such as propofol-lidocaine and isoflurane. Interestingly, thiopentone causes vasoconstriction in the normal areas of the brain and diverts blood to the ischemic idling viable but non-functional cells in the middle area called penumbra between the central non-functional area of the brain and peripherally normal viable functional brain area.

Following injury, at the cellular level, further damaging substances, such as excitatory amino acids (glutamate and aspartate) and intracellular calcium, are released; hence, excitatory amino-acid inhibitors (ketamine) as well as calcium channel blockers (Nimodipine), 21-amino-steroid (Tirilazad mesylate), Gavestinel (NMDA receptor antagonist), Remacemide (glutamate antagonist), and magnesium (calcium channel blocker) as well as Vitamin E (working against oxygen free radical induced lipid peroxidation) are tried with borderline benefits. Piracetam (Nootropil), an acyclic derivative of GABA (Gamma-Amino-Bbutyric-Acid), is used (50–200 mg/kg/day for 4–6 weeks) to improve neural transmission, with membrane stabilization, improving microcirculation and glucose metabolism with positive results on cognitive and psychological functions. Hyperbaric oxygen therapy (5–7 sittings) is used to support idling neurons to maintain the aerobic metabolism of glucose. Therefore, the neuro-protection helps reduce morbidities and mortality.

14.2.10.4 Managing posttraumatic seizures [126–132]

Recurrent convulsions/seizure episodes following head injury are called posttraumatic epilepsy (PTE) with an incidence of 15–20% in cases of SHI and 4–5% of all significant head injuries. PTE is classified as early PTE (EPTE) within the first week following trauma (occurs in 3% of cases) and late PTE (LPTE) occurring in 1% of cases. Occasionally, patients present with status epilepticus. The incidence of LPTE is higher following categories of patients: closed head injury, h/o early epilepsy, intracranial hematoma, depressed skull fracture with a dural tear, posttraumatic amnesia over 24 h, focal neurological deficits, missile injuries, alcoholics, and children.

Prophylactic anti-epileptic medications given after TBI decrease the incidence of EPTE but no significant reduction in LPTE, morbidity, and mortality. Phenytoin sodium, Levetiracetam, carbamazepine, sodium valproate, etc., are effective in EPTE and reduce the incidences of LPTE.

In patients with status epilepticus, intravenous phenytoin or levetiracetam is effective. Initially, phenytoin sodium 1.0 g (or a calculated total dose of 20 mg/kg body weight) is given at a rate of 50 mg/min and then a total daily dose of 30 mg/kg in divided doses while simultaneously monitoring the blood pressure and ECG.

In phenytoin sensitivity, sodium valproate, diazemuls 10 mg, clonazepam 1 mg, paraldehyde, magnesium sulfate, thiopentone, etc., are used. Refractory status epilepticus should be treated with IV diazepam (20 mg) or diazepam infusion (100 mg in 50 mL saline). The posttraumatic seizure disorder needs to be effectively controlled for better outcomes. Failure to control seizures even in sedated paralyzed ventilated patients may result in high metabolism beyond the cerebral oxygen supply and leading to a vicious cycle of anaerobic metabolism, lactic acidosis, and cell damage.

14.3 Head Injury Management with Algorithms: Conclusions [133–135]

In the modern world, trauma has become the leading cause of death in patients under the age of 40 years. High impact-high energy events lead to poly-trauma. About 50% of fatalities are mainly due to head injuries. In a significant number of surviving patients with moderate and severe head injuries, there are transient, long-term, or permanent psychological and physical disabilities. For the clinical management in trauma patients, based on the initial level of consciousness following resuscitation, as assessed with GCS, the severity of the head injuries is currently categorized as Minor (GCS-13–15 with overall mortality rate around 1–2%), Moderate (GCS-9–12 with mortality rate about 2–5%), and Severe (GCS-8 and less, with mortality rate of 20–40%).

The impact of trauma occurs in milliseconds during primary brain injury which mainly decides the outcome; hence, prevention of trauma is the best philosophy to avoid morbidities and mortality. The main management is carefully didactically planned and directed toward an attempt to logically prevent secondary brain injury. Primary and secondary surveys form the basis of initial management. The factors causing clinical deterioration such as hypoxia, hypocarbia, hypoxemia, hypovolemia, and hypotension are adequately treated in the NICU. Therefore, patients with SHI are mainly managed with controlled ventilation, periodic evaluations with CT scanning, ICP monitoring, cerebral protection, and neurosurgical operative procedures wherever indicated. The rapid identification and operative management of significant localized mass-producing lesions, that is, hematomas, contusions, and acute hydrocephalus are of primary concern. The combined teamwork of neurosurgeons, neuro-intensivist/neuroanesthetist, physiotherapist, neuro-radiologist, and neuro-nursing with medical and surgical efforts is of paramount importance. These efforts are directed toward the prevention of irreversible ischemic and hemorrhagic damage to the brain. Periodic planned stepwise reassessments (clinical, radiological, hematological, and biochemical) are performed to ensure recovery and to prevent deterioration in relevant parameters. These may be needed for prolonged periods following SHI. Aggressive protocol-based management is imperative for better results. With these efforts, there is a downward trend in overall trauma-related mortality (about 10–30%) and morbidity (10–40%), and therefore, still a long way to go to achieve satisfactory outcomes.

Acknowledgment We sincerely thank Mrs. Vani Sharma for her hard tireless work coordinating, preparing, and editing the manuscript as well as preparing the algorithms.

References

1. Bullock R, Chesnut RM, Clifton G, Ghajar J, Marion DW, Narayan RK, Newell DW, Pitts LH, Rosner MJ, Wilberger JE. Guidelines for the managements of severe head injury. J Neurotrauma. 1996;13:643–734.
2. Capizzi A, Woo J, Verduzco-Gutierrez M. Traumatic brain injury: an overview of epidemiology, pathophysiology, and medical management. Med Clin North Am. 2020;104(2):213–38.
3. Kelly DF, Mikas DL, Becker DP. Diagnosis and treatment of moderate and severe head injuries in adults, vol. III. 4th ed. Philadelphia: WB Saunders; 1996. p. 1618–718.
4. Procaccio F, Stocchetti N, Citerio G, Berardino M, Bretta L, Della Corte F, D'Avella D, Brambilla GL, Delfini R, Servadei F, Tomei G. Guidelines for the treatment of adults with severe head trauma (part I). Initial assessment; evaluation and pre-hospital treatment; current criteria for hospital admission; systemic and cerebral monitoring. J Neurosurg Sci. 2000;44:1–10.
5. Vella MA, Crandall ML, Patel MB. Acute management of traumatic brain injury. Surg Clin North Am. 2017;97(5):1015–30.
6. Whitaker-Lea WA, Valadka AB. Acute management of moderate-severe traumatic brain injury. Phys Med Rehabil Clin N Am. 2017;28(2):227–43.
7. Arienta C, Caroli M, Balbi S. Management of head injured patients in the emergency department: a practical protocol. Surg Neurol. 1997;48:213.
8. Brain Trauma Foundation; American Association of Neurological Surgeons; Congress of Neurological Surgeons. Guidelines for the management of severe head injury. J Neurotrauma. 2007;24(Suppl):S1–S106.
9. Mendelow AD, Teasdale G, Jennet B, Bryden J, Hessett C, Murray G. Risks of intracranial haematoma in head injuried adults. BMJ. 1983;287:1173–6.
10. Nathens AB, Cryer HG, Fildes J. The American college of surgeons trauma quality improvement program. Surg Clin North Am. 2012;92:441–54.
11. Servadi F, Teasdale G, Merry G. Defining acute mild head injury in adults: a proposal based on prognostic factors, diagnosis and management. J Neurotrauma. 2001;18(7):657–9.
12. Adams JG, et al. Traumatic brain injury (adult). In: Emergency medicine: clinical essentials. 2nd ed. Philadelphia: Elsevier; 2013.
13. Maas AI, Stocchetti N, Bullock R. Moderate and severe traumatic brain injury in adults. Lancet Neurol. 2008;7:728.
14. Nakamura N, Yamaura A, Shigemori M, Ono J, Kawamata T, Samkamoto T. Epidemiology, prevention and countermeasures against severe traumatic brain injury in Japan and abroad. Neurol Res. 2002;24:45–53.
15. Ogawa T, Kawamata T, Sakamoto T, Ono J, Tokutomi T, Nakamura N. Traumatic Coma Data Bank Project in Japan (JTCDB). Neurotraumatology. 2002;25:117–33.
16. Balestreri M, Czosnyka M, Hutchinson P, Steiner LA, Hiler M, Smielewski P, et al. Impact of intracranial pressure and cerebral perfusion pressure on severe disability and mortality after head injury. Neurocrit Care. 2006;4:8–13.
17. Bhalla T, Dewhirst E, Sawardekar A, Dairo O, Tobias JD. Perioperative management of the pediatric patient with traumatic brain injury. Paediatr Anaesth. 2012;22:627–40.

18. Brain Trauma Foundation, American Association of Neurological Surgeons, Congress of Neurological Surgeons. Guidelines for the management of severe traumatic brain injury. Blood pressure and oxygenation. J Neurotrauma. 2007;24(Suppl 1):S7.
19. Carney N, Totten AM, O'Reilly C, et al. Guidelines for the management of severe traumatic brain injury. Neurosurgery. 2017;80(1):6–15.
20. Chesnut RM, Marshall LF, Klauber MR, Blunt BA, Baldwin N, Eisenberg HM, et al. The role of secondary brain injury in determining outcome from severe head injury. J Trauma. 1993;34:216–22.
21. Gennarelli TA, Sagawa H, Wald U, Czernicki Z, Marsh K, Thompson C. Physiological response to angular acceleration of the head. In: Grossman RG, Gildenberg PL, editors. Head injury: basic and clinical aspects. New York: Raven Press; 1982. p. 129–40.
22. Gennarelli TA, Spielman GM, Langfit TW, Gildenberg PL, Harrington T, Jane JA. Influence of the type of intracranial lesion on outcome from severe head injury. J Neurosurg. 1982;56:26–36.
23. Klauber MR, Marshall LF, Toole BM. Cause of decline in head injury mortality rate in San Diego County, California. J Neurosurg. 1985;62:528–31.
24. National Institute for Clinical Excellence. Triage, assessment, investigation and early management of head injury in infants, children and adults, clinical guideline 4. London: NICE; 2003.
25. Ramamurthi B. Road accidents, epidemiology and prevention. Neurology. 1995;43:9–15.
26. Sharma RR, Lad SD, Gangwal A, Devadas RV, Joseph LM, Dev EJ, Lad S, Gosalia N. Management of severe head injury. In: Sharma BS, Mishra UK, editors. Progress in clinical neurosciences: Neurological Society of India, vol. XX. New Delhi: Creative Printers; 2005. p. 24–55.
27. Sharma RR, Pawar SJ, Devadas RV, Lad SD. Fluid and electrolyte imbalance in head injury. In: Mahapatra AK, Rajkamal, editors. A textbook of head injury. New Delhi: Modern Publishers; 2005. p. 129–44.
28. Hesdorffer DC, Ghajar J. Marked improvement in adherence to traumatic brain injury guidelines in United States trauma centers. J Trauma. 2007;63:841–7.
29. Lin K, Dulebohn SC. Ranchos Los Amigos. Treasure Island: Stat Pearls Publishing; 2017.
30. Sharshar T, Citerio G, Andrews PJ, Chieregato A, Latronico N, Menon DK, et al. Neurological examination of critically ill patients: a pragmatic approach. Report of an ESICM expert panel. Intensive Care Med. 2014;40:484–95.
31. Teasdale G, Jennett B. Assessment of coma and impaired consciousness. A practical scale. Lancet. 1974;2:81–4.
32. The Japan Society of Neurotraumatology. Guidelines for the management of severe head injury. Neurotraumatology. 2000;23(Suppl):1–51.
33. Wijdicks EF, Bamlet WR, Maramattom BV, Manno EM, McClelland RL. Validation of a new coma scale: the FOUR score. Ann Neurol. 2005;58:585–93.
34. American College of Surgeons Committee on Trauma. Resources for optimal care of the injured patient. Chicago: American College of Surgeons Committee on Trauma; 2006.
35. Bazzoli GJ, Madura, Cooper GF, et al. Progress in the development of trauma systems in the United States. Results of National survey. JAMA. 1995;273:395–401.
36. Celso B, Tepas J, Langfield-Orban B, et al. A systematic review and meta-analysis comparing outcome of severely injured patients treated in trauma centres following the establishment of trauma systems. J Trauma. 2006;60:371–8; discussion 8.
37. Eeposito TJ, Kuby A, Unfed C, et al. General surgeons and advanced trauma life support course. Chicago: American College of Surgeons; 2008.
38. Estroff JM, Foglia RP, Fuchs JR. A comparison of accidental and non-accidental trauma: it is worse than you think. Emerg Med. 2015;48:274–9.
39. Leeper WR, Leeper TJ, Yogt K, et al. The role of trauma team leaders in missed injuries: does specialty matter? J Trauma. 2013;75(3):387–90.
40. Brain Trauma Foundation, American Association of Neurological Surgeons, Congress of Neurological Surgeons. Guidelines for the management of severe traumatic brain injury. Introduction. J Neurotrauma. 2007;24(Suppl 1):S1.

41. Dash HH. Prehospital care of head injured patients. Neurology. 2008;56:415–9.
42. Davis DP. Prehospital intubation of brain-injured patients. Curr Opin Crit Care. 2008;14:142–8.
43. Matz PG, Pitts L. Monitoring in traumatic brain injury. Clin Neurosurg. 1997;44:267–94.
44. Sobuwa S, Hartzenberg HB, Geduld H, Uys C. Outcomes following prehospital airway management in severe traumatic brain injury. S Afr Med J. 2013;103:644–6.
45. Spaite DW, Bobrow BJ, Stolz U, Sherrill D, Chikani V, Barnhart B, et al. Evaluation of the impact of implementing the emergency medical services traumatic brain injury guidelines in Arizona: the excellence in prehospital injury care (EPIC) study methodology. Acad Emerg Med. 2014;21:818–30.
46. Badjatia N, Carney N, Crocco TJ, et al. Guidelines for prehospital management of traumatic brain injury 2nd edition. Prehosp Emerg Care. 2008;12(Suppl 1):S1.
47. Brain Trauma Foundation, American Association of Neurological Surgeons, Congress of Neurological Surgeons. Guidelines for the management of severe traumatic brain injury. XI. Anesthetics, analgesics, and sedatives. J Neurotrauma. 2007;24(Suppl 1):S71.
48. Davis DP, Peay J, Sise MJ, et al. Prehospital airway and ventilation management: a trauma score and injury severity score-based analysis. J Trauma. 2010;69:294.
49. Selassie AW, Zaloshnja E, Langlois JA, et al. Incidence of long-term disability following traumatic brain injury hospitalization, United States, 2003. J Head Trauma Rehabil. 2008;23:123.
50. Visca A, Faccani G, Massaro F, et al. Clinical and neuroimaging features of severely brain-injured patients treated in a neurosurgical unit compared with patients treated in peripheral non-neurosurgical hospitals. Br J Neurosurg. 2006;20:82.
51. Geijerstam JL, Britton M, Marke LA. Mild head injury: observation or computed tomography? Economic aspects by literature review and decision analysis. Emerg Med J. 2004;21:54–8.
52. Brown CV, Zada G, Salim A, et al. Indications for routine repeat head computed tomography (CT) stratified by severity of traumatic brain injury. J Trauma. 2007;62:1339.
53. Connon FF, Namdarian B, Ee JL, et al. Do routinely repeated computed tomography scans in traumatic brain injury influence management? A prospective observational study in a level 1 trauma center. Ann Surg. 2011;254:1028.
54. Geijerstam Jean-Luc AF, Sven O, Mona B. Medical outcome after immediate computed tomography or admission for observation in patients with mild head injury: randomized controlled trial. BMJ. 2006;333:465.
55. Gelernter R, Weiser G, Kozer E. Computed tomography findings in young children with minor head injury presenting to the emergency department greater than 24h post injury. Injury. 2018;49:82.
56. Haydel MJ, Jones PA, Mills TJ, et al. Indications for CT in patients with minor head injury. N Engl J Med. 2000;343:100–5.
57. Huang AP, Lee CW, Hsieh HJ, et al. Early parenchymal contrast extravasation predicts subsequent hemorrhage progression, clinical deterioration, and need for surgery in patients with traumatic cerebral contusion. J Trauma. 2011;71:1593.
58. Kaups KL, Davis JW, Parks SN. Routinely repeated computed tomography after blunt head trauma: does it benefit patients? J Trauma. 2004;56:475.
59. Thomas BW, Mejia VA, Maxwell RA, et al. Scheduled repeat CT scanning for traumatic brain injury remains important in assessing head injury progression. J Am Coll Surg. 2010;210:824.
60. McKinlay A. Controversies and outcomes associated with mild traumatic brain injury in childhood and adolescences. Child Care Health Dev. 2010;36:3.
61. National Institute for Health and Clinical Excellence. Clinical guideline 4. Head injury triage, assessment, investigation and early management of head injury in infants, children and adults. London: NICE; 2003. p. 96–7.
62. Anders N, Lars-Åke M, Jean-Lucaf G, Sven O, Mona B. Immediate computed tomography or admission for observation after mild head injury: cost comparison in randomized controlled trial. BMJ. 2006;333:469.
63. Pickering A, Harnan S, Fitzgerald P, et al. Clinical decision rules for children with minor head injury: a systematic review. Arch Dis Child. 2011;96:414.

64. Servadei F, Merry GS. Mild head injury in adults Youman's neurological surgery, vol. 4. 5th ed. Philadelphia: Saunders; 1996. p. 5065–80.
65. Contant CF, Valadka AB, Gopinath SP, Hannay HJ, Robertson CS. Adult respiratory distress syndrome: a complication of induced hypertension after severe head injury. J Neurosurg. 2001;95:560–8.
66. Cottenceau V, Masson F, Mahamid E, Petit L, Shik V, Sztark F, et al. Comparison of effects of equiosmolar doses of mannitol and hypertonic saline on cerebral blood flow and metabolism in traumatic brain injury. J Neurotrauma. 2011;28:2003–12.
67. Davison DL, Terek M, Chawla LS. Neurogenic pulmonary edema. Crit Care. 2012;16:212.
68. Perel P, Roberts I, Ker K. Colloids versus crystalloids for fluid resuscitation in critically ill patients. Cochrane Database Syst Rev. 2013;2:CD000567.
69. Pineda JA, Leonard JR, Mazotas IG, et al. Effect of implementation of a paediatric neurocritical care programme on outcomes after severe traumatic brain injury: a retrospective cohort study. Lancet Neurol. 2013;12:45.
70. Tisdall MM, Smith M. Multimodal monitoring in traumatic brain injury: current status and future directions. Br J Anaesth. 2007;99:61–7.
71. Ghajar J. Traumatic brain injury. Lancet. 2000;356:923–9.
72. Lagares A, Ramos A, Pérez-Nuñez A, et al. The role of MR imaging in assessing prognosis after severe and moderate head injury. Acta Neurochir. 2009;151:341.
73. Lingsma HF, Roozenbeek B, Steyerberg EW, et al. Early prognosis in traumatic brain injury: from prophecies to predictions. Lancet Neurol. 2010;9:543–54.
74. Marmarou A, Lu J, Butcher I, et al. IMPACT database of traumatic brain injury: design and description. J Neurotrauma. 2007;24:239–50.
75. Menon DK, Zahed C. Prediction of outcome in severe traumatic brain injury. Curr Opin Crit Care. 2009;15:437–41.
76. Miller JD, Murray S, Teasdale GM. Development of a traumatic intracranial haematoma after minor head injury. Neurosurgery. 1990;27:669–73.
77. Roozenbeek B, Lingsma HF, Lecky FE, et al. Prediction of outcome after moderate and severe traumatic brain injury: external validation of the International Mission on Prognosis and Analysis of Clinical Trials (IMPACT) and Corticoid Randomisation After Significant Head injury (CRASH) prognostic models. Crit Care Med. 2012;40:1609.
78. Skandsen T, Kvistad KA, Solheim O, et al. Prognostic value of magnetic resonance imaging in moderate and severe head injury: a prospective study of early MRI findings and one-year outcome. J Neurotrauma. 2011;28:691.
79. Brain Trauma Foundation, American Association of Neurological Surgeons, Congress of Neurological Surgeons. Guidelines for the management of severe traumatic brain injury. I. Blood pressure and oxygenation. J Neurotrauma. 2007;24(Suppl 1):S7.
80. Brain Trauma Foundation, American Association of Neurological Surgeons, Congress of Neurological Surgeons. Guidelines for the management of severe traumatic brain injury. II. Hyperosmolar therapy. J Neurotrauma. 2007;24(Suppl 1):S14.
81. Brown JB, Stassen NA, Cheng JD, et al. Trauma center designation correlates with functional independence after severe but not moderate traumatic brain injury. J Trauma. 2010;69:263.
82. Calvi MR, Beretta L, Dell'Acqua A, et al. Early prognosis after severe traumatic brain injury with minor or absent computed tomography scan lesions. J Trauma. 2011;70:447.
83. Lingsma H, Andriessen TM, Haitsema I, et al. Prognosis in moderate and severe traumatic brain injury: external validation of the IMPACT models and the role of extracranial injuries. J Trauma Acute Care Surg. 2013;74:639.
84. McNett M, Amato S, Gianakis A, et al. The FOUR score and GCS as predictors of outcome after traumatic brain injury. Neurocrit Care. 2014;21:52.
85. Schneider EB, Sur S, Raymont V, et al. Functional recovery after moderate/severe traumatic brain injury: a role for cognitive reserve? Neurology. 2014;82:1636.
86. Schnüriger B, Inaba K, Abdelsayed GA, et al. The impact of platelets on the progression of traumatic intracranial hemorrhage. J Trauma. 2010;68:881.

87. Hoffman WY. Scalp injuries and their management. In: Youmans JR, editor. Neurological surgery, vol. III. 4th ed. Philadelphia: WB Saunders; 1996. p. 1915–25.
88. Bullock MR, Chesnut R, Ghajar J, et al. Surgical management of depressed cranial fractures. Neurosurgery. 2006;58:S56.
89. Sharma RR, Chandy MJ. Shunt surgery in growing skull fractures. Report of two cases. Br J Neurosurg. 1991;5:93–8.
90. Sharma RR, Prabhu S, Parekh HC, Keogh AJ. Penetrating trans-orbital craniocerebral wind-shield glass injury. Report of two cases. Lancaster West Moorland J. 1992;1:331–4.
91. Bullock MR, Chesnut R, Ghajar J, et al. Surgical management of acute epidural hematomas. Neurosurgery. 2006;58:S7.
92. Bullock MR, Chesnut R, Ghajar J, et al. Surgical management of acute subdural hematomas. Neurosurgery. 2006;58:S16.
93. Chang EF, Meeker M, Holland MC. Acute traumatic intraparenchymal hemorrhage: risk factors for progression in the early post-injury period. Neurosurgery. 2006;58:647.
94. Cooper DJ, Rosenfeld JV, Murray L, et al. Decompressive craniectomy in diffuse traumatic brain injury. N Engl J Med. 2011;364:1493.
95. Hutchinson PJ, Kolias AG, Timofeev IS, et al. Trial of decompressive craniectomy for traumatic intracranial hypertension. N Engl J Med. 2006;375:1119.
96. Kolias AG, Kirkpatrick PJ, Hutchinson PJ. Decompressive craniectomy: past, present and future. Nat Rev Neurol. 2013;9:405.
97. Narayan RK, Maas AI, Servadei F, et al. Progression of traumatic intracerebral hemorrhage: a prospective observational study. J Neurotrauma. 2008;25:629.
98. Oertel M, Kelly DF, McArthur D, et al. Progressive hemorrhage after head trauma: predictors and consequences of the evolving injury. J Neurosurg. 2002;96:109.
99. Servadei F. Clinical value of decompressive craniectomy. N Engl J Med. 2011;364:1558.
100. Smith M. Refractory intracranial hypertension: the role of decompressive craniectomy. Anesth Analg. 2017;125:1999.
101. Adams JH. Brain damage in fatal non-missile head injury in man. In: Braakman R, editor. Handbook of clinical neurology, vol. 13. Amsterdam: Elsevier; 1990. p. 43–63.
102. Adams JH, Mitenell DE, Graham DI, Doyle D. Diffuse brain damage of immediate impact type. Brain. 1977;100:489–502.
103. Jennet B, Bond M. Assessment of outcome after severe brain damage: a practical scale. Lancet. 1975;1:480–4.
104. Rodrigues D, Mahapatra AK, Sharma RR, Lad SD, Pawar SJ. Post traumatic hydrocephalus. A study of 22 cases. In: Sharma RR, Pawar SJ, Lad SD, editors. Management of head injury in Oman. Al-Zahra Printers: Muscat; 2000. p. 100–2.
105. Sharma RR, Chandy MJ, Lad SD. Post traumatic occlusion in vertebro-basilar system. Report of two cases. Emirates Med J. 1990;8:221–5.
106. Sharma RR, Chandy MJ, Lad SD. Delayed traumatic intracerebral haematoma. Case report and review of the literature. Ann Saudi Med. 1991;11:102–5.
107. Sharma RR, Lad SD, Delmendo A. Acute traumatic subdural hygromas and trans tentorial herniation. Oman Med J. 1996;13(2):66–70.
108. Sharma RR, Mahapatra AK, Pawar SJ, Lad SD. Symptomatic calcified subdural haematomas. Case report and brief review of literature. Paediatr Neurosurg. 1999;31:150–4.
109. Sharma RR, Mujaini A, Netalkar AS. Traumatic carotico-cavernous fistula treated with balloon embolisation. Review of the literature with an illustrated case. Oman Med J. 1997;14:49–53.
110. Sharma RR, Pawar SJ, Devadas RV, Lad SD. The role of stereotactic surgery in head injury. In: Mahapatra AK, Rajkamal A, editors. A textbook of head injury. New Delhi: Modern Publishers; 2005. p. 167–86.
111. Sharma RR, Pawar SJ, Sousa J, Lad SD. Post traumatic bilateral dilated unreactive pupils in paediatric age group and long-term outcome. Abstract: 12th World Congress of Neurosurgery, 16-20 Sept. 2001, Sydney, Australia, p. 82.
112. Strich SJ. Diffuse degeneration of the cerebral white matter in severe dementia following head injury. J Neurol Neurosurg Psychiatry. 1956;19:163–74.

113. Cadena R, Shoykhet M, Ratcliff JJ. Emergency neurological life support: intracranial hypertension and herniation. Neurocrit Care. 2017;27:82.
114. Caricato A, Conti G, Della Corte F, Mancino A, Santilli F, Sandroni C, et al. Effects of PEEP on the intracranial system of patients with head injury and subarachnoid hemorrhage: the role of respiratory system compliance. J Trauma. 2005;58:571–6.
115. Howells T, Elf K, Jones PA, et al. Pressure reactivity as a guide in the treatment of cerebral perfusion pressure in patients with brain trauma. J Neurosurg. 2005;102:311.
116. Sookplung P, Siriussawakul A, Malakouti A, Sharma D, Wang J, Souter MJ, et al. Vasopressor use and effect on blood pressure after severe adult traumatic brain injury. Neurocrit Care. 2011;15:46–54.
117. Sousa J, Sharma RR, Pawar SJ, Lad SD. Role of cerebral perfusion pressure monitoring in determining the outcome in patients with severe head injuries. Results in a series of 89 patients. Pan Arab J Neurosurg. 2006;6(1):1–9.
118. Biersteker HA, Andriessen TM, Horn J, et al. Factors influencing intracranial pressure monitoring guideline compliance and outcome after severe traumatic brain injury. Crit Care Med. 2012;40:1914.
119. Bricolo AP, Pasut LM. Extradural haematoma: towards zero mortality: a prospective study. Neurosurgery. 1984;12:8–12.
120. Farahvar A, Gerber LM, Chiu YL, et al. Increased mortality in patients with severe traumatic brain injury treated without intracranial pressure monitoring. J Neurosurg. 2012;117:729.
121. Nemer SN, Caldeira JB, Santos RG, et al. Effects of positive end-expiratory pressure on brain tissue oxygen pressure of severe traumatic brain injury patients with acute respiratory distress syndrome: a pilot study. J Crit Care. 2015;30:1263.
122. Nwachuku EL, Puccio AM, Fetzick A, et al. Intermittent versus continuous cerebrospinal fluid drainage management in adult severe traumatic brain injury: assessment of intracranial pressure burden. Neurocrit Care. 2014;20:49.
123. Devlin JW, Skrobik Y, Gélinas C, et al. Clinical practice guidelines for the prevention and management of pain, agitation/sedation, delirium, immobility, and sleep disruption in adult patients in the ICU. Crit Care Med. 2018;46:e825.
124. Rajajee V, Riggs B, Seder DB. Emergency neurological life support: airway, ventilation, and sedation. Neurocrit Care. 2017;27:4.
125. Sharma A. Neuroprotection for traumatic brain injury. In: Sharma RR, Devadas RV, Mishra GP, Pawar SJ, Lad SD, editors. Current trends in neurosurgery. Muscat: Al Zahra Printers; 2004. p. 139–42.
126. Kharangate P, Sharma RR. Post traumatic epilepsy. In: Sharma RR, Pawar SJ, Lad SD, editors. Management of head injury in Oman. Muscat: Al-Zahra Printers; 2000. p. 103–7.
127. Vespa PM, Miller C, McArthur D, Eliseo M, Etchepare M, Hirt D, et al. Nonconvulsive electrographic seizures after traumatic brain injury result in a delayed, prolonged increase in intracranial pressure and metabolic crisis. Crit Care Med. 2007;35:2830–6.
128. Vespa PM, Nuwer MR, Nenov V, et al. Increased incidence and impact of nonconvulsive and convulsive seizures after traumatic brain injury as detected by continuous electroencephalographic monitoring. J Neurosurg. 1999;91:750.
129. Yang Y, Zheng F, Xu X, Wang X. Levetiracetam versus phenytoin for seizure prophylaxis following traumatic brain injury: a systematic review and meta-analysis. CNS Drugs. 2016;30:677–88.
130. Zimmermann LL, Diaz-Arrastia R, Vespa PM. Seizures and the role of anticonvulsants after traumatic brain injury. Neurosurg Clin N Am. 2016;27:499.
131. Badri S, Chen J, Barber J, et al. Mortality and long-term functional outcome associated with intracranial pressure after traumatic brain injury. Intensive Care Med. 2012;38:1800.
132. Ho KM, Honeybul S, Litton E. Delayed neurological recovery after decompressive craniectomy for severe nonpenetrating traumatic brain injury. Crit Care Med. 2011;39:2495.
133. Perel P, Arango M, et al. Predicting outcome after traumatic brain injury: practical prognostic models based on large cohort of international patients. BMJ. 2008;336:425.

134. McCredie VA, Alali AS, Xiong W, et al. Timing of withdrawal of life-sustaining therapies in severe traumatic brain injury: impact on overall mortality. J Trauma Acute Care Surg. 2016;80:484.
135. Sbordone RJ, Liter JC, Pettler-Jennings P. Recovery of function following severe traumatic brain injury: a retrospective 10-year follow-up. Brain Inj. 1995;1995(9):285.

The Paradigm Shift in the Incidence of Post-trauma Complications

15

K. L. Sampath Kumar

15.1 Introduction

In the present era, trauma is the leading cause of increasing morbidity and mortality, especially among the youth [1]. In fact, around 30% of all admissions into intensive care units of all leading hospitals are to treat the victims of trauma [2], and trauma is attributed to 10% of all deaths in tertiary care hospitals [3]. However, there have been many improvements in the management of trauma patients in the recent period. The introduction of air ambulances to carry the road traffic accident victims to the designated trauma care hospitals reduced the waiting period for the victim to be seen by the trauma care specialists. The improvements in the investigation modalities, abundant availability of ultrasound scans, and other imaging modalities improved anesthesia and surgical techniques and drastically reduced the morbidity and mortality of trauma victims [4]. At the same time, increased survival rates of the trauma victims resulted in a rapid increase in post-trauma complications (PTCs) [5, 6]. These complications may be a result of post-trauma status or a result of surgery on a trauma victim. The well-known PTCs include a deadly triad of metabolic acidosis, hypothermia, and hypercoagulopathy. These complications are controlled to some extent by immediate energetic resuscitation and damage control surgery. However, various thromboembolic complications, infection, sepsis, and various organ failure still can occur. In view of rapid improvements in trauma care, there is a perceptible shift in the incidence and the nature of PTCs now.

K. L. Sampath Kumar (✉)
Narayana Medical College, Nellore, Andhra Pradesh, India

© The Author(s), under exclusive license to Springer Nature Singapore Pte Ltd. 2024

A. Agrawal et al. (eds.), *Special Considerations in Trauma Care*,
https://doi.org/10.1007/978-981-99-9662-9_15

15.2 Discussion

Trauma is the leading cause of increasing morbidity and mortality among the youth nowadays. The road traffic accidents are the major cause of trauma. In addition, fall from high-rise buildings, urban warfare activities, and attempted homicides form the other causes of trauma. The majority of the reports indicate that more than 50% of the victims require intensive care unit admissions. Approximately 10% of the victims succumb to the trauma and its sequelae and about 25–30% of the patients suffer from PTCs [6]. However, the improvements in the shifting of the trauma victims by air ambulances to the specialized trauma hospitals reduced the waiting periods for the trauma victims and these victims are attended to, within the first Golden Hour by the trauma care specialists. Moreover, there is strict implementation of Advanced Trauma Life Support (ATLS) protocols. There is a better understanding of the pathophysiology of trauma by clinicians as a result of rapid strides in research activities. Not only the trauma centers but also the various hospitals are well equipped with ultrasound machines and various imaging modalities. In addition, there is a tremendous improvement in anesthesia techniques and surgical procedures. All these factors and the improved treatment strategies helped in decreasing mortality and morbidity rates in trauma victims. As there is an increase in the survival rates of trauma victims nowadays, there is an increase in the incidence of PTCs as these trauma survivors continue to stay in the intensive care units for longer duration and suffer from various complications [5].

Initially, most of the trauma victims suffer from the deadly triad of metabolic acidosis, coagulopathy, and hypothermia if not treated adequately. Later on, various complications can occur. These various complications may be classified under the following 12 categories [6]:

1. Acute renal failure
2. Acute respiratory distress syndrome (ARDS)
3. Cardiac arrest with cardiopulmonary resuscitation and its sequelae
4. Deep surgical site infection
5. Deep venous thrombosis (DVT)/thrombophlebitis
6. Myocardial infarction
7. Organ/space surgical site infection
8. Pneumonia
9. Pulmonary embolism
10. Stroke/cerebrovascular accident
11. Superficial surgical site infection (SSSI)
12. Systemic sepsis

Due to adequate thrombo-prophylactic measures, there is a steady decline in the incidence of pulmonary embolism. However, there is not much improvement in the incidence of DVT and superficial thrombophlebitis and they still occur as PTCs.

Most of the trauma care hospitals strictly follow the pulmonary protocols resulting in a decreased incidence of ARDS, but there is not much difference in the incidence of ventilator-associated pneumonia in post-trauma victims [7]. In addition, instead of administering large volumes of crystalloid solutions to treat post-traumatic hypotension, nowadays, permissive hypotension is practiced by limiting the fluid administration and balanced blood transfusion regimen [8].

Similarly, optimal fluid resuscitation strategies helped in the gradual decline of acute renal failure in trauma victims.

Most of the trauma victims require surgical intervention and the stress of surgery itself can increase the incidence of complications. The anesthetized brain is physiologically still awake and active hence responsive to surgical stress. It results in sympathetic overactivity and secondary activation of injury response. These two factors cause hyperinflammation, coagulopathy, immune dysfunction, and metabolic dysfunction [9, 10]. It has been proved that surgical stress induces an amplified inflammatory response in patients [11].

A patient who has been in shock and resuscitated as a result of trauma, and then operated upon, is in a precarious state. His nervous system has been disturbed originally by the original trauma, then by the low nutrient flow of blood as a result of shock, and then by the surgical procedures.

The most susceptible tissues to ischemia-reperfusion injury are the more aerobic tissues such as brain, heart, lung, and kidney. Hence, it is natural that these organs are more prone to complications after post-traumatic surgery [12].

Thus, once the body's homeostasis is disturbed, inflammatory markers rise in the circulation and alter coagulation [13], modify immunological responses [14], reduce tissue oxygen concentration [15], and thus increase the chances of infection [16]. This secondary insult results in potential multiple organ dysfunction [17].

We know that David Cuthbertson divided the body's stress response into two phases: (1) an early "ebb" phase which begins 2 h post-injury and lasts for 2–3 days and is associated with glucose intolerance and downregulation of cardiac function, tissue perfusion, and metabolic rate, and (2) a second "flow" phase lasting days and weeks, which is characterized by an upregulation of metabolism, cardiac function, higher blood glucose, and muscle wasting [18]. Therefore, a patient who sustains trauma and undergoes surgery in the so-called first phase of the "ebb" phase has a prolonged first phase resulting in prolonged glucose intolerance, diminished cardiac function, diminished tissue perfusion, and metabolic rate. Hence, these patients are more prone to multiorgan dysfunction and infection.

15.3 Age of the Patient and Complications

The age of the trauma victim is an important factor in the development of complications following trauma. "Younger the patient better the survival." Most of the younger patients are free from various medical comorbid conditions and have better immunity. In addition, they can withstand surgery better and survive for longer periods. Hence, the mortality is less, but morbidity in the form of PTCs is more [19].

It has been observed that the elderly people suffer 30% less complications than the younger individuals. It is mostly due to increased mortality as a result of trauma.

15.4 Sex of the Patient and the Complications

Recent studies on adult trauma patients admitted to hospitals in the National Trauma Data Bank of the United States of America have shown that women are less likely than men to develop inpatient complications [20, 21]. Though the exact reason is unknown, most probably, the deleterious effect of testosterone may play a role [22]. In addition, the female sex hormones may confer some immunological protection [23]. It is more so when CNS injury is present [24].

15.5 Length of Hospital Stay and Complications

By and large, both mortality and morbidity of any surgical patient are directly related to the length of hospital stay (LOS), especially in an intensive care unit. However, in the case of trauma victims, mortality is not directly related to the LOS as death occurs in trauma patients at a rate of 10% within 24 h. Hence, the dead patients have minimal LOS, whereas the morbidity in the form of complications is directly related to the LOS. Advances in prehospital care, as well as in medical and surgical care, may be responsible for the decrease in mortality rates of trauma patients allowing more severely injured patients to survive and stay in the hospital for a longer time to recover. During this prolonged stay in the hospital, the majority of the patients, approximately 50%, may suffer from PTCs [25].

15.6 Number of Complications and the Nature of Complications

The complications following trauma differ in patients who survive and in patients who do not survive. Even the number of complications also differs among survivors and non-survivors. However, pulmonary complications are the most common complications in both groups. In addition, other complications that are significantly more common in subjects who die are postoperative cardiac complications, shock or cardiorespiratory arrest, and postoperative acute myocardial infarction.

Complications that are more common in survivors are wound infection, cellulitis, decubitus ulcer, venous thrombosis, and pulmonary embolism. The prevalence of other complications is not significantly different between survivors and non-survivors.

Most of the non-survivors suffer from a single complication, such as irreversible shock, cardiopulmonary arrest, or pulmonary embolism. However, the patients with traumatic CNS injury show a higher risk of mortality and die even before suffering from any complications.

15.7 Conclusion

Trauma is a leading cause of morbidity and mortality in the present era. In spite of rapid developments in the early transportation of the victims to the designated tertiary care trauma hospitals, strict maintenance of ATLS protocols, and rapid strides in anesthesia and surgical care, morbidity in the form of PTCs does occur. Though the mortality rates are declining, the complications are increasing. The cause has been identified as increasing lengths of hospital stay of the trauma victims as more and more patients survive only to suffer from the complications. In the recent past, there has been a paradigm shift in the nature of complications following trauma as shown in various studies. Earlier, most of the trauma survivors suffered from complications such as acute renal failure, ARDS, myocardial infarction, organ space and SSSI, pneumonia, pulmonary embolism, cardiac arrest, and sepsis. Now, most of these complications are prevented by timely intervention and changes in the treatment strategies. However, the incidence of deep surgical site infection, organ space infection, DVT, and cerebrovascular catastrophe increased over time. In addition, these patients have a negative impact on the long-term quality of life of trauma patients [26].

However, one should remember that the presence of complications and the number of complications are not associated with an increased risk of mortality.

References

1. World Health Organization. Global burden of disease. http://www.cdc.gov/injury/wisqars/non-fatal.html.
2. MacKenzie EJ, Rivara FP, Jurkovich GJ, et al. The national study on costs and outcomes of trauma. J Trauma. 2007;63(supplement 6):S54–67.
3. Feliciano DV, Mattox K, Moore EE. Trauma. 6th ed. New York: McGraw-Hill; 2008.
4. Osler TM, Mukamel DB, Dick AW. Outcomes of adult trauma patients admitted to trauma centres in Pennsylvania, 2000–2009. Arch Surg. 2012;147(8):732–7.
5. Ingraham AM, Xiong W, Hemmila MR, et al. The attributable mortality and length of stay of trauma-related complications: a matched cohort study. Ann Surg. 2010;252(2):358–62.
6. Jacobson RK, Bonde A, Sillesen M. Assessment of post-trauma complications in eight million trauma cases over a decade in the USA. Trauma Surg Acute Care Open. 2021;6(1):e000667. https://doi.org/10.1136/tsaco-2020-000667.
7. Shafi S, Barnes S, Nicewander D, et al. Health care reform at trauma centers-mortality, complications, and length of stay. J Trauma. 2010;69(6):1367–71.
8. Thompson BT, Bernard GR. ARDS network (NHLBI) studies: successes and challenges in ARDS clinical research. Crit Care Clin. 2011;27:459–68. https://doi.org/10.1016/j.ccc.2011.05.011.
9. Kasotakis G, Sideris A, Yang Y, de Moya M, Alam H, King DR, Tompkins R, Velmahos G, Inflammation and Host Response to Injury Investigators. Aggressive early crystalloid resuscitation adversely affects outcomes in adult blunt trauma patients: an analysis of the glue grant database. J Trauma Acute Care Surg. 2013;74:1215–21. https://doi.org/10.1097/TA.0b013e3182826e13.
10. Anderson O, Davis R, Hanna GB, Vincent CA. Surgical adverse events: a systematic review. Am J Surg. 2013;206(2):253–62.

11. Smith SM, Vale WW. The role of the hypothalamic-pituitary-adrenal axis in neuroendocrine responses to stress. Dialogues Clin Neurosci. 2006;8(4):383–95.
12. Giannoudis PV, Dinopoulos H, Chalidis B, Hall GM. Surgical stress response. Injury. 2006;37(Suppl 5):S3–9.
13. Dobson GP, Morris JL, Davenport LM, Letson HL. Traumatic-induced coagulopathy as a systems failure: a new window into haemostasis. Semin Thromb Hemost. 2020;46(2):199–214.
14. Marik PE, Flemmer M. The immune response to surgery and trauma: implications for treatment. J Trauma Acute Care Surg. 2012;73(4):801–8.
15. Shoemaker WC, Beez M. Pathophysiology, monitoring, and therapy of shock with organ failure. Appl Cardiopulm Pathophysiol. 2010;14:5–15.
16. Anderson DJ, Chen LF, Sexton DJ, Kaye KS. Complex surgical site infections and the devilish details of risk adjustment: important implications for public reporting. Infect Control Hosp Epidemiol. 2008;29(10):941–6.
17. Choileain NN, Redmond HP. Cell response to surgery. Arch Surg. 2006;141(11):1132–40.
18. Cuthbertson DP. Symposium on 'surgery and nutrition'. Historical approach. Proc Nutr Soc. 1980;39(2):101–5.
19. Kuhne CA, Ruchholtz S, Kaiser GM, et al. Mortality in severely injured elderly trauma patients—when does age become a risk factor? World J Surg. 2005;29(11):1476–82.
20. Haider AH, Crompton JG, Oyetunji T, et al. Females have fewer complications and lower mortality following trauma than similarly injured males: a risk adjusted analysis of adults in the National Trauma Data Bank. Surgery. 2009;146(2):308–15.
21. Magnotti LJ, Fischer PE, Zarzaur BL, Fabian TC, Croce MA. Impact of gender on outcomes after blunt injury: a definitive analysis of more than 36,000 trauma patients. J Am Coll Surg. 2008;206(5):984–92.
22. Angele MK, Ayala A, Monfils BA, Cioffi WG, Bland KI, Chaudry IH. Testosterone and/or low estradiol: normally required but harmful immunologically for males after trauma-hemorrhage. J Trauma. 1998;44(1):78–85.
23. Sperry JL, Minei JP. Gender dimorphism following injury: making the connection from bench to bedside. J Leukoc Biol. 2008;83(3):499–506.
24. Bramlett HM, Dietrich WD. Neuropathological protection after traumatic brain injury in intact female rats versus males or ovariectomized females. J Neurotrauma. 2001;18(9):891–900.
25. Pape H, Remmers D, Rice J, Ebisch M, Krettek C, Tscherne H. Appraisal of early evaluation of blunt chest trauma: development of a standardized scoring system for initial clinical decision making. J Trauma. 2000;49(3):496–504.
26. Holbrook TL, Hoyt DB, Anderson JP. The impact of major in-hospital complications on functional outcome and quality of life after trauma. J Trauma. 2001;50(1):91–5.

Intracranial Pressure Monitoring in Traumatic Brain Injury

16

Raghu Samala and Ramesh Doddamani

16.1 Introduction

Raised intracranial pressure (ICP) is a common clinical condition in neurosurgical and neurological intensive care unit (ICU) setups spanning from traumatic brain injury (TBI), stroke, intracerebral hematoma (ICH), infections, and space-occupying neoplastic lesions or co-existing systemic disease. All the treatment protocols should be aimed at preventing secondary brain insult that follows primary brain injury and thus modulating the final outcomes (Fig. 16.1).

16.2 Pathophysiology of Raised ICP

16.2.1 Intracranial Compliance

The Monro-Kellie hypothesis states that the skull being an inelastic container, the sum of intracranial volumes of cerebrospinal fluid (CSF—150 mL), blood (150 mL), and brain parenchyma (1400 mL) is constant. As per this hypothesis, an increase in one of the three components leads to compensatory reduction in the other two, under physiological conditions. However, when this compensatory mechanism fails, intracranial compliance falls and there is a rapid rise of ICP. Neonates and infants may have better cranial compliance owing to non-fused sutures (Fig. 16.2).

R. Samala
Department of Neurosurgery, AIG Hospital, Hyderabad, Telangana, India

R. Doddamani (✉)
Department of Neurosurgery, All India Institute of Medical Sciences, New Delhi, India

© The Author(s), under exclusive license to Springer Nature Singapore Pte Ltd. 2024
A. Agrawal et al. (eds.), *Special Considerations in Trauma Care*,
https://doi.org/10.1007/978-981-99-9662-9_16

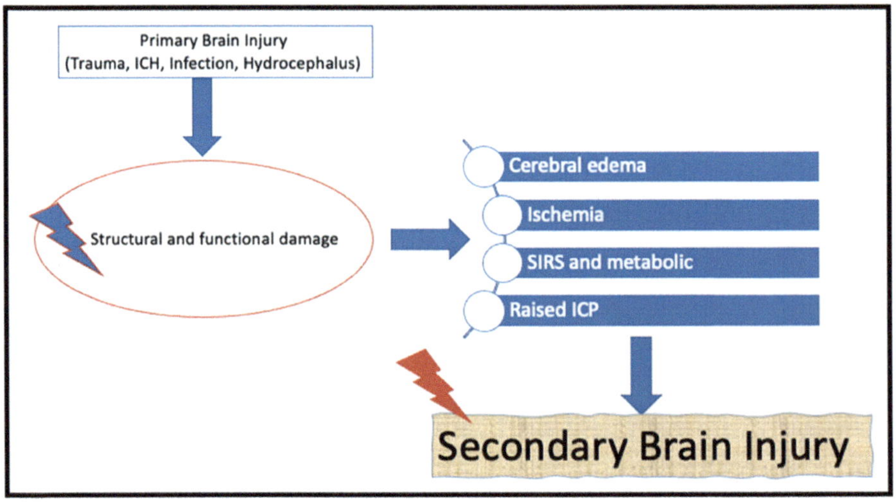

Fig. 16.1 Schematic representation of cerebral injury following initial brain insult

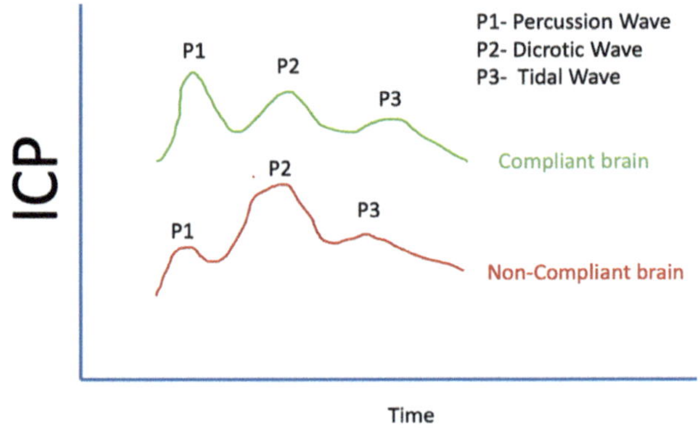

Fig. 16.2 Relationship between ICP waves and brain compliance

16.2.2 ICP Waveforms

The normal range of ICP varies with age in accordance with enlarging cranium and growing brain (Table 16.1).

Lundberg's waveforms denote ventricular pressure fluctuations and are represented by decreasing severity of ICP from A to C waves.

1. A waves or plateau waves: These waves are characterized by a steep rise of ICP from near normal range to 50 mmHg or more and then fall sharply lasting 5–20 min and are always pathological, denoting poor intracranial compliance. These waves are associated with reduced cerebral perfusion pressure (CPP) and cerebral blood flow (CBF), which, if untreated, result in poor neurological outcomes.

Table 16.1 Normal ICP range

Age	ICP (mmHg)
Infants	1.5–6
Children	3–7
Adults	10–15

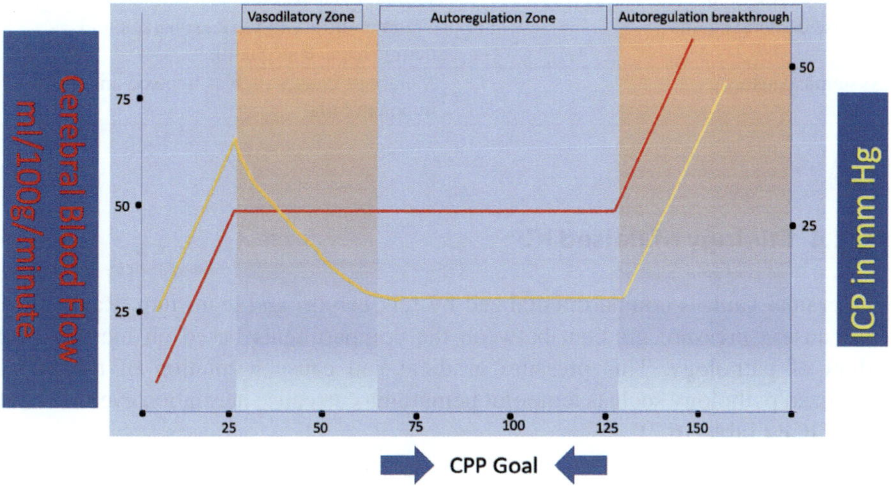

Fig. 16.3 The relation between CBF, CPP, and ICP. Note that ICP fluctuations beyond the autoregulatory zone

2. B waves: ICP rises in a crescendo manner up to 20–30 mmHg lasting 1–2 min, followed by rapid fall. These waves are associated with Cheyne-Stokes respiration and indicate failing intracranial compliance.
3. C waves: These are of limited clinical significance, associated with Traube–Hering–Mayer type variations in blood pressure, occurring at a frequency of 4–8/min and of smaller amplitude than B waves.

16.2.3 Cerebral Perfusion Pressure

CPP is defined as mean arterial pressure (MAP) minus ICP and is autoregulated between 50 and 150 mmHg. Low CPP can result in poor cerebral perfusion and ischemia, while high CPP beyond autoregulation limits can cause breakthrough hyperemia, vasogenic edema, and raised ICP. Hence, it is imperative to maintain CPP in the physiological range (Fig. 16.3).

Table 16.2 Causes of raised ICP

Pathological process	Etiology
CSF disturbances	Obstructive hydrocephalus, communicating hydrocephalus
Mass lesions	Hematoma, tumor, abscess, infarction
Venous obstruction	Cerebral venous thrombosis, trauma
Diffuse cerebral edema	Trauma, diffuse hypoxia, subarachnoid hemorrhage, encephalitis
Systemic causes	Metabolic causes such as hypoxia and hyponatremia

16.2.4 Etiology of Raised ICP

The cranial vault is compartmentalized by falx cerebri and tentorium. Raised ICP can cause a pressure gradient between the compartments based on location and extent of pathology. This pressure gradient can cause herniation of the brain. Localized pathology such as temporal hematoma can cause herniation even without raised ICP (Table 16.2).

16.2.5 What Are the Features of Raised ICP?

Depressed levels of consciousness and reflex hypertension are the two most consistent signs. Cushing's triad is a reflex phenomenon comprising hypertension, bradycardia, and irregular respiration. This is a protective mechanism noted while CPP is failing and cerebral demands are unmet. This causes increased peripheral vascular resistance and MAP. Other signs and symptoms that occur with raised ICP are vomiting, headache, papilledema, and false localizing signs such as abducens nerve palsy (Table 16.3).

16.3 Does the Patient Need ICP Monitoring?

16.3.1 ICP Monitoring

ICP monitoring is indicated when there is no clear indication for surgical intervention.

1. Severe head injury with GCS ≤8 and abnormal computed tomographic (CT) findings such as hematoma, contusion, and edema
2. Severe head injury with normal CT findings in case of
   (a) Age >40 years
   (b) Unilateral or bilateral motor posturing
   (c) Hypotension with systolic BP <90 mmHg

Table 16.3 Presentation of raised ICP

Cause	Clinical signs/symptoms
Diffuse cerebral edema	Depressed conscious level, papilledema, and signs of central herniation
Herniations	
1. Uncal herniation	Pupillary dilatation, incomplete ophthalmoplegia (oculomotor palsy), contralateral or ipsilateral motor posturing (Kernohan notch phenomenon)
2. Subfalcine herniation	Altered consciousness, asymmetric posturing, paraparesis in case of bilateral anterior cerebral artery compression, and ischemia
3. Central herniation	Coma with decerebrate or decorticate posturing
4. Cerebellar herniation	Coma with bilateral motor posturing

3. Mild to moderate injury: Usually, ICP monitoring is required; however, the clinician may decide case to case basis based on injury type
4. Reye's syndrome: Blood ammonia >300 mg/100 mL and deteriorating consciousness
5. Complex hydrocephalus: as a diagnostic tool
6. Others: Hypoxic brain injury, encephalitis, hepatic encephalopathy, and cerebral venous thrombosis
7. Tumors, spontaneous ICH, and subarachnoid hemorrhage although not routinely indicated

16.3.2 Techniques of ICP Monitoring

Several techniques are available to monitor ICP. Intraventricular fluid-filled transducer systems are considered the "gold standard." Along with measuring ICP, it provides access to intraventricular CSF allowing its drainage as a therapeutic option when ICP is raised. Intraventricular ICP monitoring is associated with a high infection rate (10–20%). Intraparenchymal catheters are easy to use and are to be calibrated before using them. Infection rates of intraparenchymal transducers are exceedingly low (1%). There are multiple devices available for measuring ICP (both direct and indirect) with various pros and cons associated with them (Tables 16.4 and 16.5).

16.3.3 Management of Raised ICP

A tiered management strategy is adopted for the management of Raised ICP in order to maintain a target CPP of above 60–70 mmHg and ICP of less than 22 mmHg (Fig. 16.4). The higher tiers of management indicate the severity and aggressive nature of the management. It is prudent to begin from the lowest tier and then escalate the management based on the patient's response. However, in severe cases

Table 16.4 Invasive modalities of ICP monitoring

Modality	Advantages	Disadvantages
Intraventricular	1. More accurate	1. Difficult to insert when there is severe edema and small ventricles
	2. Represent global ICP	2. High infection rate (10–20%)
	3. Lower cost	
	4. Can be recalibrated in situ	
	5. Can drain CSF as ICP lowering therapy	
Intraparenchymal	1. Fairly accurate	1. High cost
	2. Lower risk of infection	2. Need calibration
	3. Easier to place	3. Inability to drain CSF
		4. May not represent global ICP
Epidural	Rarely used	Less accurate and dampening effect with time
Subdural	Rarely used	Less accurate
Subarachnoid	Rarely used	Less accurate
Cerebral microdialysis	1. Allows for semicontinuous measurement at the bedside of numerous parameters	1. Time-consuming maintenance
	2. Early metabolic changes are detected before ICP raises	2. Additional costs
	3. Allow earlier therapeutic adjustments	3. Cannot represent a global insult
$PbtO_2$	1. To assist titration of medical and surgical therapies to guide ICP/CPP therapy	1. More efficacious when used along with $SjvO_2$
	2. Identify refractory intracranial hypertension and treatment thresholds	2. Represents regional metabolism
	3. Help manage delayed cerebral ischemia and selected patients for second-tier therapy	
	4. Tendency to better outcomes with combined $PbtO_2$ and ICP/CPP therapy compared to ICP/CPP therapy alone	
Jugular venous saturation ($SjvO_2$)	1. Differentiates insufficient oxygen supply due to impaired cerebral perfusion ($SjvO_2$ <50%) from reduced cerebral oxygen consumption encountered during hyperemia ($SjvO_2$ >80%)	1. More difficult to use and less reliable than $PbtO_2$ monitoring
	2. Only provide information as a part of multimodality monitoring or be used in conjunction with ICP monitoring	2. Insensitive to regional imbalances
	3. Represents local metabolism	

Table 16.5 Non-invasive modalities of ICP monitoring

Modality	Advantages	Disadvantages
Brain CT	Fastest and most cost-effective method	Radiation exposure
Brain MRI	More accurate assessment of soft tissue and cerebral substance lesions	1. Cost 2. Time-consuming
Transcranial Doppler ultrasonography	Patient bedside	Highly operator dependent
Optic nerve sheath diameter	Cheap, efficient, and not time-consuming	Optic nerve sheath diameter can be normal when optic nerve subarachnoid space is not in communication with cranial subarachnoid space
Tympanic membrane displacement	Non-invasive	Inaccurate and unreliable
Near-infrared spectroscopy	Non-invasive tool that measures cerebral oxygenation	
Continuous electroencephalography	1. Remarkably sensitive tool for detection of cerebral ischemia 2. High sensitivity to detect changes in CBF 3. Detection of convulsive and non-convulsive seizures when the patient is comatose 4. Predict outcomes and titrate treatments such as barbiturates	The severity of ICP elevation is not correlated

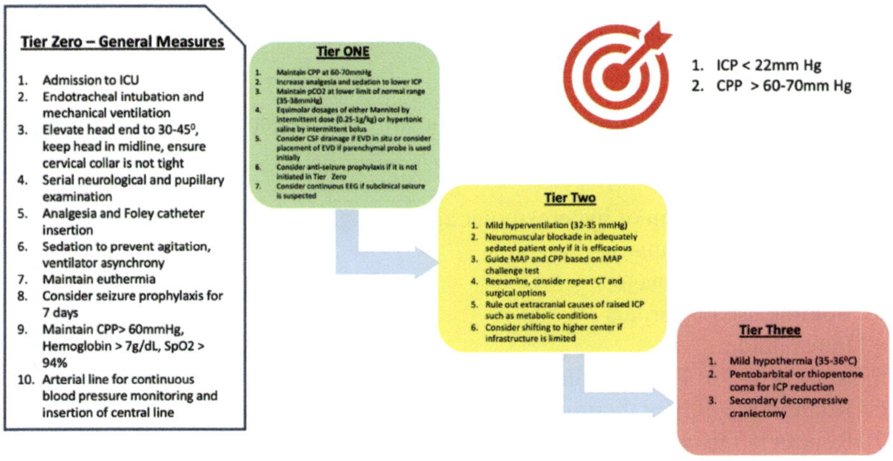

Fig. 16.4 Step-wise management of raised ICP

with raised ICP refractory to medical therapy, this tiered management can be skipped in favor of advanced treatments such as decompressive craniectomy.

Critical Neuroworsening Critical neuroworsening represents a specific situation of critical deterioration requiring emergent management. A serious deterioration can be a sudden fall in the GCS by ≥1 point, a new onset decrease in pupillary response/asymmetry, a new onset focal neurological deficit, or the development of herniation syndrome. Response to critical neuroworsening involves:

1. Emergent evaluation of the cause of worsening
2. Empiric treatment with hyperventilation and bolus of the hypertonic solution if herniation is suspected
3. Consider emergent imaging
4. Rapid escalation of treatment

16.3.4 Weaning of ICP Treatment

Rapid cessation of hyperventilation and osmotic agents can cause a rebound effect and hence should be tapered slowly.

1. Sedation holiday: Sedation holidays are required to assess patients' neurological status. For patients with ICP controlled with Tier 1 alone or Tier 1 therapy with a history of needing Tier 2 or 3 treatment, ICP must be under acceptable levels for 72 h before giving sedation holiday. Sedation holiday should be considered cautiously in patients whose ICP is controlled on Tier 2 or 3 if ICP is acceptable limits for more than 72 h.
2. ICP monitor removal: Guidelines suggest that ICP monitoring can be stopped if acceptable ICP is maintained for 72 h. ICP removal after 24 h is recommended only for patients with benign CT findings and good neurological status. However, therapeutic intensity before acceptable ICP levels strongly influences the decision of ICP removal.

Treatment Not Recommended The following treatments are not recommended for use in severe TBI:

1. Scheduled infusion of hyperosmolar agents (e.g., every 4–6 h), which should be guided by ICP status
2. Lumbar CSF drainage
3. Routine use of steroids
4. Furosemide
5. Routine use of hyperventilation (pCO_2 <30 mmHg)
6. Routine use of hypothermia below 35 °C
7. Routinely raising CPP >90 mmHg

Monitoring for Non-convulsive Status Epilepticus (NCSE) NCSE is suspected when the altered sensorium is not explained by imaging and other investigations, waxing-waning course of the sensorium, and non-improving sensorium after cessation of clinical seizure. NCSE is associated with increased cerebral metabolism and raised ICP. Therefore, ICP monitoring can be used as an adjunct to diagnose NCSE. In the presence of subtle clinical phenomena such as minor twitching of mouth, perioral or extremity twitches, and EEG features consisting of spike and wave, epileptiform discharges and spatiotemporal evolution consider NCSE as a diagnosis.

16.4 Latest Trails

BEST-TRIP trial: Six-month mortality was 39% in the pressure monitoring group and 41% in the imaging-clinical examination group. The median length of ICU stay was similar. The number of brain-specific treatments of hyperosmolar agents was higher in the imaging-clinical examination group although adverse events are similar. Survival at 14 days was better with ICP monitoring.

DECRA trial: Bifrontal decompressive craniectomy was compared with standard care. The surgical group had lower ICPs, fewer ICP interventions, and fewer ICU days. Worse outcomes were seen with decompression despite similar mortality when compared with standard care.

EUTHERM 3235: Hypothermia group had higher mortality and was less likely to survive with good outcomes than standard care (26% vs. 37%).

RESCUEicp trial: Absolute 22% reduction in mortality when compared with medical management. Better ICP controls were achieved with hemicraniectomy. Hemicraniectomy increased chances of survival but in a vegetative state or with severe disability.

16.5 Conclusions

1. Raised ICP is a major contributor to secondary brain injury.
2. Maintaining a CPP of 60–70 mmHg and ICP <22 mmHg leads to better outcomes.
3. General supportive measures should be used in all patients with severe head injury independent of ICP status.
4. Escalating treatment in a staged manner (three-tier system) increases efficacy while minimizing adverse events.
5. The use of barbiturate coma and hypothermia is associated with the highest rate of complications and should never be used as a routine/prophylactic modality of treatment.
6. Identifying worsening neurological conditions early in the ICU and initiating appropriate treatment and monitoring are essential for improved neurological outcomes.

Further Reading

Chesnut RM, Temkin N, Dikmen S, et al. A Method of managing severe traumatic brain injury in the absence of intracranial pressure monitoring: the imaging and clinical examination protocol. J Neurotrauma. 2018;35(1):54–63. https://doi.org/10.1089/neu.2016.4472.

Dunn LT. Raised intracranial pressure. J Neurol Neurosurg Psychiatry. 2002;73(Suppl 1):23–7. https://doi.org/10.1136/jnnp.73.suppl_1.i23.

Hawryluk GWJ, Aguilera S, Buki A, Bulger E, Citerio G, Cooper DJ, Arrastia RD, et al. A management algorithm for patients with intracranial pressure monitoring: The Seattle International Severe Traumatic Brain Injury Consensus Conference (SIBICC). Intensive Care Med. 2019;45(12):1783–94. https://doi.org/10.1007/s00134-019-05805-9.

Hawryluk GWJ, Rubiano AM, Totten AM, et al. Guidelines for the management of severe traumatic brain injury: 2020 update of the decompressive craniectomy recommendations. Neurosurgery. 2020;87(3):427–34. https://doi.org/10.1093/neuros/nyaa278.

Norisue Y, Fujimoto Y, Nakagawa K. Preliminary guideline- and pathophysiology-based protocols for neurocritical care. J Intensive Care. 2018;6:45. https://doi.org/10.1186/s40560-018-0316-6.

Schizodimos T, Soulountsi V, Iasonidou C, Kapravelos N. An overview of management of intracranial hypertension in the intensive care unit. J Anesth. 2020;34(5):741–57. https://doi.org/10.1007/s00540-020-02795-7.

Wettervik TS, Lenell S, Nyholm L, Howells T, Lewén A, Enblad P. Decompressive craniectomy in traumatic brain injury: usage and clinical outcome in a single centre. Acta Neurochir. 2018;160(2):229–37. https://doi.org/10.1007/s00701-017-3418-3.

Decompressive Craniectomy for Severe Traumatic Brain Injury: CSF Dynamics, Cerebral Perfusion, and Cognitive Outcome

17

Manish Agrawal, Gaurav Purohit, and Rohit Babal

17.1 Background

Traumatic brain injury (TBI) is one of the main causes of morbidity and mortality worldwide. A TBI affects roughly 69 million people globally each year. For every 100,000 people worldwide, there are 939 cases of TBI [1]. TBIs are becoming more common worldwide [2–4]. An estimated 1.5–2 million Indians endure TBIs each year, and 1 million of them die as a result [5]. External causes of TBIs include traffic accidents, falls, work-related injuries (industrial and agricultural), violence, sports injuries, and injuries from disasters. According to the National Institute of Mental Health and Neurosciences (NIMHANS) Traumatic Brain Injury (TB)I Registry, 60% of TBIs result from road crashes, 25% from falls, 10% from assaults or violence, and the rest from other causes [6]. Based on the Glasgow Coma Scale (GCS), nearly 60% of TBIs are mild, 20% are moderate, and 15–20% are severe [6]. Patients who have suffered severe TBI should be moved right away to a facility that provides neurosurgical treatment, computed tomography (CT) imaging, intracranial pressure monitoring, and intracranial hypertension medications [7].

The primary significance of a head injury lies in how much of the brain has been affected or is likely to be affected as a result. It may be damaged immediately by the disruptive mechanical force of the impact (primary injury), or it may be affected sometime later because of vasogenic edema, cytotoxic edema, intracranial hypertension, and cerebral ischemia (secondary injury). It is essential to prevent such secondary injuries using both surgical and medical measures [8, 9].

M. Agrawal (✉) · G. Purohit · R. Babal
Department of Neurosurgery, SMS Medical College, Jaipur, India

© The Author(s), under exclusive license to Springer Nature Singapore Pte Ltd. 2024

A. Agrawal et al. (eds.), *Special Considerations in Trauma Care*,
https://doi.org/10.1007/978-981-99-9662-9_17

17.2 History

The earliest discoveries about skull perforation were made during the Neolithic era (8000–5000 BC). By the fifth century BC, Hippocrates had established craniotomy as a medical practice. In the event of simple fractures or severe contusions, Hippocrates recommended completing the craniotomy within 3 days of the trauma [10]. As an Ayurvedic physician in India, Jivaka (c. 1800 BC to 500 BC), early reports mention his performing trephination on a wealthy merchant and successfully removing two worms from his brain [11]. Annandale wrote the first known report on decompressive surgery in 1894 [12]. Swiss surgeon Theodor Kocher proposed opening of the skull to release elevated intracranial pressure in the early twentieth century [13]. In 1908, the Harvey Cushing published the first case series of patients who had undergone subtemporal craniectomy for head injuries [14].

17.3 Indications

The total body volume of CSF is approximately 150–160 mL [15]. Increased intracranial pressure (ICP) is the pressure >20 mmHg in the subdural, intraventricular, or intraparenchymal compartments [16]. High ICP is the strongest predictor of neurological deterioration [17]. It is linked to a higher risk of mortality and severe disability after a TBI [16].

When an ICP is elevated, the first steps to be taken are sedation, volume resuscitation, head elevation, and normothermia. Mannitol administration, moderate hypocapnia (pCO_2 30–35 mmHg), and CSF drainage are first-line therapeutic measures that should be used (Brain Trauma Foundation 2007). As second-line treatments, high-dose barbiturates, decompressive craniectomy (DC), mild to moderate hypothermia, raising mean arterial blood pressure, and intensive hyperventilation (pCO_2 30 mmHg) are recommended when first-level measures are unable to lower ICP [7].

When it comes to lowering ICP within 48 h, DC performs better than traditional treatment [16]. DC has been shown to reduce mortality, although the implications on neurological prognosis are debatable [16]. The Monro-Kellie law underpins the reasoning for decompressive surgery. DC, with or without augmented duraplasty, is a quick and reliable method to reduce intracranial pressure and increase CBF.

As the brain bulges beyond the bony margins, it is challenging to reposition the bone flap. There is a high risk of worsened brain swelling. Primary or prophylactic DC is frequently performed during traumatic hematoma evacuation [14]. The objective is to avoid the predicted ICP rises after surgery. The decision for DC depends on the preoperative imaging findings of midline shift, effacement of basal cisterns, intraoperative brain bulge, and mass lesion >30 cc [18–20]. The majority of DCs in developing countries are primary DCs, and the treating neurosurgeon may establish appropriate indications for DC due to inadequate resources [21].

Secondary or therapeutic DC is usually done as a salvage therapy to refractory intracranial hypertension in centers with the facility of intracranial pressure monitoring [14]. A patient who has an initial injury that is compatible with acceptable

Table 17.1 Level of evidence to perform decompressive craniectomy [33]

Recommendation	
Bifrontal DC has been demonstrated to reduce ICP and length of ICU stay. However, there was no conclusive evidence for improvement in outcomes at 6 months post-severe TBI	Level IIA
A large frontotemporoparietal DC reduces mortality and improves neurological outcomes in severe TBI patients	Level IIA

recovery and whose intracranial hypertension is the predominant culprit of poor outcome is the strongest candidate for secondary DC [21]. Unless clinical worsening necessitates immediate operation, full escalation of therapy should be completed before DC [21].

Non-traumatic indications for DC include elevated ICP and epidural, subdural, or intracerebral hematoma following aneurysm surgery and uncontrolled ICP following aneurysmal subarachnoid hemorrhage when patients exhibit cerebral edema during aneurysm clipping, intraparenchymal hemorrhage, cerebral venous sinus thrombosis, or tumor-related edema [22, 23]. DC can also treat cerebral edema after cerebral infarction [24–26]. Encephalitis, toxoplasmosis, subdural empyema, Reye syndrome encephalopathy, cerebral venous, and dural sinus thrombosis are among the other reasons documented [27–32].

The updated treatment recommendations given by Brain Trauma Foundation [33] are listed in Table 17.1.

17.4 Timing

The prognosis depends on when decompressive surgery is performed. DC may be life-saving if signs of brainstem compression appear and maximal medical therapy is unable to lower ICP. Six months later, there is a significant improvement in functional outcome and a significant reduction in mortality when early decompression occurs (within 4 h of injury) [34]. Early decompression within 24 h tends to improve mortality and functional outcomes relative to decompression performed beyond 24 h [35].

17.5 Technique

In cases of diffuse brain edema, penetrating trauma, major open depressed comminuted skull fractures with underlying brain injury, lobectomy, and evacuation of an intracranial hematoma, DC can be performed.

The presence, location, and size of intracranial mass lesions, penetrating injuries, and MLS must all be considered before deciding whether the craniectomy should be bifrontal or unilateral. Decompressive hemicraniectomy and bifrontal (Kjellberg) craniectomy are the two major methods now employed to treat medically resistant cerebral edema [36, 37]. The side with the largest lesion volume or cerebral edema undergoes unilateral decompression. When diffuse brain edema occurs without lateralizing radiographic or physical signs, or when there are no or few mass lesions or MLS, bifrontal DC or unilateral DC over the non-dominant hemisphere may be performed. Ultimately, it is the surgeon's prerogative to choose one over the other.

The head of each technique is usually set on a rubber head ring. In TBI, fixation with pins is usually not indicated to speed up the procedure and prevent interference with craniotomy. Cervical spine precautions should also be taken. The jugular veins should not be compressed by a tight cervical collar or excessive head rotation, as this could cause the ICP to rise even further.

17.5.1 Decompressive Hemicraniectomy

The patient is positioned supine with the head either fixed in three-point fixation or horseshoe and rotated to the other side at about 45° to reduce the venous pressure. Carefully drawing the midline before dressing and draping the patient will reduce inadvertent transgression of the superior sagittal sinus [36, 37]. Beginning at the level of the zygoma, the incision is made in the shape of a reverse question mark. The posterior extent of the incision should be around 15 cm from McCarty's Key burr hole so that the anteroposterior axis of the craniectomy flap is 15 cm. A larger skin incision than the planned craniotomy is recommended and pinna should be avoided [21]. The incision can be adjusted to accommodate any wounds or lacerations on the scalp. The surgeon must avoid creating islands of tissue and maintain an inferior vascular pedicle to protect the scalp's blood supply [21]. Protecting the superficial temporal artery, if possible, will guarantee sufficient blood flow to the skin flap. It is cut all the way down to the skull. The myocutaneous flap that results can then be fixed with scalp hooks after being reflected anteriorly. Extending the temporalis dissection down to the zygoma will help in the nibbling of the temporal bone for adequate decompression of the herniating uncal region.

A hemicraniectomy flap that includes bone removal to the middle cranial fossa floor should ideally be large, measuring at least 12 × 15 cm [21]. By compressing the cortical surface and causing the brain's veins to herniate out through the craniectomy, more minor craniectomy flaps have the potential to injure the brain [38]. The superior extent of craniectomy should be 3–4 cm beyond the superior temporal line as compression near the vertex is not contributory to much of the intracranial pressure. Furthermore, there is crowding of the gyri near the midline, even in typical situations. Remaining a few centimeters away from the midline offers protection from injury to the venous sinuses and arachnoid granulations and reduces the risk of postcraniectomy hydrocephalus. Multiple burr holes are made which are then connected with high powered craniotome; an additional burr hole can be made above the hematoma to enable prompt decompression prior to elevating the craniectomy flap. After hemostasis is established, the temporal extent of the craniectomy should be examined and, if necessary, extended down to the middle cranial fossa floor.

Bone wax and dural tack-up sutures must be used to stop bleeding in the bone and epidural spaces, respectively, prior to opening the dura. Not long after the dura has been opened, skin closure may be necessary because an edematous brain can quickly herniate through the dural opening and prevent primary scalp closure. Any significant bleeding from the middle cranial fossa, which typically originates from the sphenoid wing or the middle meningeal artery, needs to be treated right away. In this case, a slightly more conservative temporal craniectomy can stabilize the bone, to which the dura can be attached to help stop the bleeding. Using stellate radial incisions or a C-shaped dural opening with the dural base along the frontal fossa floor, the dural opening is created.

17.5.2 Bifrontal Craniectomy

The bifrontal craniectomy, unlike DHC, allows for anterior brain swelling and is commonly utilized in cases of bifrontal contusions or diffuse cerebral edema [36, 38, 39]. Bifrontal DC has been shown to lower ICP and shorten ICU stay, but it has not been shown to improve the outcome [33].

The individual is in a supine position. Marks are made for the coronal suture and midline. A cut is made along the contralateral zygomatic arch after the patient has been prepared and draped. It begins at the level of the zygomatic arch on one side, just in front of the tragus, and runs back 2–3 cm behind the coronal suture. The cut extends all the way to the bone. After that, the myocutaneous flap is reflected over the orbital rim. Carefully remove the supraorbital nerves from the supraorbital notch on either side. If it is closed, the supraorbital notch can be opened with a tiny osteotome, which will release the supraorbital nerve. Following that, burr holes are created on both sides of the superior sagittal sinus immediately posterior to the coronal suture, in the bilateral keyholes, and in the bilateral squamous portions of the temporal bone. A Penfield 3 is inserted between the anterior and posterior burr holes to dissect the superior sagittal sinus from the surrounding bone. Once the burr holes are joined, the superior sagittal sinus must be crossed last. With Gelfoam and Surgicel, bleeding from the superior sagittal sinus can be managed after the bone flap has been elevated. After that, the craniectomy's temporal extent is extended downward to the middle fossa's floor. After achieving hemostasis, the dural opening occurs.

The anterior course of the craniectomy is followed by the dural opening, which begins at the middle fossa floor and crosses the anterior segment of the superior sagittal suture to arrive at the contralateral middle fossa floor. The dura is opened in a curvilinear manner, reaching just short of the midline. The sinus is occluded by two thick sutures wrapped around it and fastened. After that, the sinus is split. After that, the underlying falx should be divided, being cautious not to cut into the bilateral anterior cerebral arteries.

17.5.3 Dural Opening and Closure

Opening the dura gradually and cautiously is important to prevent abrupt changes in ICP. Rapidly reversing ICP can result in a Cushing reaction, which causes a loss of catecholamine support and the potential for cardiovascular collapse. The patient must be hemodynamically ready for dural opening in order for the anesthesiologist to prevent this complication. Csokay et al. [40] suggested that in order to lessen the compression of large cortical veins when the brain herniates against the dura, Gelfoam should be placed between the dura and cortex next to each large cortical vessel that travels beneath the dura. This method was referred to as vascular tunneling. Durotomy with dural slits perpendicular to the dural incision along the dural opening's perimeter may produce a comparable outcome [41]. Whether or not to evacuate the contusions/intraparenchymal hematomas should be decided by the surgeon [21].

If it is difficult to close the dura because of cerebral edema, duraplasty is done using expansile dural graft—sutured duraplasty or onlay [21]. Dural graft material options include collagen matrix products, bovine pericardium, pericranium, fascia lata, and synthetic dural replacements. The best dural substitute is up for debate [21]. Additionally, by preventing the brain from adhering to the periosteum and galea above it, these materials facilitate future dissection in the event that a cranioplasty is performed. Additionally, duraplasty enhances CSF circulation, which may lessen the risk of postoperative hygromas and wound CSF leakage.

In a hinge craniotomy, the bone is divided into multiple pieces and tied using loose threads. The edges of the bone are secured to the neighboring bone using titanium miniplate and screws. This keeps the bone flap from sinking inward toward the brain while allowing it to spread outward [42]. More research is needed to ascertain the impact of hinge craniotomy on the final result [21].

Before skin closure, an external subgaleal drain should be placed. For the galea, interrupted VICRYL sutures are mostly, and for the skin, a running nylon suture is typically used. It may be difficult to close the incision in situations of severe cerebral edema. Additional scalp elasticity is made possible by undermining the galea and making barrel-stave incisions in it. The temporalis muscle can be resected in such cases, although this should only be done as a last resort because the temporalis muscle's absence can cause significant morbidity.

The distance between the craniectomy and the base of the skull is related to the mesencephalic cisterns' visibility on postoperative CT scans, and the size of the bone flap is related to the extent of ICP reduction [34, 43]. Wherever possible, an ICP monitor should be used when the bone is replaced or following primary DC. If continuous or invasive ICP monitoring is not possible, progress should be monitored using CT imaging [21]. Unless there are limiting side effects, ICP therapy should be continued during surgery and right after DC. The medical treatment of intracranial hypertension should not be abruptly stopped or altered after DC if it successfully lowers ICP. Within 24 h following surgery, a postoperative CT scan is recommended to confirm the efficacy of DC and detect any complications.

It is possible to preserve the bone flap in a certified tissue bank or in a subcutaneous pocket in the abdomen. Resorption, rhabdomyolysis, and infection have all been linked to abdominal storage; at both storage and retrieval, an additional incision and procedure are needed. Flaps that have been contaminated should not be kept in the abdominal wall [41]. The bone flap should be treated with an antibacterial solution and cleared of any hematomas or foreign objects before being stored in tissue banks. Temperatures between −70 and −80 °C are used to keep flaps frozen until they are needed for reimplantation. This strategy may have drawbacks, such as the flap being misplaced or lost, freezer issues, and convoluted administrative requirements and agreements regarding storage services. Extended storage (months) may also worsen bone flap resorption.

17.6 Complications

Even though DC has been shown to reduce refractory intracranial hypertension as well as mortality rates, it has also been shown to increase morbidity and severe disability rates [44, 45].

Secondary brain injury, seizures, and syndrome of trephined are among the complications related to cerebral issues following DC. In the acute period after DC, there may be increased cerebral edema seen on postoperative CT scans due to a reduction of intracranial pressure leading to the refilling of previously compressed vessels causing hyperemia. The DC and duraplasty reduce ICP, allowing enough brain reperfusion and the creation of sufficient brain oxygenation to prevent subsequent damage [46]. Perfusion breakthrough hemorrhage, which can develop as a result of cerebral vasodilation and hyperemia, can induce secondary brain damage; however, this is difficult to differentiate from the natural progression of contusions that happens with or without DC. Brain herniation and injury to the brain at the craniectomy edges may occur, especially with small bone flaps. Venous compression, reduced regional blood flow, or direct brain compression can all cause infarction.

Seizures may occur in both acute and chronic stages following DC. Acute seizures can cause herniation, elevated intracranial pressure, and status epilepticus. The first week after trauma is when antiepileptics should be given to patients who have a subdural hematoma, epidural hematoma, intraparenchymal hematoma, contusion, penetrating injury, or depressed skull fracture, with a GCS score of less than 10 [41]. No guideline exists for perioperative seizure prophylaxis during secondary bone flap replacement. However, the rate of immediate postoperative seizures is high and can be reduced by avoiding the use of monopolar cautery to dissect the scalp flap (reducing heat exposure to the underlying brain) and with intraoperative use of antiepileptics, which are then continued for 7 days. If levels are subtherapeutic, patients on continued antiepileptic medication for seizures are given bolus therapy, or they are kept on their therapeutic regimen with the addition of a second drug from the intraoperative period to 1 week after surgery.

Grant and Norcross (1939) defined the Syndrome of the Trephined as a collection of symptoms that patients who had undergone DC may experience, such as dizziness, fatigability, vague discomfort at the defect site, mood swings, seizures, or occasionally motor weakness [47]. The mechanism behind this syndrome has been suggested to be related to abnormalities in CBF, atmospheric pressure's impact on the brain, and abnormalities in CSF flow [48]. The symptoms are alleviated with recumbency and mostly resolved with cranioplasty.

Yamaura et al. coined the name "sinking skin flap syndrome" after studying an extensive series of post-craniectomy patients who experienced reversible symptoms following bone flap replacement [49, 50]. Sinking of the skin flap over the dura owing to atmospheric pressure causes pressure on the underlying cortical tissue resulting in reduced compliance and gliosis, and this has been suggested as the possible mechanism for explaining the symptoms [51].

Changes in CSF dynamics can lead to complications such as hydrocephalus and hygroma. Segal et al. postulated that the atmospheric pressure and the presence of cortical scar tissue compressing the subarachnoid space and underlying cortex could change cerebral hemodynamics [52]. After a craniectomy, Plog et al. postulated that impaired arterial pulsations caused glymphatic flow impairment, which was shown to result in neurological deficits in murine models [53]. Notably, 26% of patients have hygromas. Following decompressive surgery, they frequently appear on the ipsilateral side, most likely due to changed CSF dynamics [54, 55]. There are several theories, such as pressure gradients between the hemispheres brought on by a drop in intracranial pressure and the decompression of one hemisphere, surgically altered brain anatomy, and the ruptured arachnoid that creates a one-way valve for CSF flow [56]. Hygromas usually go away on their own. In addition to being treated with lumbar punctures, either single or serial, lumboperitoneal shunts, ventriculoperitoneal shunts, or temporary continuous lumbar drainage, they can also be observed [54]. Hygromas are frequently resolved if the bone flap is replaced. Hydrocephalus affects 14–29% of people and can be either high or low pressure [55]. Programmable shunts may be considered in such instances.

Infection occurs in 2–6% of patients undergoing DC [54]. In the acute phase after DC, patients who show infection-related signs or symptoms should undergo a comprehensive fever workup, which should include CSF testing [57]. Patients with suspected infections who present later should have a complete blood work and a CT scan of the head, both with and without contrast material. Patients may need to have their incisions reopened, have their empyema evaluated, and have their debridement and irrigation treated.

Patients with endocrine disorders, the elderly, women, and those who are malnourished are more likely to experience wound dehiscence. In extreme cases, the scalp may be eroded by plates, mesh, or screws. Patients who have had reoperations and have a history of infections or wound dehiscence are more likely to experience wound dehiscence.

Resorption of contaminated bone flaps is more frequently observed in cases where the flaps were fragmented, exposed to radiation, or stored in a freezer for an extended period of time [41]. Up to 12% of patients have been reported to experience bone flap resorption following secondary bone flap replacement [58]. Frontalis muscle paralysis may result from direct damage to the facial nerve branches or from stretching them during temporalis muscle dissection. This may occur if there is a breach in the superficial fat pad or if the muscle experiences excessive traction [41].

17.7 Outcome

Cooper et al. published the DECRA (Decompressive Craniectomy in Diffuse TBI) trial in 2011 [44]. In this study, 155 patients with refractory ICP >20 mmHg for 15 min in a single hour were randomized to either maximum medical management or bifrontal DC [44]. Although DC shortened the length of stay in the intensive care unit and decreased ICP, it was also associated with more negative outcomes. The DC group, however, had a higher proportion of patients with non-reactive pupils, suggesting that these patients had herniation symptoms before treatment, which may emphasize the therapeutic benefit of the procedure. When unreactive pupil correction was used, the decompression-related damage stopped being statistically significant. This trial's small sample size and exclusive use of bifrontal DC without falx sectioning were additional drawbacks [44].

Hutchinson et al. published the RESCUEicp experiment in 2016; DC or maximum medical treatment was the two groups to which 408 TBI patients who had refractory ICP >25 mmHg for at least an hour were randomly assigned in this randomized controlled trial [10]. DC was examined as a salvage treatment for refractory intracranial hypertension in the RESCUEicp trial. Patients in the RESCUEicp trial were those who had unilateral craniectomy and intracranial hematoma. At 6 months, patients who had DC experienced lower mortality but higher rates of vegetative state compared to the medical management group [17].

Zhang et al. presented a meta-analysis that found that DC within 36 h of the original injury resulted in a superior prognosis based on 6-month Glasgow Outcome Scale scores. DC may lower mortality, ICPs, and ICU stays, but it may also raise the rate of complications, according to the meta-analysis [59].

Taylor and Associates analyzed the outcomes of early DC in the pediatric population and published the only RCT on the subject. A total of 27 infants who had a persistent elevation in intracranial pressure following TBI were randomized to either medical management or bitemporal DC. Taylor et al. concluded that early DC is more likely than maximum medical management alone to reduce ICPs and improve functional outcomes in pediatric patients with refractory ICPs. The trial's limitations, however, were its small sample size and the failure to open the dura during decompression [60]. Findings in a retrospective review by Jagannathan et al. supported the findings from Taylor et al [61].

17.8 Secondary Bone Flap Replacement

In order to protect the brain and restore the cranium's shape, cranioplasty is necessary. It has been demonstrated to enhance neurological results [21]. The timing of cranioplasty is mostly determined by the reason for craniectomy. Neoplastic invasion of the skull is one of the few reasons for immediate cranioplasty. When DC is performed for medically resistant intracranial hypertension or an intracranial infection, delayed cranioplasty is typically recommended [41]. The typical interval between a craniectomy and a cranioplasty is 6 weeks to a year [62]. The optimal time for cranioplasty (early vs. late) is uncertain due to a lack of high-quality multicenter research [21]. Vascularization of the surrounding tissues and complete healing of the prior incision are required. In addition to the patient's neurological condition and intracranial pressure being stable, there should be no indications of inflammation and no signs of cranial or systemic infection [41]. Prior to cranioplasty, patients should have their medical and surgical conditions optimized [21].

The CBF in the area of DC showed a notable improvement, according to Richard et al., and this improvement was linked to the neurological recovery following cranioplasty [63]. Using the phase contrast MRI technique, Dujovny et al. reported an increase in CSF flow after cranioplasty in a single case report [64].

A prospective observational pilot study was conducted at our institute on patients who had cranioplasty following a head injury between September 2017 and February 2018 [65]. The objective was to measure changes in CSF flow at the foramen of Magendie and aqueduct of Sylvius in patients before and after cranioplasty, as well as to examine and establish changes in trends of CBF and Mean transit time (MTT) in various cerebral regions in the bilateral hemisphere. Additionally, the cerebral hemodynamic and hydrodynamic changes were to be correlated with cognitive outcomes. A week prior to the scheduled cranioplasty procedure, cine phase cardiac gated contrast MRI studies and CT perfusion studies were performed to examine baseline cerebral hemodynamic and CSF flow, which were then compared to postoperative values (on the postoperative day 5–7). Preoperative and 1- and 6-month follow-up Montreal Cognitive Assessment (MoCA) scores were used to evaluate the cognitive status. Naresh Panwar et al. discovered that there was a statistically significant increase in CBF in the orbitofrontal cortex and total hemisphere in the ipsilateral hemisphere, while there was a statistically significant increase in CBF in the caudate nucleus, white tract fiber from sensorimotor cortex, and other areas of the contralateral hemisphere. Furthermore, a notable reduction in MTT was also observed in the contralateral thalamic region, indicating a decline in blood flow stasis. Sarubbo et al.'s findings, which also showed a decline in MTT values in the early post-cranioplasty period, are consistent with this [66]. Improved CBF in the early post-cranioplasty period, however, does not necessarily indicate a clear long-term increase, as evidenced by Sarubbo's findings of ill-sustaining improvement in CBF over a 3-month period. Decaminada et al. did, however, report that CBF improved and continued to do so for 6 months following cranioplasty [57]. The CTP protocol used and the variation in region of interest placement could be the cause of these disparities.

There is a pulsatile flow of CSF in the craniospinal cavity that corresponds to the cardiac cycle, with very little CSF being absorbed during each cycle. As the most crucial element influencing this pulsatile CSF flow is the craniospinal cavity's compliance, any alteration in compliance will be reflected in variations in the CSF flow's properties. The literature does, in fact, provide ample evidence of the changes in CSF dynamics, with studies demonstrating a notable decrease in the amplitude of the CSF pulse wave in patients who had undergone cranioplasty [67, 68].

In our study, we used phase contrast MRI to measure the change in CSF velocities and found that both the mean and peak CSF velocities measured at the foramen of Magendie and the aqueduct of Sylvius improved. It has been suggested that the cause of the change in CSF flow characteristics is the cranial cavity's decreased compliance and the increased arterial pulsatility observed following bone flap repositioning, which results in the cranium becoming a closed cavity.

Over the course of 24 weeks following cranioplasty, our study demonstrates a notable improvement in cognitive outcome. When compared to the baseline scores at 6 months, the mean scores on the MoCA demonstrated a significant improvement. Increased cerebral metabolism and glymphatic flow, as well as improved intracranial CSF dynamics and improved ipsilateral and contralateral blood flow (better CBF and lower MTT) are most likely to blame for the improvement in the neurocognitive outcome [53, 69].

17.9 Conclusion

Patients presenting with a severe head injury should be managed with medical management to prevent secondary injury to the brain. If these measures are not effective in lowering the raised ICP, or if the cerebral edema causes the brain to bulge intraoperatively, DC is a valid approach in these patients. The decision lies in the hands of the treating surgeon, based on CT findings, intraoperative surgical findings, or both. DC has been shown to be effective in lowering ICP, reducing mortality, and minimizing ICU stay. However, it is associated with significant complications including secondary brain injury caused by reperfusion, seizures, and the syndrome of trephined. Altered CSF dynamics lead can cause hygroma and hydrocephalus. Brain hemodynamics significantly improve with repositioning of the bone flap, with the ipsilateral side experiencing greater benefits. Better CSF circulation and higher CSF turnover are further benefits. Better cerebral perfusion and, more crucially, CSF dynamics could be the cause of the neurocognition improvement that has been shown in the post-cranioplasty phase.

References

1. Dewan MC, Rattani A, Gupta S, Baticulon RE, Hung YC, Punchak M, Agrawal A, Adeleye AO, Shrime MG, Rubiano AM, Rosenfeld JV, Park KB. Estimating the global incidence of traumatic brain injury. J Neurosurg. 2018;130(4):1080–97. https://doi.org/10.3171/2017.10.JNS17352.
2. WHO. Road traffic injuries. http://www.who.int/news-room/factsheets/detail/road-traffic-injuries. Accessed 17 July 2018.
3. WHO. Falls. http://www.who.int/news-room/fact-sheets/detail/falls. Accessed 17 July 2018.
4. GBD 2016 Traumatic Brain Injury and Spinal Cord Injury Collaborators. Global, regional, and national burden of traumatic brain injury and spinal cord injury, 1990–2016: a systematic analysis for the Global Burden of Disease Study 2016. Lancet Neurol. 2018;18(5):459–80. https://doi.org/10.1016/S1474-4422(18)30415-0.
5. Gururaj G. Epidemiology of traumatic brain injuries: Indian scenario. Neurol Res. 2002;24:24–8.
6. Neurotrauma Society of India. Traumatic brain injury-multi organizational Consensus Recommendations for India. 2017. https://ntsi.co.in/wp-content/uploads/2017/11/Version.pdf.

7. Badjatia N, Carney N, Crocco TJ, Fallat ME, Hennes HM, Jagoda AS, Jernigan S, Letarte PB, Lerner EB, Moriarty TM, Pons PT, Sasser S, Scalea T, Schleien CL, Wright DW, Brain Trauma Foundation; BTF Center for Guidelines Management. Guidelines for prehospital management of traumatic brain injury 2nd edition. Prehosp Emerg Care. 2008;12(Suppl 1):1–52. https://doi.org/10.1080/10903120701732052.
8. Moritz AR. Mechanisms of head injury. Ann Surg. 1943;117(4):562–75. https://doi.org/10.1097/00000658-194304000-00006.
9. Lok J, Leung W, Murphy S, et al. Intracranial hemorrhage: mechanisms of secondary brain injury. Acta Neurochir Suppl. 2011;111:63–9. https://doi.org/10.1007/978-3-7091-0693-8_11.
10. Sperati G. Craniotomy through the ages. Acta Otorhinolaryngol Ital. 2007;27(3):151–6.
11. Amar AP. Neurosurgery in India: past as prologue. World Neurosurg. 2013;79(5-6):613–4. https://doi.org/10.1016/j.wneu.2013.03.031. Epub 2013 Mar 16.
12. Annandale TN. IV - on intra-cranial surgery. Edinb Med J. 1894;June:898.
13. Kocher T. Hirnerschütterung, Hirndruck und chirurgische Eingriffe bei Hirnkrankheiten. Wien: Alfred Hölder; 1901.
14. Kolias AG, Kirkpatrick PJ, Hutchinson PJ. Decompressive craniectomy: past, present and future. Nat Rev Neurol. 2013;9(7):405–15. https://doi.org/10.1038/nrneurol.2013.106. Epub 2013 Jun 11.
15. Silverberg GD, Heit G, Huhn S, Chang SD, Bronte-Stewart H, et al. The cerebrospinal fluid production rate is reduced in dementia of the Alzheimer's type. Neurology. 2001;57(10):1763–6.
16. Sahuquillo J, Dennis JA. Decompressive craniectomy for the treatment of high intracranial pressure in closed traumatic brain injury. Cochrane Database Syst Rev. 2019;12:CD003983. https://doi.org/10.1002/14651858.CD003983.pub3.
17. Juul N, Morris GF, Marshall SB, Marshall LF. Intracranial hypertension and cerebral perfusion pressure: influence on neurological deterioration and outcome in severe head injury. The Executive Committee of the International Selfotel Trial. J Neurosurg. 2000;92(1):1–6.
18. Toutant SM, Klauber MR, Marshall LF, et al. Absent or compressed basal cisterns on first CT scan: ominous predictors of outcome in severe head injury. J Neurosurg. 1984;61:691.
19. Bullock MR, Chesnut RM, Clifton GL, et al. Management and prognosis of severe traumatic brain injury. J Neurotrauma. 2000;17:451–627.
20. Valadka AB, Gopinath SP, Robertson CS. Midline shift after severe head injury: pathophysiologic implications. J Trauma. 2000;49:1.
21. Hutchinson PJ, Kolias AG, Tajsic T, et al. Consensus statement from the international consensus meeting on the role of decompressive craniectomy in the management of traumatic brain injury. Acta Neurochir. 2019;161:1261–74. https://doi.org/10.1007/s00701-019-03936-y.
22. Fisher CM, Ojemann RG. Bilateral decompressive craniectomy for worsening coma in acute subarachnoid hemorrhage. Observations in support of the procedure. Surg Neurol. 1994;41:65.
23. Hutchinson P, Timofeev I, Kirkpatrick P. Surgery for brain edema. Neurosurg Focus. 2007;22:E14.
24. Rengachary SS, Batnitzky S, Morantz RA, et al. Hemicraniectomy for acute massive cerebral infarction. Neurosurgery. 1981;8:321.
25. Kondziolka D, Fazl M. Functional recovery after decompressive craniectomy for cerebral infarction. Neurosurgery. 1988;23:143.
26. Delashaw JB, Broaddus WC, Kassell NF, et al. Treatment of right hemispheric cerebral infarction by hemicraniectomy. Stroke. 1990;21:874.
27. Ausman JI, Rogers C, Sharp HL. Decompressive craniectomy for the encephalopathy of Reye's syndrome. Surg Neurol. 1976;6:97.
28. Schwab S, Junger E, Spranger M, et al. Craniectomy: an aggressive treatment approach in severe encephalitis. Neurology. 1997;48:412.
29. Stefini R, Latronico N, Cornali C, et al. Emergent decompressive craniectomy in patients with fixed dilated pupils due to cerebral venous and dural sinus thrombosis: report of three cases. Neurosurgery. 1999;45:626.
30. Keller E, Pangalu A, Fandino J, et al. Decompressive craniectomy in severe cerebral venous and dural sinus thrombosis. Acta Neurochir Suppl. 2005;94:177.

31. Agrawal D, Hussain N. Decompressive craniectomy in cerebral toxoplasmosis. Eur J Clin Microbiol Infect Dis. 2005;24:772.
32. Perin A, Nascimben E, Longatti P. Decompressive craniectomy in a case of intractable intracranial hypertension due to pneumococcal meningitis. Acta Neurochir. 2008;150:837.
33. Carney N, Totten AM, O'Reilly C, Ullman JS, Hawryluk GW, Bell MJ, Bratton SL, Chesnut R, Harris OA, Kissoon N, Rubiano AM, Shutter L, Tasker RC, Vavilala MS, Wilberger J, Wright DW, Ghajar J. Guidelines for the management of severe traumatic brain injury, Fourth Edition. Neurosurgery. 2017;80(1):6–15. https://doi.org/10.1227/NEU.0000000000001432.
34. Munch E, Horn P, Schurer L, et al. Management of severe traumatic brain injury by decompressive craniectomy. Neurosurgery. 2000;47:315.
35. Shah A, Almenawer S, Hawryluk G. Timing of decompressive craniectomy for ischemic stroke and traumatic brain injury: a review. Front Neurol. 2019;10:11. https://doi.org/10.3389/fneur.2019.00011. PMID: 30740085; PMCID: PMC6355668.
36. Ragel BT, Klimo P Jr, Martin JE, Teff RJ, Bakken HE, Armonda RA. Wartime decompressive craniectomy: technique and lessons learned. Neurosurg Focus. 2010;28:E2.
37. Quinn TM, Taylor JJ, Magarik JA, Vought E, Kindy MS, Ellegala DB. Decompressive craniectomy: technical note. Acta Neurol Scand. 2011;123:239–44.
38. Wagner S, Schnippering H, Aschoff A, Koziol JA, Schwab S, Steiner T. Suboptimum hemicraniectomy as a cause of additional cerebral lesions in patients with malignant infarction of the middle cerebral artery. J Neurosurg. 2001;94:693–6.
39. Kjellberg RN, Prieto A Jr. Bifrontal decompressive craniotomy for massive cerebral edema. J Neurosurg. 1971;34:488–93.
40. Csokay A, Egyud L, Nagy L, Pataki G. Vascular tunnel creation to improve the efficacy of decompressive craniotomy in post-traumatic cerebral edema and ischemic stroke. Surg Neurol. 2002;57:126–9.
41. Youmans JR, Richard Winn H. Youmans and Winn neurological surgery. 8th ed. Philadelphia: Elsevier; 2022. p. 3124–34.
42. Schmidt JH III, Reyes BJ, Fischer R, Flaherty SK. Use of hinge craniotomy for cerebral decompression. J Neurosurg. 2007;107:678–82.
43. Skoglund TS, Eriksson-Ritzen C, Jensen C, et al. Aspects on de-compressive craniectomy in patients with traumatic head injuries. J Neurotrauma. 2006;1502(23):1502–9.
44. Cooper DJ, Rosenfeld JV, Murray L, Arabi YM, Davies AR, D'Urso P, et al. Decompressive craniectomy in diffuse traumatic brain injury. N Engl J Med. 2011;364:1493–502.
45. Hutchinson PJ, Kolias AG, Timofeev I, Corteen EA, Czosnyka M, Timothy I, et al. Trial of decompressive craniectomy for traumatic intracranial hypertension. N Engl J Med. 2016;375:1119–30.
46. Reithmeier T, Speder B, Pakos P, et al. Delayed bilateral craniectomy for treatment of traumatic brain swelling in children: case report and review of the literature. Childs Nerv Syst. 2005;21:249.
47. Grant FC, Norcross NC. Repair of cranial defects by cranioplasty. Ann Surg. 1939;110:488.
48. Stiver SI, Wintermark M, Manley GT. Motor trephine syndrome: a mechanistic hypothesis. Acta Neurochir Suppl. 2008;102:273–7.
49. Yamaura A, Makino H. Neurological deficits in the presence of the sinking skin flap following decompressive craniectomy. Neurol Med Chir. 1977;17:43–53.
50. Yamaura A, Sato M, Meguro K, Nakamura T, Uemura K. Cranioplasty following decompressive craniectomy–analysis of 300 cases. No Shinkei Geka. 1977;5:345–53.
51. Stula D. The problem of the "sinking skin-flap syndrome" in cranioplasty. J Maxillofac Surg. 1982;10:142–5.
52. Segal DH, Oppenheim JS, Murovic JA. Neurological recovery after cranioplasty. Neurosurgery. 1994;34(4):729–31.
53. Plog BA, Lou N, Pierre CA, Cove A, Kenney HM, Hitomi E, Kang H, Iliff JJ, Zeppenfeld DM, Nedergaard M, Vates GE. When the air hits your brain: decreased arterial pulsatility after craniectomy leading to impaired glymphatic flow. J Neurosurg. 2019;1:1–4.

54. Guerra WK, Gaab MR, Dietz H, et al. Surgical decompression for traumatic brain swelling: indications and results. J Neurosurg. 1999;90:187.
55. Chibbaro S, Tacconi L. Role of decompressive craniectomy in the management of severe head injury with refractory cerebral edema and intractable intracranial pressure. Our experience with 48 cases. Surg Neurol. 2007;68:632.
56. Wang HK, Lu K, Liang CL, Tsai YD, Wang KW, Liliang PC. Contralateral subdural effusion related to decompressive craniecto-my performed in patients with severe traumatic brain injury. Injury. 2010;6:6.
57. Decaminada N, Pernter P, Imondi A, Tomassini A. CT perfusion evaluation of cerebral haemodynamics before and after cranioplasty. Neuroradiol J. 2008;21(4):459–71.
58. Aarabi B, Hesdorffer DC, Ahn ES, et al. Outcome following decompressive craniectomy for malignant swelling due to severe head in-jury. J Neurosurg. 2006;104:469.
59. Zhang D, Xue Q, Chen J, Dong Y, Hou L, Jiang Y, et al. Decompressive craniectomy in the management of intracranial hypertension after traumatic brain injury: a systematic review and meta-analysis. Sci Rep. 2017;7:8800. https://doi.org/10.1038/s41598-017-08959-y.
60. Taylor A, Butt W, Rosenfeld J, Shann F, Ditchfield M, Lewis E, et al. A randomized trial of very early decompressive craniectomy in children with traumatic brain injury and sustained intracranial hypertension. Childs Nerv Syst. 2001;17:154–62. https://doi.org/10.1007/s003810000410.
61. Jagannathan J, Okonkwo DO, Dumont AS, Ahmed H, Bahari A, Prevedello DM, et al. Outcome following decompressive craniectomy in children with severe traumatic brain injury: a 10-year single-center experience with long-term follow up. J Neurosurg. 2007;106:268–75. https://doi.org/10.3171/ped.2007.106.4.268.
62. Baumeister S, Peek A, Friedman A, Levin LS, Marcus JR. Management of postneurosurgical bone flap loss caused by infection. Plast Reconstr Surg. 2008;122(6):195e–208e.
63. Richaud J, Boetto S, Guell A, Lazorthes Y. Incidence des cranioplasties sur la fonction neurologique et le debit sanguin cerebral. Neuro-Chirurgie. 1985;31(3):183–8.
64. Dujovny M, Fernandez P, Alperin N, Betz W, Misra M, Mafee M. Post-cranioplasty cerebrospinal fluid hydrodynamic changes: magnetic resonance imaging quantitative analysis. Neurol Res. 1997;19(3):311–6.
65. Panwar N, Agrawal M, Sinha VD. Postcranioplasty quantitative assessment of intracranial fluid dynamics and its impact on neurocognition cranioplasty effect: a pilot study. World Neurosurg. 2019;122:96–107.
66. Sarubbo S, Latini F, Ceruti S, et al. Temporal changes in CT perfusion values before and after cranioplasty in patients without symptoms related to external decompression: a pilot study. Neuroradiology. 2014;56(3):237–43.
67. Lilja-Cyron A, Andresen M, Kelsen J, et al. Intracranial pressure before and after cranioplasty: insights into intracranial physiology. J Neurosurg. 2019;133(5):1548–58. https://doi.org/10.3171/2019.7.JNS191077.
68. Lilja-Cyron A, Andresen M, Kelsen J, Andreasen TH, Fugleholm K, Juhler M. Long-term effect of decompressive craniectomy on intracranial pressure and possible implications for intracranial fluid movements. Neurosurgery. 2020;86(2):231–40. https://doi.org/10.1093/neuros/nyz049.
69. Winkler PA, Stummer W, Linke R, Krishnan KG, Tatsch K. Influence of cranioplasty on postural blood flow regulation, cerebrovascular reserve capacity, and cerebral glucose metabolism. J Neurosurg. 2000;93:53–61.

Decompressive Craniotomy in Children 18

Nazmin Ahmed and Md. Moshiur Rahman

18.1 Introduction

Traumatic brain injury (TBI) is a global public health issue and is the largest contributor of death and disability due to trauma-related injuries followed by stroke. Therefore, both of them have a significant impact on family and economy [1, 2]. Decompressive craniectomy (DC) is a common neurosurgical technique that requires temporary exclusion of a large part of the skull to accommodate a swollen brain following TBI, stroke, and so on [3]. This surgical technique aims to immediately decrease medically refractory raised intracranial pressure. Successful DC increases the area under the scalp, which might increase the blood flow and oxygenation, thus minimizing ischemic damage, and decreases mortality as well as morbidity [4, 5]. A unilateral and/or sometimes bilateral craniotomy and dural augmentation are used. The bone can be briefly preserved in a bone bank or abdominal subcutaneous tissue if a cranioplasty is performed later [6].

The evidence about the efficacy of DC in the treatment of TBI and stroke has some conflict and some studies said it is unfavorable. For example, the DECRA study showed an increase in unfavorable outcomes after bifrontal DC with mild intracranial hypertension patients [7]. A pooled analysis of several randomized trials of stroke patients showed mortality reduction after decompressive surgery; however, many of those are disabled and require assistance with basic needs [8]. Therefore, the complications that arise due to DC or from cranioplasty in post-DC should not be ignored in the treatment of TBI or stroke. Additionally, children are

N. Ahmed
Department of Neurosurgery, Ibrahim Cardiac Hospital and Research Institute (A Centre for Cardiovascular, Neuroscience and Organ Transplant Units), Dhaka, Bangladesh

M. M. Rahman (✉)
Department of Neurosurgery, Holy Family Red Crescent Medical College Hospital, Dhaka, Bangladesh

© The Author(s), under exclusive license to Springer Nature Singapore Pte Ltd. 2024

A. Agrawal et al. (eds.), *Special Considerations in Trauma Care*,
https://doi.org/10.1007/978-981-99-9662-9_18

significantly more likely than adults to experience complications from a cranioplasty following a DC treatment, with the risk being at its highest during the first year of life [9–11]. Although commonly available reports have mostly focused the adult patients, a decompressive hinge-craniotomy is commonly utilized to prevent a cranioplasty and subsequent problems. Therefore, instead of traditional hinge craniotomy, several modified variants have been applied, such as acute subdural hematoma (ASDH) with imminent brain herniation. Studies have described and suggested taking the potential benefits of decompressive craniotomy (DCO) without bone exclusion among infants and children [3].

18.2 Indication of DECOMPRESSIVE CRANIOTOMY

Overall, DC seems to be utilized more than DCO, despite the fact that DCO is less frequent in low- and middle-income countries (LMICs). The most frequent causes include TBI, infection, ischemia, or hemorrhagic stroke, and other conditions like cancer. A clinical necessity for secondary cranial reconstruction develops after the neurosurgery [12]. Taking into account the pre-operative GCS state and the particular TBI, the three most frequent indications for a DCO were ASDH and a GCS of 9–12, ASDH with contusions and a GCS of 3–8, and ASDH with contusions and a GCS of 9–12. The least frequent symptom seems to be an extradural hematoma. Additionally, individuals with good neurology had DCO (GCS 13–15). One of the most prevalent reasons for a DCO is the existence of a subdural hematoma; however, extradural hematoma is less common. A GCS of 9–12 is the most common GCS group for which a DCO is performed. DCO is also performed among patients who have a decent neurological score (GCS 13–15) [13].

The intracerebral hemorrhage (ICH) secondary findings revealed on the CT scan are frequently used to determine the need for DCO. Patients with inconclusive indirect criteria were admitted to the ICU for ICP monitoring and were subjected to standard medical and clinical ICH therapy protocols such as mannitol, positioning, and hyperventilation. If operations fail, barbiturate coma is usually used for a set period of time, followed by DCO [14].

TBI, SAH, and hemisphere MCA infarction are the most prevalent primary events described in the literature. In other circumstances such as subdural empyema, less common applications of DC have been observed to be effective in treating refractory ICP [15], encephalitis [16], toxoplasmosis [17], and encephalopathy related to Reye's syndrome [18]. In addition to the causes mentioned above, arteriovenous malformations, hypertension, tumors, cavernous malformations, and dural arteriovenous fistulas can also result in ICH. In all of these clinical conditions, persistently increased ICP is a common feature, leading to secondary brain damage [19].

18.3 Complications of Decompressive Craniectomy in Children

Complications from a DC occur at predictable intervals after the procedure. DC is linked to a multitude of serious problems in children.

Infection There is an excessive infection frequency related to DC in the pediatric population, according to previous research. The existence of a cranial implant such as the presence of a gastrostomy, a VP shunt, and mechanical ventilation are all associated with cranioplasty-related illness [20]. In nearly 10% of patients, superficial wound infections such as necrosis, sub-galeal collections, surgical site infection (SSI), and wound breakdown occurred, whereas deeper infections such as subdural empyema and epidural abscess occurred in nearly 4% of cases [21]. A previous study observed osteomyelitis in 6% of patients nearly 2 months after the surgery [22].

Resorption The frequency of bone resorption is much higher in pediatric patients. According to the previous study conducted by Piedra et al. [23], Bowers et al. [24] and Grant et al. [25] reported resorption rates between 29.5% and 50%. Higher resorption rates were also reported by others, such as 76.9% by Beez et al. [26] and 66.7% by Martin et al. [11]. An overall rate of resorption of 36% was identified in 2013 through a systematic review [27], while another recent systematic review documented a resorption rate of 16.5% [28]. As a result, "severe" bone degradation usually necessitates a cranioplasty revision including autologous split-thickness bone grafts, synthetic materials, or exchange cranioplasties. However, this needs another surgical procedure, which exposes the individual to additional risks (especially infection), hospitalizations, and high expenditure [29, 30].

Osteolysis Osteolysis is a condition in which periprosthetic bony tissue is gradually destroyed, resulting in progressive radiolucent lines and/or cavitation at the implant–bone interface on serial radiographs [31]. According to previous studies, a substantial proportion of patients <15 years old experienced osteolysis and required revisional CP with a synthetic implant. According to several research studies, the age of patients is a crucial factor that influences calvaria growth [11]. The autologous bone flap is theoretically prone to the formation of osteolysis as the pediatric skull is undergoing a dynamic remodeling process that involves osteoclastic processes. However, animal experiments show that younger people have better osteogenic capacities while also having lower resorption rates, and the source of this age factor is mainly unknown [32]. In young children, osteolysis was also identified as a serious complication. According to research, 66.7% of patients developed osteolytic bone flaps after 6–12 months, requiring surgery to remove the osteolytic bone flap and cranioplasty with a Polymethyl Methacrylate (PMMA) or Computer-Aided Design (CAD) flap. Another study found that, after an initial bone flap cranioplasty, 29.5–50% of pediatric patients had osteolysis after a mean time interval of 4.8 months (ranging 1–36 months), or 13.3 months (ranging 2–76 months) [24, 33, 34]).

Hydrocephalus DC patients with severe TBI usually develop posttraumatic hydrocephalus and epilepsy. In 40% of the survivors, shunt-dependent posttraumatic hydrocephalus developed, requiring the placement of one subdural, one lumboperitoneal, and 12 ventriculoperitoneal shunts. Antiepileptic medications (valproic acid, phenobarbital, and phenytoin) are necessary for posttraumatic epilepsy, which occurs in 20% of children [35]. A cohort of children suffered from posttraumatic shunt-dependent hydrocephalus in 40% of cases. This rate seems to be significantly higher than the recognized incidence of posttraumatic hydrocephalus in those with severe TBI. Based on CSF dynamics and imaging studies, Marmarou and colleagues recently revealed that 20% of patients with severe TBI (GCS: 8) hydrocephalus experienced posttrauma. DC patients have a higher rate of hydrocephalus, which may simply be a reflection of the extent and pattern of damage. A DC may alter CSF dynamics and/or encourage subarachnoid scarring, which can result in hydrocephalus, especially if the surgery involves dural opening and the insertion of a large dural patch [36].

Subdural Hygroma Subdural hygroma (SDG) is a collection of cerebrospinal fluid (CSF) under the dural membrane of the brain that is devoid of blood [37]. The creation of SDG is the utmost prevalent exhibition of post-DC changes in CSF dynamics and one of the major DC consequences. Hejazi et al. found that 57.1% of individuals in a series of DC cases for severe TBI (children) developed hygroma [38]. SDGs usually cure without surgery over a period of 7–30 days, but their identification is linked to a lengthier hospital stay, a longer rehabilitation duration, and a worse neurological result [39].

CSF Leak When CSF escapes via a defect in the dura or the skull and out through the nose or ear, it is known as a CSF leak [40]. According to studies that included such data, the overall prevalence of CSF leaks related to cranioplasty was 6.8% among adults [11, 41–44]. In research focusing on children having severe TBI, Figaji et al. [45] found that after cranioplasty, 16.7% of patients had indications of CSF leak. Another study conducted in a developing nation also described a high proportion of CSF leakage [20]. Rates of CSF leakage were significantly varying between adults [46, 47] and infants [48], 5.2% and 43%, respectively. The authors of one study on DC problems in babies blamed fistula formation on the failure to properly connect the dura and scalp due to edema and suggested using a dural augmentation graft. The prognosis for unplanned CSF leaks/fistulas is usually positive, but more severe consequences, such as high intracerebral pressure, can occur [48].

18.4 DECOMPRESSIVE CRANIOTOMY Techniques for Children

A total of eight DCO methods were used, with the common (48%) lightly tying sutures with the bone flap. In a prior study, 81% of people never thinned the inner table of the bone flap, while 18% thinned it occasionally. A subgaleal wound drain is the most common complement to the DCO, whereas a cisternostomy is the least common. According to the findings, up to 49% of people use an ICP monitor during a DCO [13].

18.4.1 Floating/Hinge Craniotomy Technique

Floating/hinge craniotomy (HFDC) is a procedure that allows for some decompression while keeping the bone flap in place in a "floating" or "hinged" manner. This allows for the expansion of following cerebral edema while also avoiding the necessity for future cranioplasty. The exact technique, indications, and outcomes of this treatment are still being worked out, but it is anticipated that in some cases, HC will be a viable alternative to DC [49]. In brain edema patients, it is a relatively new and underutilized approach for achieving cerebral decompression. Although it has been utilized by neurosurgeons for several years for various other purposes, the approach was first documented by three different groups in 2007 exclusively for surgical regulation of posttraumatic therapeutically intractable high ICP [50, 51]. Later on, Park and his colleagues reported good neurological outcomes in five children, diagnosed as ASDH who underwent this innovative surgical technique with some modifications [52].

18.4.1.1 Surgical Technique

With all aseptic precautions, a large fronto-temporo-parietal craniotomy flap is planned and a question or reverse question mark incision is given depending upon the site. After dissection through subgaleal plane, the periosteum of the parietal bone is preserved to augment future duraplasty. Although its base is allowed to be partially dissected, the majority of the temporalis muscle is still significantly linked to the temporal fossa. Fronto-parieto-temporal craniotomy is carried out with the muscle hinge preserved (Fig. 18.1a). The leftover bone is rongeured to the middle cerebral fossa floor after lifting and inverting the bone flap. Dura can be incised in star shape fashion or multiple small incisions, depending upon the types of pathology addressed. Small dural incisions are then united to expose the brain surface which facilitates hematoma evacuation, securing the bleeding points and allowing expansion of the swollen brain. Utilizing preharvested pericranium and an artificial dural substitute, extensive duraplasty is carried out. Then, only three sites on the bone flap are where absorbable plates are attached (Fig. 18.1b). Following the procedure, layered closure is done respecting the anatomical plane and placement of a subgaleal drain tube in situ [52].

18.4.1.2 Advantages

In some cases, HFDC provides advantages over typical DC, such as the ability to control at least mild cerebral edema while avoiding the need for a future costly invasive cranioplasty [53]. This is especially significant in resource-constrained environments. Furthermore, unlike the standard surgical procedure of DC, there have been reports of axonal stretching being reduced following this technique. Besides this, muscle hinge prevents bone graft resorption (BGR) and SSI [52].

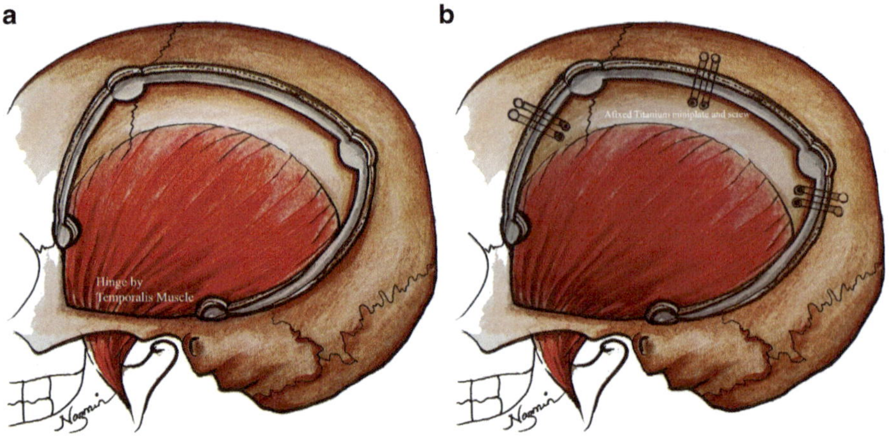

Fig. 18.1 Schematic illustration demonstrates the basic principle of HFDC, whereas temporalis muscle is allowed to be attached with a large fronto-temporo-parietal craniotomy flap which carries the hinge property (**a**), and after addressing the definitive pathology followed by dural augmentation, absorbable miniplates are attached with a bone flap which prevents sinking down the flap after controlling raised ICP (**b**)

18.4.1.3 Complications

Despite this procedure, failure to control raised ICP may necessitate the removal of the bone flap. However, a few cases may suffer from CSF hydrodynamic difficulties, which lead to the development of hydrocephalus, infection, and very rarely resorption of the autologous bone flap [54].

18.4.1.4 Outcome

HFDC can be an excellent choice for decompression, especially under 1 year of age. Park and his colleagues observed good neurological outcomes in their reported case series where none of the infants suffered from BGR or SSI in the postoperative period and exhibited ossification of the bone gap at 1-year follow-up [52].

18.4.2 Four-Quadrant Osteoplastic DCO

Four-quadrant osteoplastic DCO (FoQOsD) is a unique procedure that maintains the bone flap while obtaining enough cerebral decompression in all directions [55].

18.4.2.1 Surgical Technique

The initial surgical procedure is the same as the standard DC flap [56]. An extra burr hole is done in the center from which the bone flap becomes marked in four quadrants. The temporal craniectomy went all the way up to the zygomatic arch and to the bottom of the middle cranial fossa. After cutting the periosteum, the bone flap

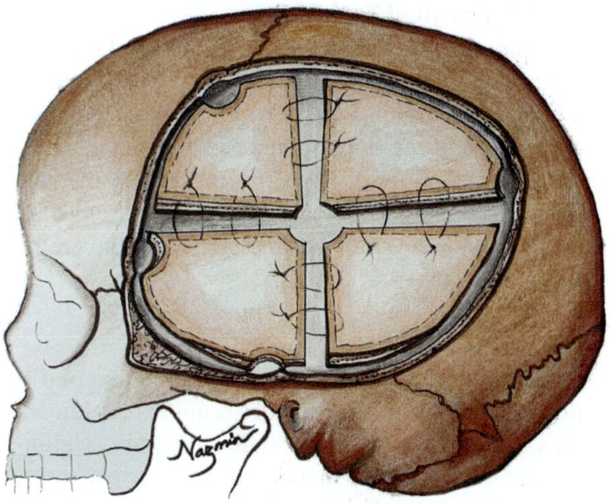

Fig. 18.2 Schematic picture showing the final appearance of FoQOsD in children

was separated into four quadrants, starting with the central burr hole. The bone flaps floated out in all four directions as the brain expanded, providing space for the expanding brain and lowering the ICP (Fig. 18.2).

18.4.2.2 Advantages

When compared to the hinge craniotomy, this surgery is more likely to provide less resistance for the brain to expand, which occurs most frequently in the middle of the opening where the stellate durotomy is performed [7]. Besides this, the tendency to develop hydrocephalus and hematoma expansion becomes minimized [56].

18.4.2.3 Outcome

Compared with standard DC procedure, Peethambaran et al. observed that SSI following the conventional DC was 30% in the conventional DC group and 20% in the FoQOsD group. In the FoQOsD group, 33% of patients developed hydrocephalus compared to 40% of patients in the DC group who survived. None of the patients in the FoQOsD group had acute neurological deterioration due to bone flap sinking onto the brain once the brain swelling had subsided.

18.4.3 Three-Pillar Expansive Craniotomy

Neurosurgeons have experimented with a range of alternative surgical procedures to achieve the benefits of a decompressive hemicraniectomy procedure without the requirement for a following cranioplasty procedure [49, 57]. The three-pillar expansive craniotomy avoids the problems discussed above while providing an effective way to regulate IH.

18.4.3.1 Surgical Technique

Initial surgical steps are the same as that of standard DC procedure. The craniotomy borders are cut in an indirect way to expand the area available for the dural and brain. At the margin of the bone flap, three small bone fragments are sutured in the inner surface of the flap in the parietal, frontal, and occipital areas simulating three pillars. The bone flap is fixed to the skull at the same location as the pillars using three absorbable skull locks in a way that assures a 5-mm space between the craniotomy flap and the skull surface. After that, layered closure is done maintaining the anatomical plane.

18.4.3.2 Advantages

The extra room generated by keeping the excised bone flap 5 mm above its anatomic position allows for further brain expansion with this method. A cranial plate with a 5-mm offset accommodates the brain swelling that happens in patients with ischemic stroke [58]. While the three-pillar expansive craniotomy is not intended to replace a DC, it may reduce the need for one in some cases and add another tool to the toolbox for the management of IH after brain traumatic injury, brain ischemic stroke, and even postoperative elevated ICP due to rehemorrhage or cerebral edema [59].

18.4.3.3 Complications

Compared with standard DC procedure, reported complications in this method are subdural effusion and postoperative hydrocephalus [59].

18.4.4 Greenstick Fracture Hinge Craniotomy Technique

18.4.4.1 Surgical Technique

Following a large question mark or reverse question mark scalp incision, subgaleal dissection allows the galeo-cutaneous flap to retract antero inferiorly. The temporal muscle is allowed to be attached to the temporal fossa. After that, multiple burr holes are done and connected with each other to create a large fronto-temporo-parietal craniotomy flap sparing the temporal base. Meanwhile, a hinge-craniotomy is done with a greenstick fracture made at the temporal base. Several dural hitches are given to prevent epidural hemorrhage. The pathology is addressed after the dural opening. Duraplasty is done, and a hinge-bone flap is placed in situ without fixation (Fig. 18.3).

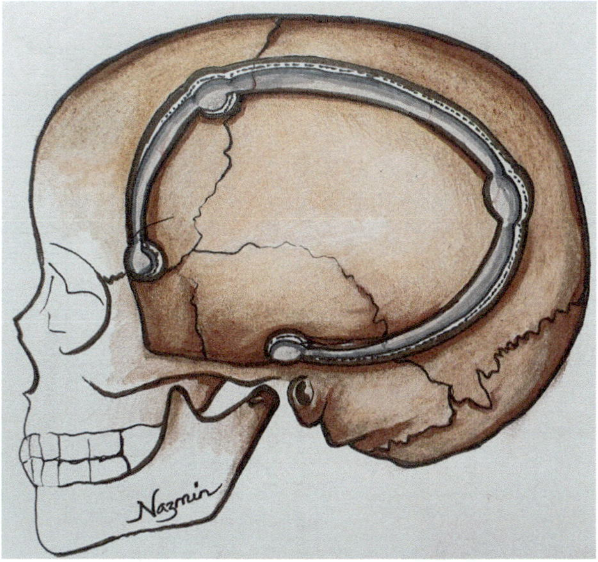

Fig. 18.3 Schematic illustration demonstrates the appearance of the bone flap in the Greenstick fracture hinge craniotomy technique

18.5 Complications and Outcome

After a DCO, a variety of problems and negative outcomes might occur (Table 18.1). The most prevalent infections are superficial infections, which include hydrocephalus, subdural effusions, and different infections such as meningitis [6]. The belief that DCO provides insufficient ICP control is perhaps the most common explanation for its low popularity. DCO, on the contrary, has been found in multiple studies to be equivalent to DC in the control of ICP. Kano et al. compared DCO and DC in 58 patients with TBI and stroke over the course of 7 years [57]. In terms of postoperative mRS or GOS, there was no distinction between the two groups. In addition, no patients in the DCO group had a bone flap infection compared to six in the DC arm. However, due to high ICP, two patients in the DCO group required a later DC. The authors concluded that using DCO with ICP monitoring afterward could be a viable substitute for DC. Their advice appears to be based on real-world experience and is consistent with the findings of our analysis. A new broad scoping assessment on the topic of DCO presents an early indication that the efficiency of DC versus DCO is clinically equivalent [49]. Polin et al. have identified a 28.5% prevalence of hydrocephalus [69]. Guerra et al. observed subdural effusions in 26%, infection in 2%, and hydrocephalus in 14% [70]. In another study, Aarabi et al. found 25% of subdural effusions among 50 cases [71]. Spontaneous resolution was observed among all patients, and bone resorption and bone flap infection were also common [72, 73].

Table 18.1 Reported cases of DCO techniques in children to date

Author and year	Pt	Age	Sex	Indication	DCO techniques	Intraoperative complications	Postoperative complications	Outcome
Kjellberg and Prieto [60]	6	4–17 years	4M, 2F	TBI; brain trauma	Bifrontal DCO	NM	Expressive dysphasia	Survived most of them were neurologically and mentally normal. Some required chronic care
Du Plessis [61]	7	9–18 years	4M, 3F	Sclerosteosis	Bifrontal, posterior fossa, lumboperitoneal	Blood loss from bone	Pseudomeningocele, posterior headache, cardiac arrest	Good mostly, Loss of review, one death
Cho et al. [62]	10	2–14 months	7M, 3F	Acute shaken baby syndrome where ICP >30 mmHg	Bifrontal DCO—5 pt, Unilateral F-T-P DCO—5 pt	Bridging vein rupture-4 pt Sagittal sinus rupture-1 pt	Cortical atrophy, cerebral infarction, SDH	Excellent recovery—2 pt Nondisabling deficit—3 pt Severe motor or cognitive deficit—4 pt Vegetative—1 pt
Figaji et al. [63]	5	6–12 years	3M, 2F	Severe TBI	Unilateral F-T-P DCO—3 pt	NM	Nothing significant	Nondisabling deficit—4 pt Motor or cognitive deficit—1 pt
Martínez-Lage et al. [64]	3	1–13 years	1M, 2F	Brain contusions and ASDH	Bilateral temporo-parietal Craniotomies	Minimal ventricular problems	Nothing significant	Resolution of symptoms
Mracek et al. [65]	1	8 years	M	ASDH	Osteoplastic DCO	NM	Nothing significant	Favorable outcome
Wani et al. [66]	3	6–18 years	3 M	ASDH, malignant MCA infarction	F-T-P DCO	NM	Hydrocephalus	Improvement after ventriculo-peritoneal (VP) shunt, one patient died

Nguyen and Lew [67]	9	3–17	2M, 7F	epidural hematoma, contusion, ASDH, hemorrhage	Craniotomy for hematoma evacuation and EVD placement	CSF leak from nose	Behavioral challenges	All had a good recovery
Yokota et al. [68]	1	4 months	M	Abusive head Trauma, ASDH	Greenstick fracture hinge decompressive craniotomy	No	No	Survived ICP <20 mmHg
Park et al. [52]	5	2–20 months	NM	ASDH	HFDC	NM	CSDH, subcutaneous fluid collection	Excellent recovery—2 pt No significant disability—1 pt Slight disability—1 pt Moderate disability—1 pt
Wang et al. [59]	16	2–18 years	11M, 5F	Ischemic stroke, head injury	Three-pillar expansive craniotomy	NM	Subdural effusion, hydrocephalus	Two children died

Pt patient, *M* male, *F* female, *NM* not mentioned, *ICP* intracranial pressure, *TBI* traumatic brain injury, *ASDH* acute subdural hematoma, *DCO* decompressive craniotomy, *F-T-P* fronto-temporo-parietal, *HFDC* hinge and floating decompressive craniotomy, *SDH* subdural hematoma

18.6 Future Research

Patients with TBI and stroke urgently require cost-effective surgical treatment, particularly in LMICs, where the relevant burden is increasing. DCO is a common technique that is most typically used to treat an ASDH. A number of techniques are now being utilized to reattach the bone flap to the cranium, the most popular of which is lightly tying sutures to the bone flap. There is a lot of interest around the world regarding the usefulness of DCO over DC; however, further research is needed. Neurosurgery procedures are often expensive, thus making them unaffordable for the majority of the patients from LMICs. Therefore, more research is required regarding the more cost-effective techniques of neurosurgery. Additional research would be required to reduce post-craniotomy problems, influencing factors, patient performance improvement, and patient risk. Evidence suggests that patients who have had a craniotomy or have had a brain tumor endure severe post-surgical pain; however, there are no guidelines for treating the pain developed. Little research has been done on the complexities of post-craniotomy, postbrain tumor pain, and how it affects people. The quality of life of post-craniotomy patients has to be studied more extensively in order to enhance the outcome of existing methods.

18.7 Conclusion

DCO provides some important advantages over DC and is also more suitable for LMICs. It also creates access to reach the desired area of the neurosurgeon, such as blood vessels, tumors, and any other area within the skull. To overcome the complications related to DCO, it is critical to advance the currently existing craniotomy procedures. More steps should be taken to understand the post-craniotomy situations of patients in order to develop timely interventions and standardize treatment to improve functional outcomes.

References

1. Go AS, Mozaffarian D, Roger VL, Benjamin EJ, Berry JD, Blaha MJ, Dai S, et al. Heart disease and stroke statistics - 2014 update: a report from the American Heart Association. Circulation. 2014;129(3):80. https://doi.org/10.1161/01.cir.0000441139.02102.80.
2. Gorelick PB. The global burden of stroke: persistent and disabling. Lancet Neurol. 2019;18(5):417–8. https://doi.org/10.1016/S1474-4422(19)30030-4.
3. Schirmer CM, Ackil AA, Malek AM. Decompressive craniectomy. Neurocrit Care. 2008;8(3):456–70. https://doi.org/10.1007/s12028-008-9082-y.
4. Reithmeier T, Löhr M, Pakos P, Ketter G, Ernestus RI. Relevance of ICP and $PtiO_2$ for indication and timing of decompressive craniectomy in patients with malignant brain edema. Acta Neurochir. 2005;147(9):947–52. https://doi.org/10.1007/s00701-005-0543-1.
5. Stiefel MF, Heuer GG, Smith MJ, Bloom S, Maloney-Wilensky E, Gracias VH, Sean Grady M, Leroux PD. Cerebral oxygenation following decompressive hemicraniectomy for the treatment of refractory intracranial hypertension. J Neurosurg. 2004;101(2):241–7. https://doi.org/10.3171/jns.2004.101.2.0241.

6. Faleiro RM, Faleiro LCM, Caetano E, Gomide I, Pita C, Coelho G, Brás E, Carvalho B, Gusmão SNS. Decompressive craniotomy: prognostic factors and complications in 89 patients. Arq Neuropsiquiatr. 2008;66(2B):369–73. https://doi.org/10.1590/S0004-282X2008000300017.
7. Adeleye A, Azeez A. Decompressive Craniectomy bone flap hinged on the temporalis muscle: a new inexpensive use for an old neurosurgical technique. Surg Neurol Int. 2011;2(1):150. https://doi.org/10.4103/2152-7806.86227.
8. Alexander P, Heels-Ansdell D, Siemieniuk R, Bhatnagar N, Chang Y, Fei Y, Zhang Y, McLeod S, Prasad K, Guyatt G. Hemicraniectomy versus medical treatment with large MCA infarct: a review and meta-analysis. BMJ Open. 2016;6(11):e014390. https://doi.org/10.1136/bmjopen-2016-014390.
9. Frassanito P, Massimi L, Caldarelli M, Tamburrini G, Di Rocco C. Complications of delayed cranial repair after decompressive craniectomy in children less than 1 year old. Acta Neurochir. 2012;154(5):927–33. https://doi.org/10.1007/s00701-011-1253-5.
10. Frassanito P, Tamburrini G, Massimi L, Peraio S, Caldarelli M, Di Rocco C. Problems of reconstructive cranioplasty after traumatic brain injury in children. Childs Nerv Syst. 2017;33(10):1759–68. https://doi.org/10.1007/s00381-017-3541-8.
11. Martin KD, Franz B, Kirsch M, Polanski W, Von Der Hagen M, Schackert G, Sobottka SB. Autologous bone flap cranioplasty following decompressive craniectomy is combined with a high complication rate in pediatric traumatic brain injury patients. Acta Neurochir. 2014;156(4):813–24. https://doi.org/10.1007/s00701-014-2021-0.
12. Zheng F, Hao X, von Spreckelsen N, Stavrinou P, Timmer M, Goldbrunner R, Cao F, et al. Early or late cranioplasty following decompressive craniotomy for traumatic brain injury: a systematic review and meta-analysis. J Int Med Res. 2018;46(7):2503–12. https://doi.org/10.1177/0300060518755148.
13. Mohan M, Horsfall HL, Solla DJF, Robertson FC, Adeleye AO, Teklemariam TL, Khan MM, et al. Decompressive craniotomy: an international survey of practice. Acta Neurochir. 2021;163(5):1415–22. https://doi.org/10.1007/s00701-021-04783-6.
14. Mehan ND, Wagner KE, Ullman JS. Decompressive craniotomy and craniectomy for brain trauma. Curr Surg Rep. 2016;4(8):4. https://doi.org/10.1007/s40137-016-0151-4.
15. Wada Y, Kubo T, Asano T, Senda A, Isono M, Kobayashi H. Fulminant subdural empyema treated with a wide decompressive craniectomy and continuous irrigation - case report. Neurol Med Chir. 2002;42(9):414–6. https://doi.org/10.2176/nmc.42.414.
16. Schonewille WJ, Tuhrim S, Stacy C. Craniectomy: an aggressive treatment approach in severe encephalitis. Neurology. 1997;49(5):1476. https://doi.org/10.1212/WNL.49.5.1476.
17. Agrawal D, Hussain N. Decompressive craniectomy in cerebral toxoplasmosis. Eur J Clin Microbiol Infect Dis. 2005;24(11):772–3. https://doi.org/10.1007/s10096-005-0017-7.
18. Eghwrudjakpor PO, Allison AB. Decompressive craniectomy following brain injury: factors important to patient outcome. Libyan J Med. 2010;5(1):1–6. https://doi.org/10.4176/091104.
19. Mitchell P, Gregson BA, Vindlacheruvu RR, David Mendelow A. Surgical options in ICH including decompressive craniectomy. J Neurol Sci. 2007;261(1-2):89–98. https://doi.org/10.1016/j.jns.2007.04.040.
20. Waqas M, Ujjan B, Hadi YB, Najmuddin F, Laghari AA, Khalid S, Bari ME, Bhatti UF. Cranioplasty after craniectomy in a pediatric population: single-center experience from a developing country. Pediatr Neurosurg. 2017;52(2):77–9. https://doi.org/10.1159/000452808.
21. Kurland DB, Khaladj-Ghom A, Stokum JA, Carusillo B, Karimy JK, Gerzanich V, Sahuquillo J, Marc Simard J. Complications associated with decompressive craniectomy: a systematic review. Neurocrit Care. 2015;23(2):292–304. https://doi.org/10.1007/s12028-015-0144-7.
22. Anto D, Manjooran R, Aravindakshan R, Lakshman K, Morris R. Cranioplasty using autoclaved autologous skull bone flaps preserved at ambient temperature. J Neurosci Rural Pract. 2017;8(4):595–600. https://doi.org/10.4103/jnrp.jnrp_270_17.
23. Piedra MP, Thompson EM, Selden NR, Ragel BT, Guillaume DJ. Optimal timing of autologous cranioplasty after decompressive craniectomy in children. J Neurosurg Pediatr. 2012;10(4):268–72. https://doi.org/10.3171/2012.6.PEDS1268.

24. Bowers CA, Riva-Cambrin JAY, Hertzler DA, Walker ML. Risk factors and rates of bone flap resorption in pediatric patients after decompressive craniectomy for traumatic brain injury. J Neurosurg Pediatr. 2013;11(5):526–32. https://doi.org/10.3171/2013.1.PEDS12483.
25. Grant GA, Jolley M, Ellenbogen RG, Roberts TS, Gruss JR, Loeser JD. Failure of autologous bone-assisted cranioplasty following decompressive craniectomy in children and adolescents. J Neurosurg. 2004;100(2):163–8. https://doi.org/10.3171/ped.2004.100.2.0163.
26. Beez T, Munoz-Bendix C, Ahmadi SA, Steiger HJ, Beseoglu K. From decompressive craniectomy to cranioplasty and beyond—a pediatric neurosurgery perspective. Childs Nerv Syst. 2019;35(9):1517–24. https://doi.org/10.1007/s00381-019-04303-z.
27. Rocque BG, Amancherla K, Lew SM, Lam S. Outcomes of cranioplasty following decompressive craniectomy in the pediatric population: a systematic review. J Neurosurg Pediatr. 2013;12(2):120–5. https://doi.org/10.3171/2013.4.PEDS12605.
28. Malcolm JG, Mahmooth Z, Rindler RS, Allen JW, Grossberg JA, Pradilla G, Ahmad FU. Autologous cranioplasty is associated with increased reoperation rate: a systematic review and meta-analysis. World Neurosurg. 2018;116:60–8. https://doi.org/10.1016/j.wneu.2018.05.009.
29. Fodstad H, Love JA, Ekstedt J, Fridén H, Liliequist B. Effect of cranioplasty on cerebrospinal fluid hydrodynamics in patients with the syndrome of the trephined. Acta Neurochir. 1984;70(1–2):21–30. https://doi.org/10.1007/BF01406039.
30. Halani SH, Chu JK, Malcolm JG, Rindler RS, Allen JW, Grossberg JA, Pradilla G, Ahmad FU. Effects of cranioplasty on cerebral blood flow following decompressive craniectomy: a systematic review of the literature. Neurosurgery. 2017;81(2):204–16. https://doi.org/10.1093/neuros/nyx054.
31. Chiang PP, Burke DW, Freiberg AA, Rubash HE. Osteolysis of the pelvis: evaluation and treatment. Clin Orthop Relat Res. 2003;417:164–74. https://doi.org/10.1097/01.blo.0000096816.78689.e5.
32. Gosain AK, Gosain SA, Sweeney WM, Song LS, Amarante MTJ. Regulation of osteogenesis and survival within bone grafts to the calvaria: the effect of the dura versus the pericranium. Plast Reconstr Surg. 2011;128(1):85–94. https://doi.org/10.1097/PRS.0b013e31821740cc.
33. Gruber R, Peter R, Hora J. The prognosis of cranioplasty following large craniectomy in children. Eur J Pediatr Surg. 1988;43(6):375–83. https://doi.org/10.1055/s-2008-1043488.
34. Reid Gooch M, Gin GE, Kenning TJ, German JW. Complications of cranioplasty following decompressive craniectomy: analysis of 62 cases. Neurosurg Focus. 2009;26(6):1–7. https://doi.org/10.3171/2009.3.FOCUS0962.
35. Kan P, Amini A, Hansen K, White GL, Brockmeyer DL, Walker ML, Kestle JRW. Outcomes after decompressive craniectomy for severe traumatic brain injury in children. J Neurosurg. 2006;105(5):337–42. https://doi.org/10.3171/ped.2006.105.5.337.
36. Marmarou A, Abd-Elfattah MA, Foda KB, Yoshihara M, Yamamoto T, Tsuji O, Zasler N, Ward JD, Young HF. Posttraumatic ventriculomegaly: hydrocephalus or atrophy? A new approach for diagnosis using CSF dynamics. J Neurosurg. 1996;85(6):1026–35. https://doi.org/10.3171/jns.1996.85.6.1026.
37. Almenzalawy MA, Essa AEA, Ragab MH. Subdural hygroma: different treatment modalities and clinical outcome. Open J Mod Neurosurg. 2019;9(3):208–20. https://doi.org/10.4236/ojmn.2019.93020.
38. Hejazi N, Witzmann A, Fae P. Unilateral decompressive craniectomy for children with severe brain injury. report of seven cases and review of the relevant literature. Eur J Pediatr. 2002;161(2):99–104. https://doi.org/10.1007/s00431-001-0864-x.
39. Honeybul S, Kwok M. Incidence and risk factors for post-traumatic hydrocephalus following decompressive craniectomy for intractable intracranial hypertension and evacuation of mass lesions. J Neurotrauma. 2012;29(10):1872–8. https://doi.org/10.1089/neu.2012.2356.
40. Schievink WI. Spontaneous spinal cerebrospinal fluid leaks and intracranial hypotension. JAMA J Am Med Assoc. 2006;295(19):2286–96. https://doi.org/10.1001/jama.295.19.2286.
41. Shamim MS, Qadeer M, Murtaza SG, Bari ME, Sobani ZA, Zafar SN, Bilal N, Enam SA. Cranioplasty after decompressive craniectomy: an institutional audit and analy-

sis of factors related to complications. Surg Neurol Int. 2011;2(1):123. https://doi.org/10.4103/2152-7806.85055.
42. Godil SS, Shamim MS, Enam SA, Qidwai U, Qadeer M, Sobani ZA. Cranial reconstruction after decompressive craniectomy: prediction of complications using fuzzy logic. J Craniofac Surg. 2011;22(4):1307–11. https://doi.org/10.1097/SCS.0b013e31821c6d37.
43. Woertgen C, Rothoerl RD, Schebesch KM, Albert R. Comparison of craniotomy and craniectomy in patients with acute subdural haematoma. J Clin Neurosci. 2006;13(7):718–21. https://doi.org/10.1016/j.jocn.2005.08.019.
44. Huang YH, Lee TC, Chen WF, Wang YM. Safety of the nonabsorbable dural substitute in decompressive craniectomy for severe traumatic brain injury. J Trauma. 2011;71(3):533–7. https://doi.org/10.1097/TA.0b013e318203208a.
45. Figaji AA, Fieggen AG, Argent A, Peter JC. Surgical treatment for 'brain compartment syndrome' in children with severe head injury. S Afr Med J. 2006;96(9 Pt 2):969–75. https://pubmed.ncbi.nlm.nih.gov/17077927/.
46. Bao YH, Liang YM, Gao GY, Pan YH, Luo QZ, Jiang JY. Bilateral decompressive craniectomy for patients with malignant diffuse brain swelling after severe traumatic brain injury: a 37-case study. J Neurotrauma. 2010;27(2):341–7. https://doi.org/10.1089/neu.2009.1040.
47. Jiang JY, Wei X, Li WP, Wen Hui X, Zhang J, Bao YH, Ying YH, Luo QZ. Efficacy of standard trauma craniectomy for refractory intracranial hypertension with severe traumatic brain injury: a multicenter, prospective, randomized controlled study. J Neurotrauma. 2005;22(6):623–8. https://doi.org/10.1089/neu.2005.22.623.
48. Adamo MA, Drazin D, Waldman JB. Decompressive craniectomy and postoperative complication management in infants and toddlers with severe traumatic brain injuries. J Neurosurg Pediatr. 2009;3(4):334–9. https://doi.org/10.3171/2008.12.PEDS08310.
49. Layard Horsfall H, Mohan M, Indira Devi B, Adeleye AO, Shukla DP, Bhat D, Khan M, et al. Hinge/floating craniotomy as an alternative technique for cerebral decompression: a scoping review. Neurosurg Rev. 2020;43(6):1493–507. https://doi.org/10.1007/s10143-019-01180-7.
50. Goettler CE, Tucci KA. Decreasing the morbidity of decompressive craniectomy: the tucci flap. J Trauma. 2007;62(3):777–8. https://doi.org/10.1097/TA.0b013e31802ee55e.
51. Schmidt JH, Reyes BJ, Fischer R, Flaherty SK. Use of hinge craniotomy for cerebral decompression: technical note. J Neurosurg. 2007;107(3):678–82. https://doi.org/10.3171/JNS-07/09/0678.
52. Park YS, Kogeichi Y, Haku T, Kim TK, Yokota H, Nakagawa I, Motoyama Y, Nakase H. Hinge and floating decompressive craniotomy for infantile acute subdural hematoma: technical note. Childs Nerv Syst. 2021;37(1):295–8. https://doi.org/10.1007/s00381-020-04942-7.
53. Kolias AG, Viaroli E, Rubiano AM, Adams H, Khan T, Gupta D, Adeleye A, et al. The current status of decompressive craniectomy in traumatic brain injury. Curr Trauma Rep. 2018;4(4):326–32. https://doi.org/10.1007/s40719-018-0147-x.
54. Gutman MJ, How E, Withers T. The floating anchored craniotomy. Surg Neurol Int. 2017;8(1):130. https://doi.org/10.4103/sni.sni_460_16.
55. Vankipuram S, Sasane SV, Chandra A, Ojha BK, Singh SK, Srivastava C, Jaiswal S, Bajaj A, Jaiswal M. A comparative analysis between four-quadrant osteoplastic decompressive craniotomy versus conventional decompressive craniectomy for traumatic brain injury. World Neurosurg. 2020;135:393–404. https://doi.org/10.1016/j.wneu.2019.12.004.
56. Peethambaran AK, Valsalmony J. Four-quadrant osteoplastic decompressive craniotomy: a novel technique for decompressive craniectomy avoiding revision cranioplasty after surgery. Neurology. 2012;60(6):672–4. https://doi.org/10.4103/0028-3886.105221.
57. Kano T, Kurosaki S, Wada H. Retrospective analysis of hinge technique for head trauma or stroke. Neurol Med Chir. 2012;52(11):816–21. https://doi.org/10.2176/nmc.52.816.
58. Stoner KE, Abode-Iyamah KO, Grosland NM, Howard MA. Volume of brain herniation in patients with ischemic stroke after decompressive craniectomy. World Neurosurg. 2016;96:101–6. https://doi.org/10.1016/j.wneu.2016.08.095.

59. Wang Y, Han Y, Chen M, Wang H. Three-pillar expansive craniotomy: a new surgical technique for cerebral decompression in children. Childs Nerv Syst. 2021;37(5):1723–8. https://doi.org/10.1007/s00381-021-05073-3.
60. Kjellberg RN, Prieto A. Bifrontal decompressive craniotomy for massive cerebral edema. J Neurosurg. 1971;34(4):488–93. https://doi.org/10.3171/jns.1971.34.4.0488.
61. Du Plessis JJ. Sclerosteosis: neurosurgical experience with 14 cases. J Neurosurg. 1993;78(3):388–92. https://doi.org/10.3171/jns.1993.78.3.0388.
62. Cho DY, Wang YC, Chih CS. Decompressive craniotomy for acute shaken/impact baby syndrome. Pediatr Neurosurg. 1995;23(4):192–8. https://doi.org/10.1159/000120958.
63. Figaji AA, Fieggen AG, Peter JC. Early decompressive craniotomy in children with severe traumatic brain injury. Childs Nerv Syst. 2003;19(9):666–73. https://doi.org/10.1007/s00381-003-0804-3.
64. Martínez-Lage JF, Vilar AR-E, Pérez-Espejo MA, Almagro MJ, Pedro JRDS, Murcia MF. Shunt-related craniocerebral disproportion: treatment with cranial vault expanding procedures. Neurosurg Rev. 2006;29(3):229–35. https://doi.org/10.1007/s10143-006-0022-z.
65. Mracek J, Choc M, Mork J, Vacek P, Mracek Z. Osteoplastic decompressive craniotomy-an alternative to decompressive craniectomy. Acta Neurochir. 2011;153(11):2259–63. https://doi.org/10.1007/s00701-011-1132-0.
66. Wani AA, Ramzan AU, Tanki H, Malik NK, Dar BA. Hydrocephalus after decompressive craniotomy: a case series. Pediatr Neurosurg. 2013;49(5):287–91. https://doi.org/10.1159/000363701.
67. Nguyen HS, Lew S. Equestrian-related traumatic brain injury in the pediatric population. Pediatr Neurosurg. 2016;51(6):279–83. https://doi.org/10.1159/000446402.
68. Yokota H, Sugimoto T, Nishiguchi M, Hashimoto H. Greenstick fracture-hinge decompressive craniotomy in infants: illustrative case and literature review of techniques for decompressive craniotomy without bone removal. Childs Nerv Syst. 2019;35(9):1491–7. https://doi.org/10.1007/s00381-019-04177-1.
69. Polin RS, Shaffrey ME, Bogaev CA, Tisdale N, Germanson T, Bocchicchio B, Jane JA. Decompressive bifrontal craniectomy in the treatment of severe refractory posttraumatic cerebral edema. Neurosurgery. 1997;41(1):84–94. https://doi.org/10.1097/00006123-199707000-00018.
70. Guerra WK, Welch MR, Gaab HD, Mueller JU, Piek J, Fritsch MJ. Surgical decompression for traumatic brain swelling: indications and results. J Neurosurg. 1999;90(2):187–96. https://doi.org/10.3171/jns.1999.90.2.0187.
71. Aarabi B, Hesdorffer DC, Ahn ES, Aresco C, Scalea TM, Eisenberg HM. Outcome following decompressive craniectomy for malignant swelling due to severe head injury. J Neurosurg. 2006;104(4):469–79. https://doi.org/10.3171/jns.2006.104.4.469.
72. Britt RH, Hamilton RD. Large decompressive craniotomy in the treatment of acute subdural hematoma. Neurosurgery. 1978;2(3):195–200. https://doi.org/10.1097/00006123-197805000-00001.
73. Sánchez-Carpintero R, Aguilera S, Idoate M, Bejarano B. Temporal lobectomy in acute complicated herpes simplex encephalitis: technical case report. Neurosurgery. 2008;62(5):E1174. https://doi.org/10.1227/01.neu.0000325885.00033.c3.

Posttraumatic Stress Disorder 19

Chirag Solanki and Iti Shukla

19.1 Introduction

A traumatic event sets off a complex series of issues, physical as well as mental. The psychological distress after the confrontation of a traumatic event is variable, the most common being fear-based context or anxiety. Diagnostic and Statistical Manual of Mental Disorders (DSM) classifies many other phenotypic manifestations under trauma and stress-related disorders other than psychological distress. Posttraumatic stress disorder (PTSD) is one of the neurological sequelae of trauma to be classified as the psychological impact of trauma. The widely accepted definition of PTSD consists of persistent anxiety and related symptoms after exposure to a traumatic event. It is not uncommon to misdiagnose PTSD as a postconcussion disorder, other psychiatric sequelae like personality disorder, adjustment disorder, or posttraumatic degenerative disorders like dementia. Therefore, trauma physicians must suspect and diagnose this condition early and treat it accordingly. Timely diagnosis and appropriate management of PTSD are likely to improve the quality of life of the patient.

19.2 Epidemiology

The prevalence rate of PTSD in the general population is 7.8%. In comparison, it ranges from 10% to 27% in patients with mild traumatic injury, as defined by the Glasgow coma scale of 13–15 [1]. It is pretty similar to the rates of PTSD on other traumatic injuries [1]. Surprisingly, the prevalence is much lower, around 3%, in

C. Solanki (✉)
Marengo CIMS Hospital,, Ahmedabad, Gujarat, India

I. Shukla
Sterling Hospital, Ahmedabad, Gujarat, India

© The Author(s), under exclusive license to Springer Nature Singapore Pte Ltd. 2024
A. Agrawal et al. (eds.), *Special Considerations in Trauma Care*,
https://doi.org/10.1007/978-981-99-9662-9_19

patients with severe TBI [2]. This data was based on DSM-IV criteria, but limited data is available based on recently published DSM-V-TR. Based on DSM-V, the World Mental Health Survey in 24 countries showed an overall prevalence of 3.9%, although the numbers varied substantially among countries [3]. Accordingly, military veterans and people in occupations with a higher likelihood of traumatic exposure are expected to have higher incidence rates of PTSD. Studies have shown that gender has some influence on the development of PTSD, wherein male gender appears to be protective for the development of PTSD (prevalence rates in males vs females: 4–5.4% vs 8–11%) [3]. The exact reasons for such an association are not clear.

19.3 Diagnosis

As per DSM, the diagnostic criteria for PTSD are different for age groups: children <6 years, children >6 years, adolescents, and adults. In the present chapter, the diagnostic criteria for PTSD in adults are presented, and interested readers may look into the DSM manual for the diagnostic criteria for other age groups. Adults with PTSD can be diagnosed using the following DSM-V-TR criteria:

(a) A traumatic event should have been exposed to.
(b) Intrusion symptoms linked to a traumatic incident are present.
(c) Continuous avoiding of situations or people connected to the traumatic experience.
(d) Adverse changes brought on by the traumatic event in terms of thoughts and mood.
(e) Notable changes in reactivity and arousal related to the traumatic experience.
(f) Over a month has passed since the onset of symptoms.
(g) These symptoms produce a significant amount of distress or functional impairment.
(h) Medical conditions or drug effects on the body cannot be the cause of the disturbance.

19.4 Etiology and Pathophysiology

The etiology of PTSD can be classified into two accounts: neurobiological and behavioral. The neurobiological component of PTSD suggests that the neural circuits likely mediate the abnormalities in implicit learning. The neurobiological changes considered to cause this issue are as follows [4]:

- There is an inability to suppress attention to stimuli related to trauma because of inadequate frontal inhibition.
- The response of conditioned fear and reaction to potential threats occurs because of the excessive response of the amygdala.

- The inability to distinguish between safe and unsafe environments occurs secondary to the disturbances in the hippocampal function.

The behavioral part includes processing the previous traumatic event as a current threat due to active implicit memories of that event [5]. Therefore, any impending threat is appraised as the memory of the previous traumatic event, generating anxious behavior.

The following are the pathophysiological aspects of PTSD observed in several studies on neuroimaging.

- Atrophy of the hippocampus and anterior cingulate cortex, although inconsistently in PTSD patients, has been found in some of the structural imaging studies. Some have considered it either a stress-induced change or the reduced volume as a pre-trauma vulnerability factor [6].
- There is increased regional blood flow in the right superior temporal and parietal region. In addition, angular gyri white matte, prefrontal lobes, and anterior cingulate show reduced functional anisotropy [7].

19.5 Risk Factors of PTSD

The presentation of PTSD may be ambiguous, and the presence of risk factors for PTSD may help in the diagnosis of PTSD.

- Risk factors before the traumatic event: Marital status and gender are the strongest demographic predictors, with a higher risk of developing PTSD in women who are divorced or widowed [8].
  - Temperamental: Personality trait with negative responses like anxiety or depressed mood and premorbid trait impulsivity.
  - Environmental: Exposure to previous trauma, lower socioeconomic status, lower education, ethnic or racist discrimination, and family history of psychiatric illness.
  - Genetic and physiological: Epigenetic factors influence the susceptibility to PTSD, modestly inheritable, especially in twins.
- Peri-traumatic risk factors:
  - Environmental: varies according to the degree of trauma, perceived threat to one's life, personal injury, and interpersonal violence. For women, rape and sexual harassment/molestation are risk factors, while for men, battlefield veterans or those who have witnessed death or severe injury to someone can pose a risk of development of PTSD.
- Posttrauma risk factors:
  - Temperamental: After-trauma acute stress disorder development, negative evaluations, and improper coping mechanisms.

  - Environmental: The presence or experience of additional stressors following an initial traumatic event and inadequate social support in a later period may cause PTSD [9].
- Poor cognition: The pre-existing cognitive disturbances may reduce the capability of coping with stressors and make them vulnerable to PTSD [10].
- In case of patients with TBI, they are prone to develop PTSD after 6 months after injury [11]:
  - If they experience acute stress disorder, depression, or anxiety within a week of injury.
  - If they had a prior history of psychiatric disorders.
  - If they remembered the earlier traumatic events negatively.

19.6 Clinical Presentation of PTSD [12]

- Intrusion symptoms:
  - Repeated, unprovoked, bothersome, and upsetting memories of the traumatic incident in the past. They interrupt the patient's tasks and are abrupt and unwelcome.
  - Distressing nightmares or dreams about the traumatic event that occurs frequently.
  - Dissociative behavior is when someone acts or experiences an event as though it were happening right now, reoccurring like a flashback. Contact with current reality is weakened and, in severe situations, may be lost entirely.
  - Cues related to trauma can initiate intense physiological reactivity and psychological distress.
- Persistent avoidance:
  - A person constantly tries to avoid thoughts or feelings associated with the traumatic event.
  - Similarly, one tries to avoid situations or activities that might cause a recollection of the traumatic event.
- Maladaptive changes in cognition and mood:
  - Posttraumatic amnesia should be ruled out as the cause of the inability to remember a crucial component of the trauma.
  - Dysfunctional, persistent, and overly generalized beliefs about oneself, others, and the world.
  - Recurring and skewed blame thoughts.
  - Reduced interest in activities that are still accessible despite a physical impairment.
  - Feeling alienated or detached from other people.
  - Persistent lack of happy feelings.
  - Self-destructive conduct.
- Maladaptive changes in arousal and reactivity:
  - Sleep disturbances (initiation or maintenance)
  - Anger outbursts and irritability

- Lack of concentration
- Hypervigilance: constant perception of danger
- Exaggerated startle response

19.7 Differential Diagnosis of PTSD

- Adjustment disorder:
  - The stressor may be of mild or moderate severity as well, unlike PTSD.
  - The criteria for symptom stressors or symptom patterns do not meet that of PTSD criterion A.
- Acute stress disorder:
  - Unlike PTSD, the symptom pattern in acute stress disorder is restricted to a duration of 3 days to 3 months,
- Anxiety disorders and obsessive-compulsive disorder (OCD):
  - The frequent intrusive thoughts that fit the OCD criteria have nothing to do with traumatic experiences.
  - The traumatic event has nothing to do with the dissociative symptoms of panic disorder, arousal, avoidance, irritability, and anxiety of generalized anxiety disorder.
- Major depressive disorder:
  - It may or may not be preceded by a traumatic event.
  - It may co-exist with PTSD.
- Attention-deficit/hyperactivity disorder (ADHD):
  - In ADHD, symptom onset is before age 12 and not associated with exposure to trauma.
  - In PTSD, attention and concentration disruptions are attributable to hypervigilance and startle response.
- Personality disorders:
  - The interpersonal difficulties may not be associated with exposure to trauma.
- Dissociative disorders:
  - The dissociative symptoms may not be related to PTSD.

19.8 Evaluation of Symptoms

- Screening for PTSD: Self-reported questionnaires like PTSD may be used for screening patients suspected to have PTSD. The advantage is that it requires a short duration, and the clinician's involvement is not mandatory to complete the questionnaire. Self-reporting tends to be inaccurate and has poor specificity, so it should not be used as a diagnostic tool.
- Diagnostic tests:
  - Neuropsychological evaluation:

    It provides a detailed description of cognitive and emotional disturbances. In the presence of a pre-existing moderate or severe TBI, it may prove to be the diagnostic test.

- Structured interviews:
  It is the "gold standard" and test of choice for the diagnosis of PTSD. The drawback of the test is that the clinician's interview requires a long time to complete. Also, as inter-rater variability may exist, formally trained clinicians are essential for test reliability. The tools used in structural interviews are the Scale for DSM-V [13] and the Structured Clinical Interview for DSM-5 Disorders—Clinician Version (SCID-5-CV) [14].

19.9 Management of PTSD

19.9.1 Cognitive-Behavioral Treatment

The common fear structures and reactions serve as a template for appropriate and successful action in response to real-world threats, which makes them essential for survival. Specific pathological components are present in the traumatic memory in PTSD, according to the emotional processing theory. These unhealthy fear patterns could get in the way of everyday activities. They contain several stimulus components mistakenly interpreted as harmful, aberrant reflex physiological arousal, and behavioral responses.

- Exposure therapy:
  In a safe and encouraging setting, exposure therapy increases exposure to stimuli linked to traumatic events, which effectively lessens symptoms. Decreasing one of the main factors that sustain PTSD aids in preventing the negative reinforcement of cognitive and behavioral avoidance in response to memories or reminders of the traumatic events. Constantly being exposed to the trauma memory in the mind can also help people learn to distinguish between the past and the present and realize that thinking about trauma is not the same as experiencing it.
- Cognitive therapy:
  Experiences that lessen excessive fear and irrational expectations of harm are the goal of cognitive therapy. The patient benefits from cognitive therapy by gaining realistic viewpoints on the traumatic event and its memories. Although they employ different methods and varying levels of exposure, exposure and mental therapies, both aim to address the negative thoughts.

19.9.2 Solution-Focused Brief Therapy (SFBT) [15–17]

It is a method that works well for crises and trauma. People are helped by solution-focused (SF) interventions, which offer a secure and comforting therapeutic alliance. In addition to assisting patients to develop proper coping mechanisms and competencies, SFBT helps them balance their strong emotions in reaction to memories of traumatic experiences. It assists by creating small, gradual steps for the near future. SF interventions lessen the possibility of recurrent traumatization, increase an individual's resilience, and lessen distress.

According to the SFBT approach, people with PTSD are capable of overcoming hardship and growing, and they have the resources to lead more fulfilling lives. This idea is used with the patients during the discussion to help them become more resilient and capable of handling the fallout from a traumatic event, ultimately contributing to a fulfilling future and healthy living.

19.9.3 Pharmacotherapy

- Drugs acting on gamma-aminobutyric acid (GABA)-benzodiazepine receptor complex:
  - Benzodiazepines act on these receptors and help reduce anxiety. Gabapentin, a GABA analog, is also found to be beneficial. The GABA agonist, baclofen, is found to improve PTSD symptoms significantly.
  - The benzodiazepines are considered to provide temporary relief of symptoms. On the contrary, they may delay recovery or cause rebound and dependence.
- Drugs acting on norepinephrine(NE) and serotonin receptors:
  - There is a role of norepinephrine in chronic stress causing increased arousal to stress, PTSD, modulation of encoding memory, and the role of serotonin in anxiety; drugs acting on these receptors are used for PTSD.
  - Propranolol, a centrally acting beta-blocker, reduces autonomic hyperarousal and significantly reduces PTSD symptoms.
  - The two-receptor agonist, clonidine, by acting on NE cell bodies in locus coeruleus, reduces NE release centrally in the brain and benefits patients with PTSD. Prazosin, a centrally acting one blocker, reduces frontal lobe metabolism. Prazosin is considered for patients with PTSD, especially those who have nightmares, sleep disturbances, and daytime anxiety.
  - An anti-anxiety drug, buspirone, a serotonin agonist, is shown to improve PTSD and anxiety symptoms.
  - Cyproheptadine, an antihistamine with an antagonist effect on $5\text{-HT}_{2A\text{-}2B\text{-}2C}$ receptors, is also considered helpful for PTSD with nightmares.
  - Selective serotonin reuptake inhibitors, paroxetine, and sertraline are approved for the treatment of PTSD. Although fluvoxamine and escitalopram are also found to be effective, these agents have fewer anticholinergic side effects but higher sexual side effects.
  - A newer class of antidepressants with dual-uptake inhibitors, nefazodone, trazodone, and venlafaxine, tend to improve nightmares, sleep, and depressive symptoms, as well as other symptoms of PTSD.
- Tricyclic and monoamine oxidase (MAO) inhibitor antidepressants:
  - Tricyclic antidepressants affect the NE system and also have an anticholinergic effect, the reason behind side effects, like imipramine, have a positive effect on PTSD. Similarly, MAO inhibitor like phenelzine also improves PTSD symptoms.
  - On the contrary, amitriptyline, a tricyclic antidepressant, is not shown to have significant benefits for PTSD.

- Mood stabilizers:
  - Originally developed as antiepileptics, drugs such as carbamazepine, topiramate and tiagabine, phenytoin, and levetiracetam with mood stabilizing effects are helpful in PTSD by improving global function and intrusive and depressive symptoms.
- Atypical antipsychotic medications:
  - Atypical antipsychotics and neuroleptics (like olanzapine and quetiapine) due to metabolic and other potential side effects are only considered for predominant psychotic symptoms like irritability, anger, and aggression, if present, in PTSD.

19.9.4 Neuromodulation

Combining neuromodulation therapies with other treatment options is being investigated for PTSD that is resistant to treatment. By improving prefrontal inhibitory control over the amygdala, neuromodulation seeks to lessen the overreaction to unpleasant memories associated with trauma. It happens frequently that PTSD and major depressive disorder are linked. PTSD symptoms may also improve as a result of improvements in depressive symptoms. PTSD symptoms may be lessened if neuromodulation is used in conjunction with psychotherapy to improve extinction recall.

19.10 Transcranial Magnetic Stimulation (TMS)

When comparing the right dorsolateral prefrontal cortex (DLPFC) to the left, it has been demonstrated that TMS helps PTSD patients [18]. In general, the majority of the studies have shown significant benefits of TMS in PTSD as compared to sham stimulation and also when comparing the effect before and after stimulation [19–21]. The targets of the brain (e.g., G. DLPFC, dorsomedial prefrontal cortex, and medial prefrontal cortex) and the stimulation parameters employed in each study differed considerably. At intensities between 80% and 120% of the motor threshold, the TMS settings varied from 1 to 20 Hz. Although therapeutic responses were different TMS settings that used high and low frequency, a more significant effect was found with low frequency [22, 23]. TMS in combination with psychotherapy is shown to have substantial benefits compared to TMS alone [24–27]. The advantage of TMS is that it is a non-invasive therapy with minimal side effects like headache, insomnia, or mood disturbances, which can be managed by pharmacotherapy.

19.11 Transcranial Direct Current Stimulation (TDCS)

Though it substitutes constant low-energy direct current for TMS electromagnetic pulses, TDCS is a safe, non-invasive treatment that works similarly to TMS. It restores regular connectivity between malfunctioning neurons by changing local electrical activity in the target region of the brain. Most studies have demonstrated notable advantages of TDCS despite the paucity of available data [28–31]. The available studies have used different targets (e.g., prefrontal cortex, temporal cortex, etc.) without conclusive evidence of the superiority of one over the other. The same applies to the stimulation parameters, that is, current intensity, thresholds, and session duration, used in TDCS.

19.12 Vagus Nerve Stimulation (VNS)

The US Food and Drug Administration (USFDA) has approved implantable VNS devices for treatment-resistant. VNS may be particularly useful for stress-related psychiatric disorders by blocking sympathetic and immune responses to stressors and enhancing brain plasticity and cognition [32–36]. Another advantage is that transcutaneous cervical VNS (tcVNS) is an effective non-invasive technique. It also has a role in the rehabilitation of PTSD patients, apart from being an adjunct to exposure therapy.

19.13 Deep Brain Stimulation (DBS)

Unlike MS and TDCS, the DBS is an invasive procedure that modifies both local and distant neural activity by delivering an electric current to the deep regions of the brain through implanted electrodes. The USFDA has previously approved the DBS through a humanitarian exemption for major depressive disorder, Tourette syndrome, and obsessive-compulsive disorder (OCD); however, its overall use in psychiatric indications has been modest. Research on using DBS to target the basolateral nucleus of the amygdala (BLA) is ongoing. As of right now, DBS is still an experimental treatment for PTSD, with only a few case reports available.

19.14 Consequences of PTSD

Those suffering from PTSD experience significant impairment in physical, mental, social, and occupational functioning. The quality of life is also impaired. This impaired functioning also impacts the interpersonal, developmental, and educational spheres, resulting in low-income family and social relationships, absenteeism from work, decreased success in the workplace and school, and reduced income.

19.15 Conclusion

PTSD is a significant health issue faced by patients following a traumatic event. It significantly affects these patients' quality of life, taking a toll on physical, mental, personal, social, and occupational aspects of well-being. Identifying and diagnosing the issue early in the course of the disease is essential to start early treatment and achieve better outcomes. To date, cognitive behavioral therapy, along with pharmacotherapy, remains the mainstay of the treatment of PTSD. The neuromodulation therapies are reserved for pharmaco-resistant cases, with TMS being the most commonly used treatment option.

References

1. Kim E, Lauterbach EC, Reeve A, Arciniegas DB, Coburn KL, Mendez MF, et al. Neuropsychiatric complications of traumatic brain injury: a critical review of the literature (a report by the ANPA Committee on Research). J Neuropsychiatry Clin Neurosci. 2007;19(2):106–27.
2. American Psychiatric Association, editor. Diagnostic and statistical manual of mental disorders. 5th ed. Washington: American Psychiatric Association; 2022.
3. American Psychiatric Association. Trauma- and stressor-related disorders. In: Diagnostic and statistical manual of mental disorders. Washington: American Psychiatric Association Publishing; 2022.
4. Sherin JE, Nemeroff CB. Post-traumatic stress disorder: the neurobiological impact of psychological trauma. Dialogues Clin Neurosci. 2011;13(3):263.
5. Ehlers A, Clark DM. A cognitive model of posttraumatic stress disorder. Behav Res Ther. 2000;38(4):319–45.
6. Gilbertson MW, Shenton ME, Ciszewski A, Kasai K, Lasko NB, Orr SP, et al. Smaller hippocampal volume predicts pathologic vulnerability to psychological trauma. Nat Neurosci. 2002;5(11):1242–7.
7. Schuff N, Zhang Y, Zhan W, Lenoci M, Ching C, Boreta L, et al. Patterns of altered cortical perfusion and diminished subcortical integrity in posttraumatic stress disorder: a MRI study. NeuroImage. 2011;54(S1):S62.
8. Kessler RC, Sonnega A, Bromet E, Hughes M, Nelson CB. Posttraumatic stress disorder in the National Comorbidity Survey. Arch Gen Psychiatry. 1995;52(12):1048–60.
9. Brewin CR, Andrews B, Valentine JD. Meta-analysis of risk factors for posttraumatic stress disorder in trauma-exposed adults. J Consult Clin Psychol. 2000;68(5):748–66.
10. Parslow RA, Jorm AF. Pretrauma and posttrauma neurocognitive functioning and PTSD symptoms in a community sample of young adults. Am J Psychiatry. 2007;164(3):509–15.
11. Gil S, Caspi Y, Ben-Ari IZ, Koren D, Klein E. Does memory of a traumatic event increase the risk for posttraumatic stress disorder in patients with traumatic brain injury? A prospective study. Am J Psychiatry. 2005;162(5):963–9.
12. Larson EB, Belanger HG. Recognizing manifestations of posttraumatic stress disorder in patients with traumatic brain injury. In: Zollman FS, editor. Manual of traumatic brain injury. New York: Springer; 2021. p. 150–6.
13. Clinician-Administered PTSD Scale for DSM-5 (CAPS-5) - PTSD: National Center for PTSD [Internet]. [cited 2022 Jul 17]. Available from: https://www.ptsd.va.gov/professional/assessment/adult-int/caps.asp.
14. First MB. Structured clinical interview for DSM-5 disorders—clinician version (SCID-5-CV). Arlington: American Psychiatric Association Publishing; 2015.
15. Froerer A, Cziffra-Bergs J, Kim JS, Connie EE. Solution-focused brief therapy with clients managing trauma. Oxford: Oxford University Press; 2018. p. 1–252.
16. Bannink FP. Solution-focused brief therapy. J Contemp Psychother. 2007;37(2):87–94.
17. Babu S, Ramesh B. Solution focused brief therapy in the indian context: a review. In: International Conference on Solution Focused Practices. 2016.
18. Boggio PS, Rocha M, Oliveira MO, Fecteau S, Cohen RB, Campanhã C, et al. Noninvasive brain stimulation with high-frequency and low-intensity repetitive transcranial magnetic stimulation treatment for posttraumatic stress disorder. J Clin Psychiatry. 2010;71(8):992–9.

19. Nam DH, Pae CU, Chae JH. Low-frequency, repetitive transcranial magnetic stimulation for the treatment of patients with posttraumatic stress disorder: a double-blind, Sham-controlled study. Clin Psychopharmacol Neurosci. 2013;11(2):96–102.
20. Philip NS, Barredo J, Aiken E, Larson V, Jones RN, Tracie Shea M, et al. Theta-burst transcranial magnetic stimulation for posttraumatic stress disorder. Am J Psychiatry. 2019;176(11):939–48.
21. Watts BV, Landon B, Groft A, Young-Xu Y. A sham controlled study of repetitive transcranial magnetic stimulation for posttraumatic stress disorder. Brain Stimul. 2012;5(1):38–43.
22. Kozel FA, van Trees K, Larson V, Phillips S, Hashimie J, Gadbois B, et al. One hertz versus ten hertz repetitive TMS treatment of PTSD: a randomized clinical trial. Psychiatry Res. 2019;273:153–62.
23. Cohen H, Kaplan Z, Kotler M, Kouperman I, Moisa R, Grisaru N. Repetitive transcranial magnetic stimulation of the right dorsolateral prefrontal cortex in posttraumatic stress disorder: a double-blind, placebo-controlled study. Am J Psychiatry. 2004;161(3):515–24.
24. Isserles M, Shalev AY, Roth Y, Peri T, Kutz I, Zlotnick E, et al. Effectiveness of deep transcranial magnetic stimulation combined with a brief exposure procedure in post-traumatic stress disorder–a pilot study. Brain Stimul. 2013;6(3):377–83.
25. Osuch EA, Benson BE, Luckenbaugh DA, Geraci M, Post RM, McCann U. Repetitive TMS combined with exposure therapy for PTSD: a preliminary study. J Anxiety Disord. 2009;23(1):54–9.
26. Kozel FA, Motes MA, Didehbani N, DeLaRosa B, Bass C, Schraufnagel CD, et al. Repetitive TMS to augment cognitive processing therapy in combat veterans of recent conflicts with PTSD: a randomized clinical trial. J Affect Disord. 2018;229:506–14.
27. Fryml LD, Pelic CG, Acierno R, Tuerk P, Yoder M, Borckardt JJ, et al. Exposure therapy and simultaneous repetitive transcranial magnetic stimulation: a controlled pilot trial for the treatment of posttraumatic stress disorder. J ECT. 2019;35(1):53–60.
28. van't Wout-Frank M, Shea MT, Larson VC, Greenberg BD, Philip NS. Combined transcranial direct current stimulation with virtual reality exposure for posttraumatic stress disorder: feasibility and pilot results. Brain Stimul. 2019;12(1):41–3.
29. van't Wout M, Longo SM, Reddy MK, Philip NS, Bowker MT, Greenberg BD. Transcranial direct current stimulation may modulate extinction memory in posttraumatic stress disorder. Brain Behav. 2017;7(5):681.
30. Saunders N, Downham R, Turman B, Kropotov J, Clark R, Yumash R, et al. Working memory training with tDCS improves behavioral and neurophysiological symptoms in pilot group with post-traumatic stress disorder (PTSD) and with poor working memory. Neurocase. 2015;21(3):271–8.
31. Ahmadizadeh MJ, Rezaei M, Fitzgerald PB. Transcranial direct current stimulation (tDCS) for post-traumatic stress disorder (PTSD): a randomized, double-blinded, controlled trial. Brain Res Bull. 2019;153:273–8.
32. Bansal V, Ryu SY, Lopez N, Allexan S, Krzyzaniak M, Eliceiri B, et al. Vagal stimulation modulates inflammation through a ghrelin mediated mechanism in traumatic brain injury. Inflammation. 2012;35(1):214–20.
33. Borovikova LV, Ivanova S, Zhang M, Yang H, Botchkina GI, Watkins LR, et al. Vagus nerve stimulation attenuates the systemic inflammatory response to endotoxin. Nature. 2000;405(6785):458–62.
34. Schomer AC, Nearing BD, Schachter SC, Verrier RL. Vagus nerve stimulation reduces cardiac electrical instability assessed by quantitative T-wave alternans analysis in patients with drug-resistant focal epilepsy. Epilepsia. 2014;55(12):1996–2002.
35. Peña DF, Engineer ND, McIntyre CK. Rapid remission of conditioned fear expression with extinction training paired with vagus nerve stimulation. Biol Psychiatry. 2013;73(11):1071–7.
36. PeñA DF, Childs JE, Willett S, Vital A, McIntyre CK, Kroener S. Vagus nerve stimulation enhances extinction of conditioned fear and modulates plasticity in the pathway from the ventromedial prefrontal cortex to the Amygdala. Front Behav Neurosci. 2014;8:327.

Rehabilitation Aspects in Trauma Patients

20

Rishabh Kumar Rana

20.1 Introduction

Thousands of years ago, Chinese people employed Cong Fu, a movement technique to alleviate pain, while Greeks used gymnastics to treat and prevent diseases. However, it was not until late in the fifteenth century that Mercurialis suggested gymnastics as a preventative and restorative therapy in 1569. The first use of the word "rehabilitation" was perhaps used for the first time in these treatises [1].

The first definition of the word "rehabilitation" was given by the British Council for Rehabilitation in 1944 as "the whole range of services from the time of the onset of the individual's disability to the point at which he is restored to normal activity or the nearest possible approach to it" [2].

Prior to the 1944 definition, however, a past President of the United States certainly had a role to play, as documented in the detailed account by Richard Emery et al. It gives us a glimpse of how young Franklin Delano Rosevelt, who would go on to become the 32nd US president, was treated in Warm Springs when he was infected with polio and relied heavily on the local natural resources to fully recover and walk without crutches or braces. This was possibly the starting point for the significance of rehabilitation. And indeed, it is well documented as one of the possible reasons for his victory owing to the models he developed through his own experience in warm springs across the country for other polio-afflicted patients. Also, his recovery is remarkable and notable as in those times it was easy for anyone with any disability to be ridiculed and sidelined by society [3].

R. K. Rana (✉)
Department of Preventive and Social Medicine/Community Medicine, Shaheed Nirmal Mahto Medical College and Hospital, Dhanbad, Jharkhand, India; https://drrishabhkumarrana.com

© The Author(s), under exclusive license to Springer Nature Singapore Pte Ltd. 2024
A. Agrawal et al. (eds.), *Special Considerations in Trauma Care*, https://doi.org/10.1007/978-981-99-9662-9_20

20.2 Historical Perspective

It was the Renaissance period that aimed to rehabilitate the wartimes disabled individuals. Two books of the times "De humani corporis fabrica" (On the Fabric of the Human Body) and "De Arte Gymnastica" (The Art of Gymnastics) detailed many aspects of human anatomy and were keen on improving the lives of persons with disability. They also talked about medical gymnastics for the prevention of disabilities. They were detailed about various rehabilitative options to keep oneself functional if they had disabilities [4, 5]. Another name of repute in the same era was a French surgeon, tasked with caring for soldiers, popularly known as the "Barber Surgeon." He is considered by many as the father of surgery. He promoted the use of prosthetics which were light in weight and made of leather and wood [6, 7].

After the Renaissance in the seventeenth century, noted works by the French physician Nicolas Andry de Bois-Regard (1658–1742) who linked medical rehabilitation with correct exercise in his seminal work "Traité d'orthopédie" (Treatise on Orthopaedics,1741). He gave the term Orthopedics and asserted the role of health in the maintenance of health [8].

In his work "Gymnastique Médicinale et Chirurgicale," Tissot (1747–1826) later went on to establish how timely movement was necessary for quick surgical healing, contrary to the popular belief in those times, which was more inclined toward bed rest, in his work "Gymnastique Médicinale et Chirurgicale." His work documented rehabilitative management for hemiplegic patients [9].

The above-quoted works met with stiff resistance as they were not as per the popular belief of those times. It took many other individuals to convince their contemporaries about the rehabilitative models proposed, the role of exercise, and so on [4].

The "Muscle sense," which links the nervous system, muscles, and the brain, was first described by Charles Bell in the nineteenth century. Bell's work helped to improve our understanding of the feedback system. While works by Johannes Karl Eugen Alfred Goldscheider and Fulgence Raymond were definitive in understanding the management of disabled patients and the successful implementation of various functional rehabilitation techniques [10].

As we move ahead in time, in the 1920s, Zander Rooms in Massechutes General Hospital needed special mention. The wars were the biggest source of the disabled needing rehabilitative service, while the rise of polio in those times was another reason for the rise in demand for rehabilitative service. The Zander Rooms hosted many machines and instruments and were afterward enriched with UV therapy and hydrotherapy facilities. In a re-educational context, the Zander room's equipment served as tools to support the performance of human body movements [11].

In the European hemisphere, a new concept rose to prominence known as the Bobath Concept, which faced hurdles. The Bobath concept in 1948 emphasized that the whole rehabilitative management of the patient involves everyone linked with the patient, from his family to carers, from medical specialists to other health workers, to guarantee a daily, all-day treatment. It was perhaps among the first approaches that prompted the definition as given in the earlier portion to take its current form.

In modern medicine, the Bobath concept has been applied to cerebral palsy, stroke, and cardiac patients for best outcomes [12].

Rapid mobilization of surgical patients in the absence of contraindications has now emerged as one of the cornerstones of rehabilitative postsurgical treatment. Gradually, from the 1950s onward, the philosophy of structured movement experienced a boost [13].

In their work, Nancy et al. further went on to clarify the various principles of rehabilitation. She further argued that in traditional medical management, the physician assumes an authoritative role while the patient is a passive receiver. She explains how, in the rehabilitation model, the emphasis lies on the disability instead of the person, on the handicap that has been produced. The patient has an active role in learning to maximize his potential with his diminished abilities while minimizing the impairments and disabilities. The physician plays a double role, acting on the medical model to minimize the disease and acting as a teacher, facilitator, and coordinator with the rehabilitation team. Emphasis is on the two components: interrelationships and interaction. A whole list of possible members is given, ranging from physicians, nurses, physical therapists, occupational therapists, psychologists, language pathologists, and social workers, with their detailed roles. This work nicely sums up the principles of rehabilitation after trauma for various settings and is in sync with the earlier quoted Bobath Concept [14].

20.3 Problem Statement

As per the World Health Organization (WHO), "Rehabilitation is the care needed when a person is experiencing or is likely to experience limitations in everyday functioning due to aging or a health condition, including chronic diseases or disorders, injuries, or traumas" [15].

According to the most recent research, rehabilitation is most commonly required in disorders such as muscular-skeletal disorders, neurological disorders, sensory impairments, mental disorders, chronic respiratory diseases, cardiovascular diseases, and neoplasms. Among musculoskeletal disorders according to the hierarchy of prevalence are these disorders: Low back pain, neck pain, fractures, other injuries, osteoarthritis, amputation, and rheumatoid arthritis are the major ones requiring rehabilitation, while, among neurological disorders, cerebral palsy, stroke, traumatic brain damage, Alzheimer's disease, spinal cord trauma, Parkinson's disease, multiple sclerosis, motor neuron disease, and GB syndrome are the major disorders needing rehabilitation. In 2020, estimates suggested that 2.41 billion people with a wide range of medical conditions need rehabilitation as a result of these diseases, which require rehabilitation. This number is only going to go up by all estimates due to the long-term illness/prolonged consequence of COVID-19. Trauma encompasses a wide range of ailments which can be mental, social, or physical, ranging from emotional conflicts and stress to fractures [16].

Rehabilitation plans for rehabilitative strategies: Rehabilitation is advised for COVID-19 patients who present with respiratory failure in order to improve health outcomes during the acute phase of care. There are, however, a number of clinical manifestations that might necessitate rehabilitation outside of acute care, like (a) post-intensive care syndrome, (b) complications from acute illness in COVID-19 like ischemic stroke and ischemic heart stroke, and (c) post-COVID-19 conditions including fatigue, shortness of breath, and, in some cases, loss of cognitive functions.

Rehabilitation for people experiencing severe problems or a protracted course of post-COVID-19: Most likely, the condition necessitates the use of interventions that are person-centered, all-inclusive, and multidisciplinary and are delivered in close coordination with primary healthcare and a number of medical specialties. Advice on resumed activities, breathing exercises, exercise therapy, psychological interventions, cognitive training, rehabilitation for communication and swallowing issues, and occupational rehabilitation are just a few examples of rehabilitation interventions [17].

20.4 Rehabilitative in Musculoskeletal Disorders (Need for a Framework Based on Various Aspects)

Primarily, rehabilitation is given as physiotherapy in most musculoskeletal fracture cases.

Generally, it is done with the aim of maximizing autonomous efficiency and minimizing complications such as wound bacterial infection, deep vein thrombosis, pulmonary emboli, and hip dislocation (for hip replacements). For example, in cases of hip replacement, the activities of daily living (ADL) instruction, gait training, transfer training, and therapeutic exercise make up the four parts of the physiotherapy rehabilitation program [18]. Following physiotherapy as the rehabilitation therapy, the other modality given is occupational therapy. There is a new concept of prehabilitation as well. Evidence regarding the outcomes is more inclined toward the previous functional status [19].

20.5 Various Facets of Rehabilitation

Ongoing through this short narrative about one disorder of the musculoskeletal system, it is obvious that a framework is a must so that it can be decided what should be the core values around which rehabilitation services will depend. What competencies will be required? What activities need to be prioritized? What beliefs are needed to move ahead, which is best in the interests of patients and caregivers? Also, it is important to understand that rehabilitation, being a team effort, needs resources in the form of appropriate infrastructure, trained manpower, and economic capacity to hire the services, upkeep the logistics, and maintain them for a long period of time. Indeed, such is the scenario where resources at hand and the economy decide the quality of rehabilitation programs, as evidenced by Jesus et al. in their work. They put forward their argument as a "chasm in rehabilitation" as evidenced by (1) the absence of rehabilitation in global quality of care reports; (b) concerns about care quality in low- and middle-income countries (LMICs) have been ignored by rehabilitation-specific literature; and (c) structural issues with the healthcare and rehabilitation delivery systems. As is known, most systems in LMIC are in shambles, riddled with corruption, poor data quality, and upkeep, along with other issues [20, 21].

20.6 The WHO Rehabilitation Competencies Framework RCF (An Ideal Solution for All Settings)

A competency framework that harmonizes rehabilitation competencies and captures the breadth of rehabilitation activities, provides a common language, and is applicable to both low- and high-resource settings is urgently needed. As mentioned, there are various aspects to the proper functioning of rehabilitation across resource settings of two extremes. The competency framework attempts to provide answers to these questions. What are the fundamental values, beliefs, skills, behaviors, tasks, activities, and knowledge required by the rehabilitation workforce? The framework is novel because it aims to include all rehabilitation professions, specializations, and settings. This will be good for all rehabilitation service providers, including workers from audiology, occupational therapy, physical and rehabilitation medicine, physiotherapy, prosthetics and orthotics, psychology, rehabilitation nursing, speech and language therapy, and researchers [22].

20.7 What Is in the RCF? [23]

The Rehabilitation Competency Framework (RCF) is a patient-centric model that conveys the anticipated or desired *performance of the rehabilitation workforce* across professions, specializations, and settings to enable the provision of high-quality care and services (Fig. 20.1). The "adopt and adapt" methodology, which allows competency framework developers to adopt the structure and language of the RCF and adapt the content to their situation and needs, is primarily used to facilitate the development of context-specific competency frameworks. RCF is useful to all rehabilitation specialists, services, and settings; the core values and beliefs and competencies, as well as the behaviors through which these are expressed, can be considered cross-cutting and applicable to all rehabilitation workers. The activities and the tasks might vary according to specialization. The RCF should only be contextualized using the activities and tasks that are pertinent to the workforce of the developing organization. The whole work has been divided into five thematic domains, namely: (1) Practice; (2) Professionalism; (3) Education; (4) Development, Management, and Leadership; and (5) Research.

Each domain includes four core values and beliefs: (1) competencies, and the behaviors through which they are expressed; (2) activities; (3) the tasks that they encompass; and (4) knowledge and skills.

Competencies vary for the five domains.

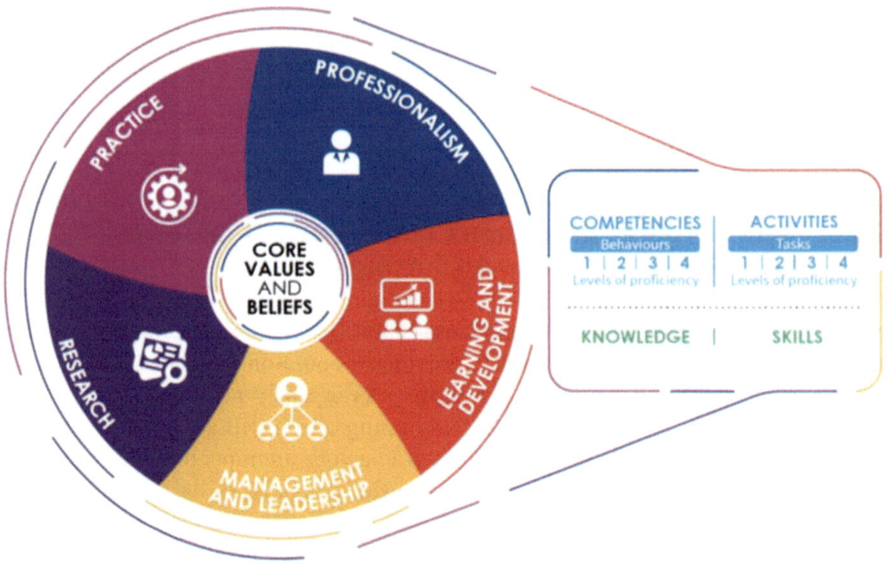

Fig. 20.1 WHO Competency Framework [23] (available at https://www.who.int/multi-media/details/rehabilitation-competency-framework)

For the *first domain of practice, five* competencies are (Fig. 20.1)

C1. Places the person and their family at the center of practice

C2. Establishes a collaborative relationship with the person and their family

C3. Communicates effectively with the person, their family, and their healthcare team

C4. Adopts a rigorous approach to problem-solving and decision-making

C5. Works within the scope of practice and competence, while the listed activities are

A1. Obtaining informed consent for rehabilitation

A2. Documenting information

A3. Conducting rehabilitation assessments

A4. Developing and adapting rehabilitation plans

A5. Referring to other providers

A6. Implementing rehabilitation interventions

A7. Evaluating progress toward desired outcomes

A8. Discharging and ensuring appropriate continuity of care

The rehabilitation workers are supposed to be working as an independent, to grade their work, various levels of practice proficiencies have been assigned, level 4 being the highest where he can work autonomously and can (1) prescribe rehabilitation interventions, (2) make decisions regarding rehabilitation plans, and (3) has a specialist level of relevant knowledge and skills that are applied when working with people with highly complex needs and their families. Similar roles have been given for other competencies and thematic areas.

20.8 What Exists in the Indian Context of Community Settings/Resource-Constrained Settings?

As can be seen after going through the framework, it is quite exhaustive and of recent origin!!! Readers must be inquisitive about what is going on currently in cases of rehabilitation needed after trauma. What is happening in our hinterlands? What is happening to those who were afflicted by floods, who suffered mental trauma after the death of near and dear ones, what is happening to those who lost everything in disasters of natural origin, etc.? It is also a paradigm shift from the earlier accepted community-based rehabilitation (CBR) and its shortcomings in the Indian context as evidenced in terms of inadequate knowledge about competencies which is affecting the service delivery coupled with poor capacity building [24].

In 1976, the World Health Assembly passed a resolution endorsing and promoting the incorporation of rehabilitation into all tiers of health care, particularly primary care. Plans for rehabilitation must be individualized, goal-oriented, and achievable. A person's interests, age, gender, financial situation, and home environment must be considered while creating a plan. A long-term vision with short-term targets is required due to the lengthy nature of rehabilitation [25]. It has been documented that in India prior to the 1980s, people with disabilities (PWDs) were largely considered non-significant members of society, and their management was mostly focused on treatment aspects. Such management reinforces a culture of dependency. Through education and training, the need to integrate PWDs into society was recognized in the 1980s. The government and rehabilitation organizations realized that they needed to mobilize local resources and support to keep disability rehabilitation programs running during the Decade of Disabled Persons (1983–1992). It was understood that the culture of dependency is directly causing a huge loss in the workforce and that the model needs a change [26]. The earliest intervention by the Government of India was started as the District Rehabilitation Center Project. (1985). This was slowly leveraged up with the establishment of various national institutes and regional rehabilitation centers. The Persons with Disability Act, passed in 1995, was a robust act that further paved the way for the better integration of rehabilitation courses into the national framework. In 2000, GOI launched District Disability Rehabilitation Centers. This was further enhanced with the launch of the National Policy for Persons with Disability in 2005 [27].

20.8.1 WHO CBR Program 2010

WHO published a document describing CBR in 2010. In addition to the PWD's own initiatives, those of their families, communities, and the pertinent governmental and non-governmental health, educational, vocational, social, and other services, CBR is implemented through a collaborative effort between all of these groups. CBR is delivered within the community using predominantly local resources. It has five key components: health, education, livelihood, social, and empowerment [28, 29]. An exhaustive review done by Valentia Lemmi et al. published in 2015 proved the effectiveness of CBR on various fronts spanning various countries with limited resource settings, including India, ranging from arthritis, Chronic Obstructive Pulmonary Disease (COPD), schizophrenia, and dementia [30]. To date in India, various government initiatives have been launched with a focus on five components of CBR and effects have been visible on the ground as we can see more PWDs coming into the mainstream and giving their maximum in building the nation. Most published evidence suggests that CBR was in India in its early infancy till now [31]: (a) lack of cooperation from families of persons with disabilities, (b) engagement in helping CBR workers by the government agencies deal with problems they experience, let alone intervene in any way, and (c) a shortage of trained manpower, logistics, including funding resources for the processes to be done on the ground, has been cited as the major barriers for the program's success in India. One of the bottlenecks documents has been running of the different ministries in the vertical stream. The two ministries, the Ministry of Social Justice and Empowerment and the Ministry of Health and Family Welfare, are running vertically, whereas any patient facing trauma needing rehabilitation services first visits the hospitals for all rehabilitative needs [32].

After COVID-19, with all the focus shifting toward the pandemic, it will be no wonder if the CBR initiatives still stay in their infancy. With the effects of long-term COVID-19, which for many patients might end up with trauma in various aspects such as stress, post-recovery from ICU admission, lung damage, diabetes, and so on, in all these conditions, patients might need rehabilitation as well [17]. Now is the right time for Governments to imbibe both the CBR and RCF and adopt a comprehensive policy for best results. A matrix taken from the CBR guidelines has been included in the text as Fig. 20.2 for enhanced reading of the concept [33].

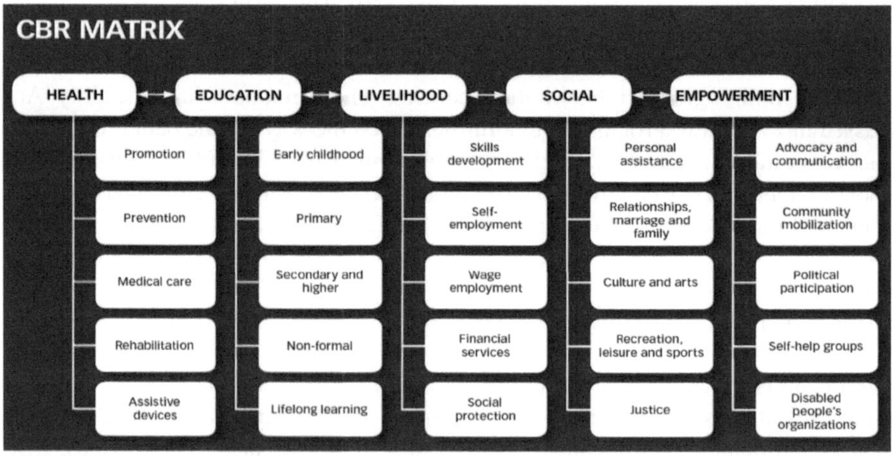

Fig. 20.2 Community-based matrix eliciting how health, education, livelihood, societal incorporation, and empowerment play a key role in rehabilitation services for all patients needing rehabilitation services after any trauma [33]

20.9 Way Ahead !!

With the Rehabilitation Framework coming up, we need a more balanced approach with a focus on intercoordinated medical teams and social structure with willpower from policymakers at the top for the best possible outcome. Prioritizing resources such as money, trained and motivated manpower, and supplies of various logistics needed is a crucial consideration. Priority-wise resolution of major problems such as lack of available evidence, poor coordination among the government and non-governmental organizations, lack of a defined community-level approach, low expertise and capability for service distribution, and nonexistent models to emulate best practices needs to be addressed for achieving desired outcomes. A multisectoral strategy that incorporates social integration efforts, health and education programs, and vocational training possibilities are essential components of rehabilitation services. The primary health care system must play an important role as both a provider and a supporter, engaging in initiatives such as early identification of impairments and provision of basic interventions, referrals to specialized services such as physical, occupational, and speech therapies, prosthetics and orthotics, and corrective surgeries. As cited earlier, rural health in India plays a pivotal role in overall healthcare delivery. This role is mostly played by primary healthcare settings in facilities such as health subcenter, primary healthcare centers, and health wellness centers spread across the country. These centers are providers and supporters of health as a package; therefore, for rehabilitation services to penetrate the last mile individual, the primary health care system must play an important role. All efforts must be ensured so that the staff attending these centers are able to understand the competencies they are required to have and understand the thematic expertise that is demanded in their jobs for them to provide optimum services. Making classrooms, facilities, and instructional materials more accessible is a crucial step in creating a more inclusive educational system for individuals of all abilities. This is one of the most significant steps toward a more inclusive educational system. Creative, context-specific solutions may allow the child with multiple or severe disabilities to attend school, even if they require considerable additional support. To guarantee that people of all ages who are disabled have access to education and job opportunities in their local communities, it is crucial to coordinate efforts with the employment and labor sectors. This encompasses adolescents and adults. The Government of India has been promoting various schemes that have been designed keeping in mind the above-cited core principles. Be it the reservation policy in various vacancies for PWDs, "Divyang" friendly hospital entrances as mandated by the Kayakalp program, toilets that are easy for PWDs in various government-run public facilities such as railways, religious places, and so on. These initiatives have still not taken place effectively across the country. More monitoring, more proactiveness, more inclusion, and more innovative research, perhaps, is the best way forward. The WHO's latest initiative "Rehabilitation in health system: A call to action 2030" has been suggested as further reading for health systems revamp, to incorporate rehab services in a way that the CBR and RCF can be imbibed in health systems across countries.

References

1. Dreeben O. Introduction to physical therapy for physical therapist assistants. In: Development of the physical therapy profession. Sudbury: Jones & Bartlett Publishers; 2007. p. 3–22.
2. Gensini GF, Conti AA. Rehabilitation in the elderly: differentiated strategies and objectives? Ital Heart J. 2003;4:73S–5S.
3. Verville RE, Ditunno JF. Franklin Delano Roosevelt, polio, and the warm springs experiment: its impact on physical medicine and rehabilitation. PMR. 2013;5:3–8.
4. Conti AA. Reconstructing medical history: historiographical features, approaches and challenges. Clin Ter. 2011;162:133–6.
5. Mercurialis H. De Arte Gymnastica Libri Sex, in Quibus Exercitationum Omnium Vetustarum Genera-et.../Hieronymi Mercurialis.
6. Popa CC, Marinescu AA, Mohan AG, et al. Remember: Ambroise Paré (1510-1590) - message for young surgeons. Romanian J Morphol Embryol. 2018;59:637–40.
7. Thurston AJ. Paré and prosthetics: the early history of artificial limbs. ANZ J Surg. 2007;77:1114–9.
8. de Boisregard A. L'orthopédie ou l'art de prévenir et de corriger dans les enfants les difformités du corps. Alix, 1741.
9. Tissot C-J. Gymnastique médicinale et chirurgicale. Bastian, 1780.
10. Opitz JL, Folz TJ, Gelfman R, et al. The history of physical medicine and rehabilitation as recorded in the diary of Dr. Frank Krusen: Part 1. Gathering momentum (the years before 1942). Arch Phys Med Rehabil. 1997;78:442–5.
11. Lippi D, Conti AA. Storia della Medicina per il Corso di Laurea triennale in Fisioterapia. CLUEB Bologna, Italy, 2007.
12. Cosmacini G, Sironi VA. La mia baracca: storia della fondazione Don Gnocchi. Laterza, 2004.
13. Macchi C, Fattirolli F, Lova RM, et al. Early and late rehabilitation and physical training in elderly patients after cardiac surgery. Am J Phys Med Rehabil. 2007;86:826–34.
14. Cobble N, Burks JS. Introduction to principles of rehabilitation. J Neuroeng Rehabil. 1990;4:181–5.
15. Krug E, Cieza A. Strengthening health systems to provide rehabilitation services. Bull World Health Organ. 2017;95:167.
16. Cieza A, Causey K, Kamenov K, et al. Global estimates of the need for rehabilitation based on the Global Burden of Disease study 2019: a systematic analysis for the Global Burden of Disease Study 2019. Lancet. 2020;396:2006–17.
17. WHO.int. Rehabilitation needs of people recovering from COVID-19: Scientific brief, 29 November 2021. https://www.who.int/publications/i/item/WHO-2019-nCoV-Sci-Brief-Rehabilitation-2021.1. Accessed 31 July 2022.
18. Bitar AA, Kaplan RJ, Stitik TP, et al. Rehabilitation of orthopedic and rheumatologic disorders. 3. Total hip arthroplasty rehabilitation. Arch Phys Med Rehabil. 2005;86:56–60.
19. Lucas B. Does a pre-operative exercise programme improve mobility and function post-total knee replacement: a mini-review. J Orthop Nurs. 2004;8:25–33.
20. Jesus TS, Hoenig H. Crossing the global quality chasm in health care: where does rehabilitation stand? Arch Phys Med Rehabil. 2019;100:2215–7.
21. Gans BM. Evolving models of rehabilitation-related patient safety and quality: PIECES. Arch Phys Med Rehabil. 2018;99:1033–4.
22. Mills J-A, Cieza A, Short SD, et al. Development and validation of the WHO rehabilitation competency framework: a mixed methods study. Arch Phys Med Rehabil. 2021;102:1113–23.
23. WHO.int. Rehabilitation competency framework. rehabilitation competency framework; 2021, p. 2–23.
24. Gale L, Gillis S, Grills N. Determining the vocational competencies required to deliver community-based rehabilitation and inclusive development services in India. Disabil Rehabil. 2021:1–15.

25. Srivastava AK. Rehabilitation of rural disabled — an experience. J Physio-Occup Ther Rehabil. 1976;1:23–8.
26. Srivastava AK, Baipai P. Community-based rehabilitation: the Indian perspective. World Fed Occup Ther Bull. 2005;52:39–44.
27. Kumar S, Roy G, Kar S. Disability and rehabilitation services in India: issues and challenges. J Family Med Prim Care. 2012;1:69.
28. Khasnabis C, Heinicke Motsch K, Achu K, et al. Community-based rehabilitation: CBR guidelines. 1st ed. Geneva: World Health Organization; 2010.
29. www.afri-can.org. Afri-can.org. 2022. Community_Based_Rehabilitation_Protocol. 2012, p. 3–23.
30. Iemmi V, Kumar KS, Blanchet K, et al. Community-based rehabilitation for people with physical and mental disabilities in low- and middle-income countries. Cochrane Database Syst Rev 2017; 2017: CD010617. DOI: https://doi.org/10.1002/14651858.CD010617.pub2.
31. Sanjay PK. A brief overview of community based rehabilitation for severe mentally ill: an Indian perspectives. Int J Indian Psychol. 2021;9:1461–8.
32. Senjam S, Singh A. Addressing the health needs of people with disabilities in India. Indian J Public Health. 2020;64:79.
33. WHO.int. Community based rehabilitation 2010. Community-based rehabilitation: CBR guidelines., https://www.who.int/publications/i/item/WHO-2019-nCoV-Sci-Brief-Rehabilitation-2021.1. Accessed 29 July 2022.

Further Reading

Community Based Rehabilitation 2010 Who.int. 2022. Community-based rehabilitation: CBR guidelines. https://www.who.int/publications/i/item/9789241548052. Accessed 31 July 2022.

Kayakalp Guidelines Qi.nhsrcindia.org. 2022. http://qi.nhsrcindia.org/sites/default/files/Kayakalp_2021%20%28with%20eco%20friendly%29.pdf. Accessed 31 July 2022.

Lemmi, V., Gibson, L., Blanchet, K., Kumar, K., Rath, S., Hartley, S., Murthy, G., Patel, V., Weber, J. and Kuper, H., 2015. Community-based rehabilitation for people with disabilities in low- and middle-income countries: a systematic review. Campbell Syst Rev, 11(1), pp. 1-177.

Rehabilitation in health systems: a call to action 2030. Rehabilitation 2030 Call for an action plan. https://www.who.int/multi-media/details/rehabilitation-in-health-systems-guide-for-action. Accessed 31 July 2022.

Who.int. 2022. Rehabilitation Competency Framework. [online]. https://www.who.int/multi-media/details/rehabilitation-competency-framework.

Community Integration and Holistic Rehabilitation for Traumatic Brain Injuries

21

Vinoth Rajendran, Ankit Mittal, and Neeti Rustagi

21.1 Introduction

One of the leading causes of mortality and disability worldwide is traumatic brain injury (TBI), sometimes known as the "silent pandemic" [1, 2]. According to an estimate, every year, 69 million people (95% confidence interval (CI): 64–74 million) experience TBI incidents. Further, low and middle-income countries experience around three times as many TBI instances as high-income countries [1]. TBI is a complex condition of significant public health importance. TBI can have a variety of negative physical, cognitive, and emotional effects that need specialized care. The physical and emotional effects of TBI can last for a very long time, which increases the financial and health care burden [3]. The chronic health condition that results from the long-term effects of TBI comprises several neurological conditions, such as epilepsy, stroke, and neurodegenerative disease [4]. The diversity of TBI and the use of overly simplified approaches for describing its initial type and severity impede efforts to individualize treatment. To maximize recovery outcomes, people with TBI need rehabilitation therapies tailored to their requirements as well as community-based nonmedical interventions. Throughout the whole recovery process, both the TBI patient and their social support systems should have access to rehabilitation services, and the services needed will change as per the patient's needs [5]. Recent advancements in TBI rehabilitation include task-specific training for cognitive decline, computer-assisted cognitive rehabilitation, visual-spatial and visual scanning techniques, and body weight-supported treadmill training for motor deficits [6].

V. Rajendran · A. Mittal · N. Rustagi (✉)
Department of Community Medicine and Family Medicine, All India Institute of Medical Sciences (AIIMS), Jodhpur, India

© The Author(s), under exclusive license to Springer Nature Singapore Pte Ltd. 2024

A. Agrawal et al. (eds.), *Special Considerations in Trauma Care*,
https://doi.org/10.1007/978-981-99-9662-9_21

21.2 An Overview of Rehabilitation After Traumatic Brain Injury

Broadly speaking, rehabilitation entails "a problem-solving educational process aimed at reducing disability and handicap experienced as a result of disease or injury" [6, 7]. The objective is to assist individuals in returning to their pre-injury level of functioning as much as possible within the confines of any lingering physical, functional, or cognitive limitations [6]. Post-TBI, rehabilitation should start early at the level of acute care [8]. TBI has long-lasting impacts, and patients and their families frequently need constant care and assistance for the rest of their lives. When continual support and supervision are made accessible to individuals who need it, rehabilitation has the best long-term results [8]. Studies show that undergoing rehabilitation at the earliest stages of TBI enhances cognition, perception, and motor recovery and resulted in shorter lengths of stay (LOS) in rehabilitation facilities [9, 10]. Figure 21.1 shows the schematic representation of the rehabilitation after traumatic brain injuries [8].

Rehabilitation services, where available can be institution-based, outreach programs or community-based integration. The different types of rehabilitation serve a particular purpose as they help in the patient's recovery with the common goal of assisting them in leading a healthy and active lifestyle. The salient features differentiating among various types of rehabilitation services are provided in Table 21.1.

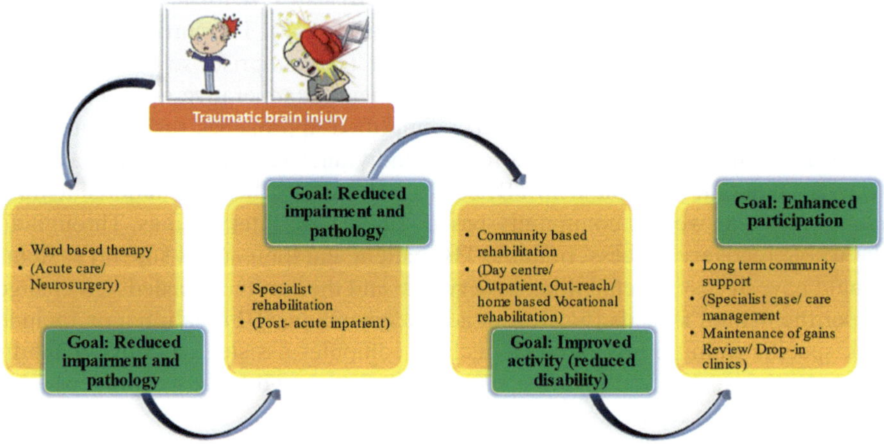

Fig. 21.1 Schematic representation of rehabilitation after traumatic brain injury (Adapted from source)

Table 21.1 Differentiating between community-based rehabilitation from other types of rehabilitation

	Rehabilitation services		
	Institutional based	Outreach services	Community-based
Location	Residential setting, or hospital	Homes of people with disabilities	Home setting, community
Accessibility of services	Located usually in urban centers, inaccessible to individuals in outlying areas	Limited accessibility	Accessible to all
Cost of treatment	High cost	Moderate to high cost	Low cost
Socio-economic status	Not considered	Considered	Considered
Active involvement of family/ community	Not done	Usually limited	Family and community are actively involved Community groups assist the families of disabled people
Services	Special assessments using specialized equipment along with skilled treatment and surgical interventions	Primarily focus on the disabled person and their family	Promotes removal of physical and attitudinal barriers and ensures participation in school, work, leisure, social, and political activities within the community
Skilled personal care	Yes	Yes	No
Shortcomings	Little consideration is given to the person's family and community, or other relevant social factors Lack of qualified personnel in a specialized institution	Generally, education and vocational training are not included	Improper care due to lack of health care personnel Limitation of local resources and unreliability of community

21.3 Community-Based Rehabilitation

Primary healthcare and community-based strategies were prioritized in the "Alma Ata Declaration" in the year of 1978 as "Health for All," which emphasized health as the fundamental right of humans. WHO established "community-based rehabilitation" (CBR) as per Alma Ata's principle to provide access to rehabilitative services for the person with disabilities in their community, utilizing locally available resources. CBR is a plan for all persons with disabilities to get rehabilitation, equitable access to opportunities, and social inclusion [11]. To achieve independent and better social integration, and equal access to health, education, and employment opportunities for individuals with disabilities after any trauma, including those of

TBI, CBR must be implemented with cumulative efforts at each level, that is, individual, family, and community.

Guidelines targeting establishing and implementing CBR programs that must be followed are highlighted in Box 21.1 [11].

Box 21.1 Guidelines for Establishing and Implementing CBR Programs

1. Inclusive: All phases and levels of CBR programs, including initial program design and execution, must involve people with disabilities. They need to play specific decision-making roles for their involvement in these programs.
2. Quality of Life: The main goal of activities in the CBR program is enhancing the "Quality of Life" for those having disabilities.
3. Positive attitude: Encouraging the community to support and take part in activities for CBR by fostering positive attitudes toward those with disabilities.
4. Assistance: Support for everyone, including the elderly, those with leprosy or epilepsy, persons with various types of impairments (physical, sensory, psychological, and mental), and anybody else who could be designated by the community as needing particular assistance.
5. Gender-sensitive: Women and girls should be considered while planning for any activity.
6. Decentralization: CBR programs need to have the flexibility to be able to function locally and within their context. Multiple models of CBR are recommended to address varying socio-economic contexts and individual community's needs. CBR with such flexibility will ensure the involvement of the community and will further lead to the development of program models that are specific to individual places
7. Intersectoral coordination: Delivery services under CBR programs should have coordination at the local level. The service should be provided to people with disabilities through a "single window." This will make the services easier and more accessible for them, as they may not understand the roles and specializations that are required in their rehabilitation. Also, the person with a disability is usually only concerned about the place and person to approach for a specific problem and is not concerned with the interventions required in totality for fulfilling his life as a community member. This proposed single window will play the role of a hub for all concerned departments and sectors involved in the process

Successful integration of TBI patients demands the community to recognize that people with disabilities (PWDs) and limitations have equal rights as others irrespective of their altered or limited capacity. A system approach in this regard will involve technology, service delivery, and community involvement along with cooperation with organizations of people working with TBI. "The Standard Rules on the

Equalization of Opportunities for Persons with Disabilities" conceptualized by the United Nations in 1993 form the basis for the policy directions. These rules are categorized into "Preconditions for Equal Participation," "Target Areas for Equal Participation," and "Implementation Measures" [12].

These rules provide policy directions to countries to safeguard equitable opportunities for PWDs to show their participation in society resulting in greater outcomes from their participation These rules emphasize that rehabilitation programs at the national level should have the principles of equality and community participation at the center of it and should include them in the goals of it. This will again be in line with recommendations—"that individuals be involved in their rehabilitation, that services be available in the local community, and that advocacy groups be included in national programme planning."

21.4 Community-Based Rehabilitation (CBR) Framework in India

In India, the "Ministry of Social Justice and Empowerment," the nodal ministry, is concerned with the planning of rehabilitative amenities for all PWDs. To support social inclusion and empowerment of PWDs, the Department of "Empowerment of Persons with Disabilities (Divyangjan)" was established under this Ministry in May 2012. It oversees all the development goals for PWDs as a nodal agency.

The process of empowering PWDs is accepted as a multi-disciplinary process that addresses a diverse range of issues, including social integration, early identification, intervention, education, health, and vocational training. The Department envisions an inclusive and safe society with the mission of empowerment:

Vision—"To build an inclusive society where equal opportunities are provided for the growth and development of Persons with Disabilities so they can lead productive, safe, and dignified lives."

Mission—"To empower Persons with Disabilities, through its various Acts/Institutions/Organizations and Schemes for rehabilitation and to create an enabling environment that provides such persons with equal opportunities, protection of their rights, and enables them to participate as independent and productive members of society."

On February 10, 2006, the Indian government developed and released the "National Policy for Persons with Disabilities," to foster an environment that gives such individuals equal chances for the defense of their rights and full engagement in society.

Only one ministry or even one sector cannot carry out CBR. To establish CBR for people with traumatic brain injuries, the "Ministry of Social Justice and Empowerment" works in conjunction with the following Ministries: "Ministry of Home Affairs," "Ministry of Health and Family Welfare," "Ministry of Rural Development," "Ministry of Housing and Urban Affairs," "Ministry of Youth Affairs

& Sports," "Ministry of Railways," "Ministry of Science & Technology," "Ministry of Statistics & Programme Implementation," "Ministry of Labour," "Ministry of Panchayati Raj," "Ministry of Women & Child Development," "Ministry of Education," "Ministry of Road Transport & Highways," "Ministry of Public Enterprises," and "Department of Revenue" (Fig. 21.2)

The successful application of the CBR along with education, vocational, psychosocial, and other services is primarily dependent on PWDs, their families, organizations, and communities. CBR has a positive impact on society as a whole by enabling people, groups, and communities to fulfill their fundamental requirements, have access to health and education, fight poverty, and have a source of income. A comprehensive CBR program contributes toward the health, education, and livelihood of disabled patients alongside their social integration and empowerment in more than one way as detailed in the CBR matrix (Fig. 21.3) [13]. All the stakeholders operating in various disciplines must form alliances to share duties and make use of their comparative advantages for CBR to be implemented successfully. The "Asia Pacific Development Centre on Disability" focuses on "environment" as an integrated component to empower persons with disabilities by making their voice heard toward removing obstacles in information & communication, laws & processes, attitudes & biases, and their physical environment.

The "Ministry of Social Justice and Empowerment" of the Government of India launched the District Disability Rehabilitation Centre (DDRC) with the aim of providing comprehensive services to individuals having disability from rural regions [14]. For services such as identifying PWDs, raising awareness, early detection and intervention, providing/fitting, monitoring, and repairing assistive devices,

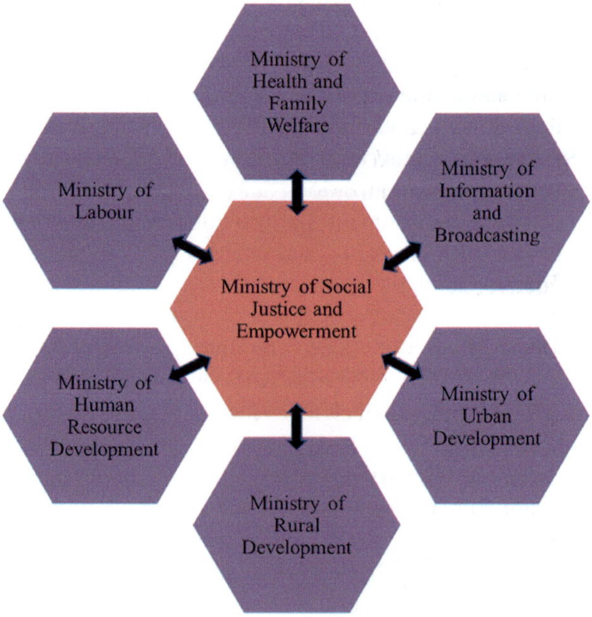

Fig. 21.2 Intersectoral coordination among the Ministries to establish community-based rehabilitation for trauma patients

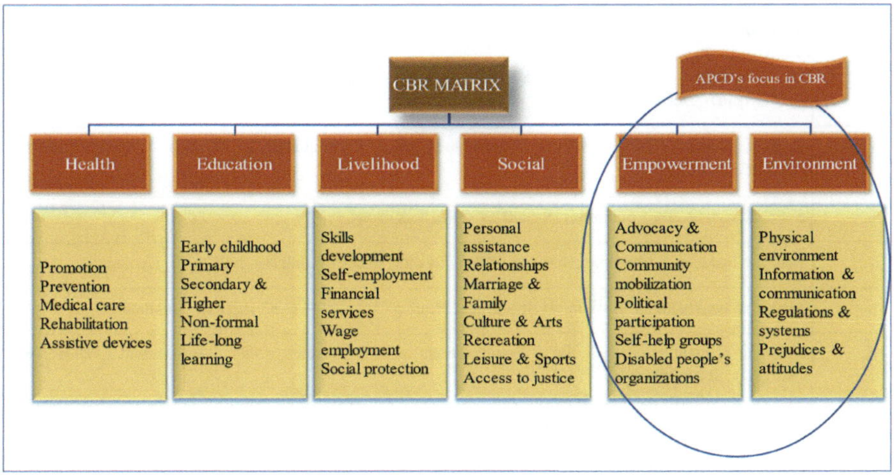

Fig. 21.3 CBR matrix

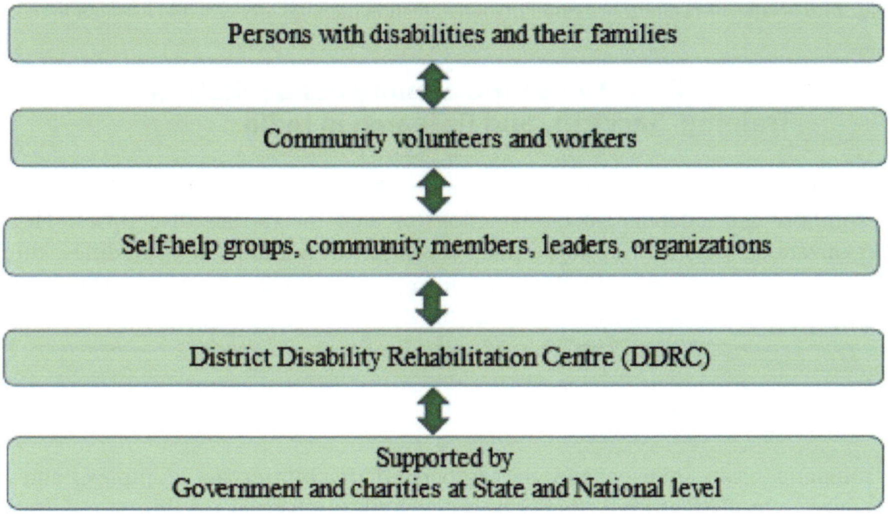
Persons with disabilities and their families
Community volunteers and workers
Self-help groups, community members, leaders, organizations
District Disability Rehabilitation Centre (DDRC)
Supported by
Government and charities at State and National level

Fig. 21.4 Community-based rehabilitation continuum in India

therapeutic services including speech therapy, physiotherapy, etc., facilitating disability certificates, bus passes, and other concessions/facilities for PWDs, these units have a group of rehabilitation professions. Figure 21.4 outlines the community-based rehabilitation continuum currently existing in India.

S. No.	National Institutes
i.	Pt. Deendayal Upadhyaya National Institute for Persons with Physical Disabilities (PDUNIPPD), Delhi.
ii.	Swami Vivekanand National Institute of Rehabilitation Training and Research (SVNIRTAR), Cuttack.
iii.	National Institute for Locomotor Disabilities (NILD), Kolkata.
iv.	National Institute for the Empowerment of Persons with Visual Disabilities (NIEPVD), Dehradun.
v.	Ali Yavar Jung National Institute of Speech and Hearing Disabilities (AYJNISHD), Mumbai
vi.	National Institute for the Empowerment of Persons with Intellectual Disabilities (NIEPID), Secunderabad.
vii.	National Institute for Empowerment of Persons with Multiple Disabilities (NIEPMD), Chennai.
viii.	Indian Sign Language Training and Research Centre, New Delhi.
ix.	National Institute of Mental Health Rehabilitation (NIMHR), Sehore, Madhya Pradesh.

Fig. 21.5 National Institutes for disability rehabilitation training, services, and research in India

21.5 National Institutes for Disability Rehabilitation Training, Services, and Research in India

Nine National Institutes are working on disability rehabilitation in India. These institutions are independent organizations created for various disabilities. These organizations work to develop human resources in the field of disabilities, offer rehabilitative services to PWDs, and do research and development. These nine National Institutes are shown in Fig. 21.5.

21.6 Conclusion

Traumatic brain injuries and the associated disabilities are complex, and it requires a multi-factorial approach to developing effective rehabilitation strategies. Rehabilitation, rather than an outcome, is the process where those having disabilities and those supporting them decide what services they require to improve their involvement in all facets of daily life. The rehabilitation services aim to assist the individual, family, and community in comprehending all the disabilities caused by brain injury and to learn how to help an injured person recover as many abilities as possible. With unbiased odds for the highest contribution in the totality of societal components of life, CBR promotes individuals with disabilities living as equal citizens in their communities and exercising their fundamental right to human rights.

21.7 Summary

TBI can have a variety of negative physical, cognitive, and emotional effects that need specialized care. Rehabilitation following TBI is a complex, challenging, and creative process for all trauma patients including TBI as it may involve various disabilities and is primarily focused on complete community reintegration. To maximize recovery outcomes, people with TBI need rehabilitation therapies tailored to their requirements as well as community-based nonmedical interventions. CBR refers to an approach for the rehabilitation, opportunity equality, and social inclusion of all individuals with disabilities. The principles that are ensured for the development and implementation of CBR programs include inclusive of all PWDs, improving quality of life, positive attitude, providing assistance, gender-sensitive activities, decentralization of CBR programs, and intersectoral coordination of various sectors. In India, the "Ministry of Social Justice and Empowerment" is the nodal ministry to plan rehabilitation services for all PWDs which provides CBR by intersectoral coordination with various other Ministries. The CBR matrix explains the comprehensive CBR program that contributes toward the health, education, and livelihood of disabled patients alongside their social integration and empowerment in more than one way. The "Ministry of Social Justice and Empowerment" of the Government of India launched the DDRC with the aim of providing comprehensive services to individuals having disability from rural regions.

References

1. Dewan MC, Rattani A, Gupta S, Baticulon RE, Hung YC, Punchak M, et al. Estimating the global incidence of traumatic brain injury. J Neurosurg. 2018;130(4):1080–97.
2. Vaishnavi S, Rao V, Fann JR. Neuropsychiatric problems after traumatic brain injury: unraveling the silent epidemic. Psychosomatics. 2009;50(3):198–205.
3. Singaravelu Jaganathan K, Sullivan KA. Traumatic brain injury rehabilitation: an exercise immunology perspective. Exerc Immunol Rev. 2022;28:90–7.
4. Wilson L, Stewart W, Dams-O'Connor K, Diaz-Arrastia R, Horton L, Menon DK, et al. The chronic and evolving neurological consequences of traumatic brain injury. Lancet Neurol. 2017;16(10):813–25.
5. Al Yazeedi W, Venkatachalam L, Al Molawi S, Al Kuwari F. Traumatic brain injury rehabilitation: an overview. In: Traumatic Brain Injury. London: IntechOpen; 2014.
6. Chua KSG, Ng YS, Yap SG, Bok CW. A brief review of traumatic brain injury rehabilitation. Ann Acad Med. 2007;36(1):31–42.
7. Khan F, Baguley IJ, Cameron ID. Rehabilitation after traumatic brain injury. Med J Aust. 2003;178(6):290–5.
8. Turner-Strokes L. Rehabilitation following acquired brain injury: concise guidance. Clin Med. 2003;4(1):61–5.
9. Blackerby WF. Intensity of rehabilitation and length of stay. Brain Inj. 1990;4(2):167–73.
10. Barnes MP. Rehabilitation after traumatic brain injury. Br Med Bull. 1999;55(4):927–43.
11. WHO. Community-based rehabilitation for and with people with disabilities: 1994 joint position paper, 1994.

12. WHO. The UN standard rules on the equalization of opportunities for persons with disabilities: NGO responses to the implementation of the rules on medical care, rehabilitation, support services and personnel training: regional reports. World Health Organization; 2002.
13. WHO. Compilation of community-based rehabilitation practices in the WHO South-East Asia Region. WHO Regional Office for South-East Asia; 2013.
14. District Disability Rehabilitation Centre; 2022. https://niepid.nic.in/DDRCs.php.

GPSR Compliance

The European Union's (EU) General Product Safety Regulation (GPSR) is a set of rules that requires consumer products to be safe and our obligations to ensure this.

If you have any concerns about our products, you can contact us on ProductSafety@springernature.com

In case Publisher is established outside the EU, the EU authorized representative is:

Springer Nature Customer Service Center GmbH
Europaplatz 3
69115 Heidelberg, Germany

Batch number: 08998951

Printed by Printforce, the Netherlands